A–Z
of Haematology

A–Z
of Haematology

Barbara J. Bain
MB BS FRACP FRCPath
Reader in Diagnostic Haematology
Honorary Consultant Haematologist
Department of Haematology
St Mary's Hospital Campus
Imperial College Faculty of Medicine
London

Rajeev Gupta
MB ChB PhD MRCP MRCPath
Clinical Research Fellow
Section of Gene Function and Regulation
The Institute of Cancer Research
London

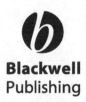

Blackwell
Publishing

First published 2003 by Blackwell Publishing Ltd

Library of Congress Cataloging-in-Publication Data

Bain, Barbara J.
    A-Z of haematology/Barbara Bain.
        p. ; cm.
    ISBN 1-40510-322-1
    1. Hematology—Dictionaries.
    [DNLM: 1. Hematology—Dictionary—English.   WH 13 B162a 2003]   I. Title.
    RB145 .B245 2003
    616.15'003—dc21

                                                                    2002007250

ISBN 1-4051-0322-1

A catalogue record for this title is available from the British Library

Set in 8.5/10.5 Times by Graphicraft Limited, Hong Kong

Commissioning Editor: Maria Khan
Editorial Assistant: Elizabeth Callaghan
Production Editor: Charlie Hamlyn
Production Controller: Kate Charman

For further information on Blackwell Publishing, visit our website:
http://www.blackwellpublishing.com

Contents

Preface

In this A–Z of Haematology we have sought to be as comprehensive as possible, but we have nevertheless given particular emphasis to recent advances in molecular haematology. We have detailed the important genes that have been implicated in haematological neoplasms and in constitutional haematological disorders. Blood transfusion, haemostasis and thrombosis and immunology have not been neglected. We have provided the reader with a complete list of the molecules that have been assigned a Cluster of Designation (CD) number, with descriptions of their functions and patterns of expression in health and disease. Because of the emphasis we have given to the scientific basis of haematology and related disciplines we believe that this work will be useful not only to haematologists but also to research scientists and to biomedical scientists working in diagnostic laboratories. Those working in cancer cytogenetics and immunophenotyping will also find it a valuable repository of relevant knowledge. The very existence of such a book is indicative of the fact that a book still remains a highly convenient reference source. However, for those who wish to seek further information electronically we have provided a list of some of the more useful of the many websites available.

It will be helpful to the reader to know some of the conventions we have followed. All human genes are designated as recommended by the human genome project, in upper case italics with Greek letters being replaced by their Roman equivalent. Approved names are given but where a gene is better known to haematologists by another name, we have mainly used that name in further discussion. We have indicated how gene names (and some protein names) are derived from a longer descriptive phrase by means of bold print plus underlining of the relevant letters, e.g. *PLZF*—**P**romyelocytic **L**eukaemia **Z**inc **F**inger. However, **bold print without underlining** is used for another purpose, to indicate that there is a relevant entry in the book. In order to avoid tedium, words and phrases that are used very frequently, e.g. 'acute myeloid leukaemia' are not generally cross referenced in this manner.

We wish to thank those who have helped with the provision of illustrations: the publisher of the late Professor M. Bessis, Professor D. Catovsky, Dr W. Gedroyc, Miss C. Hughes, Mr R. Morilla, Ms L. Phelan, Ms Julia Pickard and the Cytogenetics Department at Hammersmith Hospital, Professor A. Polliack, Professor Lorna Secker-Walker, The North Trent Cytogenetics Service at Sheffield Childrens Hospital, the Kennedy Galton Institute and the United Kingdom Cancer Cytogenetics Group.

Barbara J. Bain and Rajeev Gupta

Online Resources

General haematology

American Society of Hematology **www.hematology.org**

British Society for Haematology **www.blacksci.co.uk/uk/society/bsh**
(use this site to access PubMed, Centers of Disease Control and Institute of Biomedical Science)

European Hematology Association **www.ehaweb.org**

British Committee for Standards in Haematology guidelines **www.bcshguidelines.com/**
(use this site to access *Cells of the Blood, Haematological Malignancy Diagnostic Service* and *Hematology Digital Image Bank*)

Haematologists in Training **www.hit.gb.com/**
(use this site to access *MRC Leukaemia Trials* and an on line medical dictionary through *doctors' guide to internet* and *Guide to Internet Resources on Haematological Malignancies*)

Other general haematology **www.bloodline.net**

Chromosomes, genes and proteins—molecular haematology

Cytogenetics in haematology

Genetics and cytogenetics in Haematology **www.infobiogen.fr/services/chromcancer/**

Online Mendelian Inheritance in Man **www.ncbi.nlm.nih.gov/omim/**

Cardiff Human Gene Mutation Data Base **www.uwcm.ac.uk/uwcm/mg/hgmd0.html**

Sources of probes for molecular genetic studies: Vysis **www.vysis.com/hematology**
and Q-Biogene (previously Oncor) **www.cambio.co.uk/starfish/**

Human proteins website **www.ncbi.nlm.nih.gov/prow**

Websites of antibody manufacturers

   http://serotec.oxi.net/asp/index.html

   www.bdbiosciences.com

   www.vectorlabs.com

Realtime PCR www.cgr.otago.ac.nz/SLIDES/7700/SLD001.HTM

Chemokine review **http://www.path.sunysb.edu/courses/syllabus/chemkin.htm**

Cytokine minireviews **http://www.rndsystems.com/asp/g_sitebuilder.asp?BodyId=2**

Haemoglobinopathies and thalassaemias

http://globin.cse.psu.edu

Thrombosis and haemostasis

The International Society on Thrombosis and Haemostasis **www.med.unc.edu/isth/welcome**
The World Federation of Hemophilia **www.wfh.org**

Blood transfusion

American Association of Blood Banks **www.aabb.org**

British Blood Transfusion Society **www.bbts.org.uk**
(use this site to access British blood transfusion guidelines)

National Blood Service **www.blood.co.uk**

Serious Hazards of Transfusion **http://www.shot.demon.co.uk**

Malaria

http://www.rph.wa.gov.au/labs/haem/malaria/

Haematological neoplasms

General **http://cancerweb.ncl.ac.uk/cancernet.html**
(use this site to access an online medical dictionary)

http://www.cancerindex.org/clinks2.htm

The British National Lymphoma Investigation **www.bnli.ucl.ac.uk/**

Lymphoma Forum **www.lymphoma.org.uk/lymphoma.htm**

The Leukaemia Research Fund **www.dspace.dial.pipex.com/lrf-/**

The UK Myeloma Forum **www.ukmf.org.uk**

American Association for Cancer Research **www.aacr.org**

(use this site for access to the five journals published by the AACR)

Abstracts and journals

Entrez PubMed **www.ncbi.nlm.nih.gov/**
Blood **www.bloodjournal.org/**
Haematologica **www.haematologica.it/main.html**
Online flow cytometry cases **www.flowcases.org**
British Medical Journal **www.bmj.com**

Teaching sites

www.hematology.org (click on educational materials)
www.haem.net
http://pathy.med.nagoya-u.ac.jp/atlas/doc/atlas.html
www-medlib.med.utah.edu/WebPath/webpath.html

A

α alpha, the first letter of the Greek alphabet, often used to designate polypeptide chains

α₁ antitrypsin a **serpin** which inactivates **neutrophil elastase**; mutation of the gene encoding α₁ antitrypsin can lead to production of a protein that inhibits coagulation pathway proteases and leads to a bleeding disorder

α **chain** (i) the alpha globin chain which is essential for formation of haemoglobins A, A₂ and F (ii) the heavy chain of immunoglobulin A; two alpha chains combine with two light chains (in a single molecule either kappa or lambda) to form a complete immunoglobulin molecule (iii) part of the αβ T-cell receptor, a surface membrane structure in T lymphocytes which permits antigen recognition

α **error** a statistically significant difference when no real difference exists; e.g. if the results of two treatment strategies are statistically different with a probability of $P = 0.05$ there is a 1 in 20 chance that there is no real difference

α **globin cluster** the cluster of genes on chromosome 16 that includes the genes encoding ζ, α2 and α1 chains (Fig. 1)

α **globin gene** the *HBA* genes, gene map locus 16p13.3, encoding the **α globin chain** of **haemoglobin**; there are two α globin genes, designated α2 and α1, on each chromosome 16

Figure 1 α **and** β **globin gene clusters**.
The alpha and beta globin gene clusters on chromosomes 11 and 16 respectively. The β cluster has an upstream locus control region (LCR) and ε, ᴳγ, ᴬγ, δ and β genes; there is one pseudogene, ψβ. The α cluster has an upstream H40 regulatory region and ζ, α₂ and α₁ globin chain genes; there are two pseudogenes, ψζ and ψα.

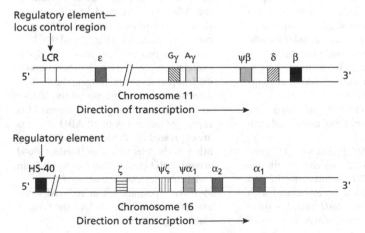

1

α heavy chain disease a plasma cell dyscrasia characterized by secretion of the heavy chain of **immunoglobulin A**

α naphthyl acetate esterase (ANAE) an enzyme belonging to the **non-specific esterase** group of enzymes, strongly expressed in cells of the monocytic and megakaryocytic lineages

α naphthyl butyrate esterase (ANBE) an enzyme belonging to the **non-specific esterase** group of enzymes, strongly expressed in cells of the monocytic lineage

α satellite DNA repeat sequences at the **centromere** of a **chromosome**; the sequences differ between chromosomes, permitting the development of **centromeric probes** that identify different chromosomes

α thalassaemia a group of thalassaemias characterized by deletion or, less often, altered structure and reduced function of one or more of the α globin genes (*see also* **α thalassaemia trait**, **haemoglobin H disease** and **haemoglobin Bart's hydrops fetalis**) (Fig. 2)

α thalassaemia trait a minor haematological abnormality resulting from deletion of one or two of the four α globin genes; includes **heterozygosity** and **homozygosity** for α^+ **thalassaemia**, when one of two α genes on a chromosome is deleted, and heterozygosity for α^0 **thalassaemia**, when both α genes on a single chromosome are deleted (*see* Fig. 2)

A an abbreviation for the purine, adenine

ABC7 a gene, gene map locus Xq13, encoding **A**TP **B**inding **C**assette transporter **7**, a **mitochondrial** protein, mutation of which can cause **sideroblastic anaemia** with spino-cerebellar ataxia

aberrant diverging from normal, e.g. expression of an antigen which is inappropriate for a lineage

abetalipoproteinaemia inherited absence of beta lipoproteins, associated with **acanthocytosis**

ABI1 a gene, **Ab**l-**I**nteractor **1**, gene map locus 10p11.2, which contributes to the *MLL-ABI1* fusion gene in M4 acute myeloid leukaemia associated with t(10;11)(p11.2;q23); *ABI1* encodes spectrin SH3 domain-binding protein 1, which

is a widely expressed component of a multi-protein complex that negatively regulates cellular responses to various mitogenic signals

ABL a gene, Abelson murine leukaemia viral oncogene homologue 1, gene map locus 9q34; cellular homologue of *v-abl*, a gene in the **Abe**lson murine leukaemia retrovirus which is involved in some murine leukaemias; encodes a non-receptor tyrosine kinase; *ABL* contributes to:
- the *BCR-ABL* fusion gene in t(9;22)(q34;q11) associated with chronic granulocytic leukaemia and with Philadelphia-positive acute lymphoblastic and acute myeloid leukaemias
- the *ETV6-ABL* fusion gene in chronic myeloid leukaemias, acute myeloid leukaemia and acute lymphoblastic leukaemia associated with t(9;12)(q34;p13) and variant translocations

Both *BCR-ABL* and *ETV6-ABL* are inhibited by the ABL tyrosine kinase inhibitor, imatinib mesylate (STI571)

ABL is amplified by segmental jumping translocations in some patients with therapy-related acute myeloid leukaemia

abnormal localization of immature precursors (ALIP) location of **myeloblasts** and **promyelocytes** in the centre of the intertrabecular space rather than adjacent to trabeculae or surrounding arterioles

ABO blood group system a blood group system in which A and B alleles at the ABO locus at 9q34 encode specific glycosyltransferases that modify a precursor disaccharide (Fig. 3 and Table 1, p. 4); this precursor is part of a glycoprotein or glycolipid which, when unmodified, expresses the H antigen; the O allele does not encode a functional transferase so that homozygosity for O means H is expressed but not A or B; ABO antigens are expressed on all blood cells and many other body cells (see also **Bombay blood group**); ABO chimaerism can result from constitutional mosaic trisomy 9

abortion spontaneous or induced termination of pregnancy before the fetus is viable, e.g. before 28 weeks

Figure 2 α thalassaemias.

The terminology applied to the alpha thalassaemias; most of the alpha thalassaemias result from deletion of one or both alpha genes at a locus and in some cases the zeta gene is also deleted; α^+ thalassaemia indicates that there is one remaining alpha gene at the locus whereas α^0 thalassaemia indicates that both genes at a locus are deleted; in the case of $-\alpha^{3.7}$ the remaining gene at the locus is an $\alpha 2\alpha 1$ fusion gene; non-deletional thalassaemia refers to the less common alpha thalassaemias resulting from mutation rather than deletion of an alpha gene, the gene being designated α^T, e.g. α^{Tsaudi}.

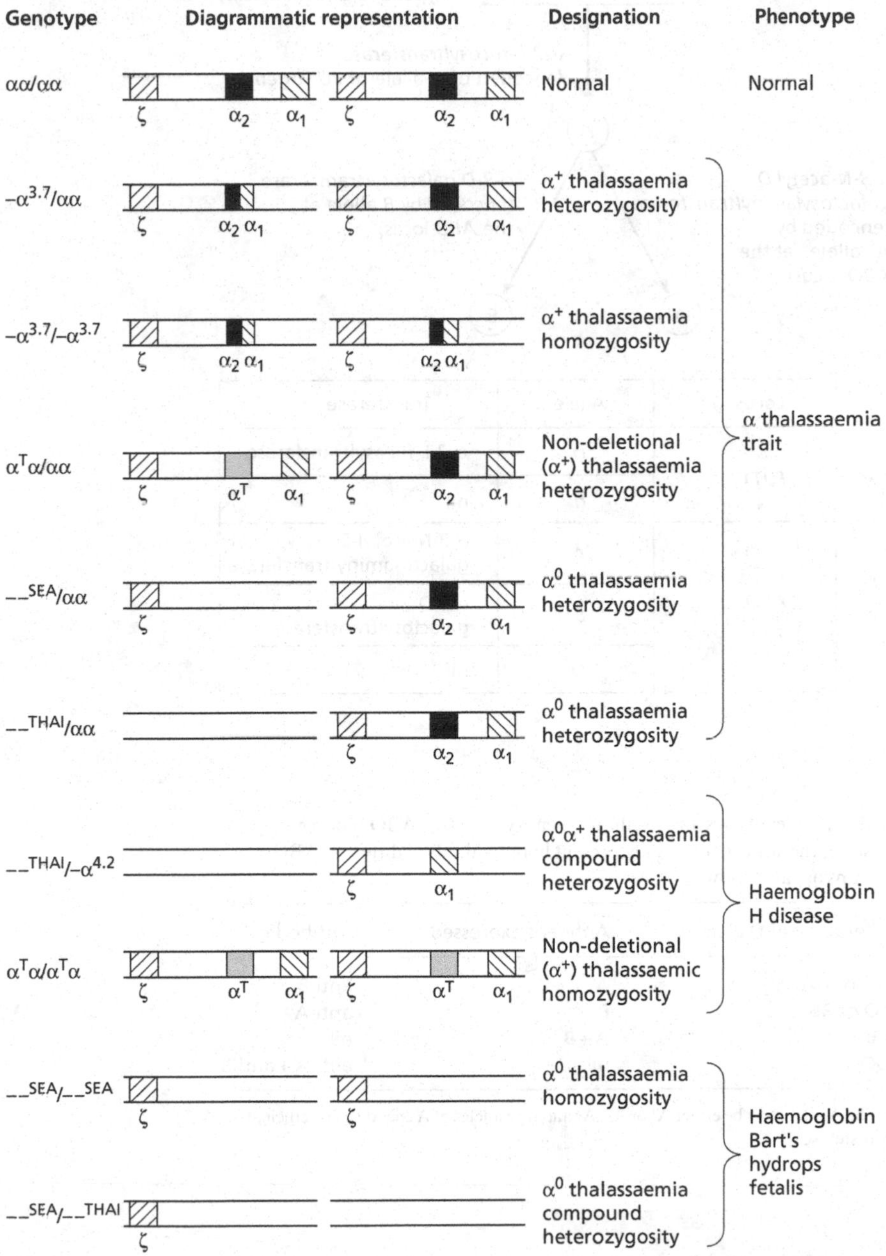

Genotype	Diagrammatic representation	Designation	Phenotype
$\alpha\alpha/\alpha\alpha$		Normal	Normal
$-\alpha^{3.7}/\alpha\alpha$		α^+ thalassaemia heterozygosity	
$-\alpha^{3.7}/-\alpha^{3.7}$		α^+ thalassaemia homozygosity	
$\alpha^T\alpha/\alpha\alpha$		Non-deletional (α^+) thalassaemia heterozygosity	α thalassaemia trait
$--^{SEA}/\alpha\alpha$		α^0 thalassaemia heterozygosity	
$--^{THAI}/\alpha\alpha$		α^0 thalassaemia heterozygosity	
$--^{THAI}/-\alpha^{4.2}$		$\alpha^0\alpha^+$ thalassaemia compound heterozygosity	Haemoglobin H disease
$\alpha^T\alpha/\alpha^T\alpha$		Non-deletional (α^+) thalassaemic homozygosity	
$--^{SEA}/--^{SEA}$		α^0 thalassaemia homozygosity	Haemoglobin Bart's hydrops fetalis
$--^{SEA}/--^{THAI}$		α^0 thalassaemia compound heterozygosity	

Figure 3 ABO antigens.
The formation of ABO antigens: (a) formation of H antigen and formation of A and B
antigens from H; (b) the loci, the alleles and the transferases involved in the formation
of ABO antigens. * The A^2 allele encodes a less efficient transferase that does not
utilize types 3 and 4 disaccharide; A^3 and A^x also encode less efficient transferases.

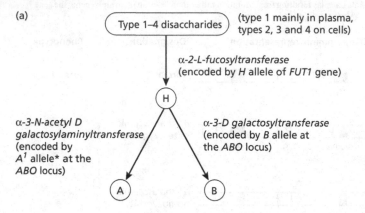

(a)

Type 1–4 disaccharides — (type 1 mainly in plasma, types 2, 3 and 4 on cells)

α-2-L-fucosyltransferase
(encoded by *H* allele of *FUT1* gene)

H

α-3-N-acetyl D
galactosylaminyltransferase
(encoded by
A^1 allele* at the
ABO locus)

α-3-D galactosyltransferase
(encoded by *B* allele at
the *ABO* locus)

A   B

(b)

Locus	Allele	Transferase
FUT1	H	α-2-L-fucosyltransferase
	h	nil
ABO	A	α-3-N-acetyl-D-galactosaminyltransferase
	B	α-3-D galactosyltransferase
	O	nil

Table 1 Genotypes and resultant phenotypes of the ABO blood group
system; the antibodies usually present in individuals of different ABO
groups are also shown.

Alleles* at ABO locus	Antigens expressed	Antibodies
AO or AA	A	anti-B
BO or BB	B	anti-A
AB	A + B	nil
OO	nil	anti-A + anti-B

* The A allele may be either A^1 or A^2; A^2 and rare alleles of A encode a less efficient
transferase.

Figure 4   An acanthocyte and a discocyte.
Scanning electron micrographs of an acanthocyte and a normal shaped red cell, a discocyte.

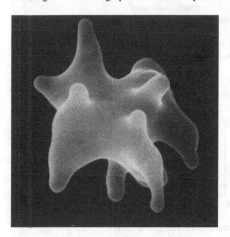 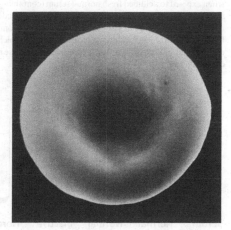

absorbance   the degree of absorption of light

acaeruloplasminaemia   an inherited, autosomal recessive condition, resulting from mutation in the caeruloplasmin gene on chromosome 3q, and consequent deficiency of caeruloplasmin ferroxidase; there is iron overload with low serum iron, normal **transferrin** concentration and moderately elevated **serum ferritin**

acanthocyte   an erythrocyte covered with a small number of spicules of variable length, thickness and shape (Fig. 4)

acanthocytosis   the presence of **acanthocytes**

accelerated phase   a term used to describe a more aggressive phase of **chronic granulocytic leukaemia**

accuracy   the closeness of a measured value to the true value

acentric   having no **centromere**; acentric chromosomes cannot become attached to the **mitotic spindle** and consequently may not be present in either daughter nucleus

ACHE   a gene, gene map locus 7q22, alleles of which encode the Yt^a and Yt^b antigens of the Cartwright blood group system, these antigens being expressed on **GPI**-linked Acetylcholinesterase

achlorhydria   absence of gastric acid secretion, a feature of **pernicious anaemia**

acid   (i) a hydrogen-containing substance that yields a free hydrogen ion and a cation on dissociation (ii) having a low pH

acidified serum test   *see* **acid lysis test**

acid-fast bacillus (AFB)   a microorganism, usually a bacillus of the genus Mycobacteria, um, which, when stained with a Ziehl–Neelsen stain, retains its colour when exposed to acid

acid lysis test   a test for **paroxysmal nocturnal haemoglobinuria** and type II **congenital dyserythropoietic anaemia** (Fig. 5)

acidophilic   having an affinity for acid dyes such as eosin

acidosis   having a blood pH less than 7.35

acid phosphatase   this is a generic term for an enzyme that works optimally at acid pH to release phosphate groups from complex molecules, e.g. from the serine, threonine and tyrosine residues of proteins; they are usually fairly target specific; many lymphoid and myeloid cells have acid phosphatase activity that is demonstrable cytochemically (*see also* **alkaline phosphatase**)

aCML   **atypical chronic myeloid leukaemia**

acquired   not present at birth; the term generally implies a condition or characteristic that is not inherited

Figure 5   The acid lysis test.
The principle of the acid lysis test (Ham test) is that some of the patient's cells lyse when exposed to acidified fresh normal serum (containing complement), conveying a pink or red colour to the supernatant of the centrifuged test sample; lysis does not occur when the serum has not been acidified or when complement in the serum has been inactivated by prior heating. Normal red cells, which are not susceptible to complement-induced lysis in acidified serum, do not lyse in any of these circumstances.

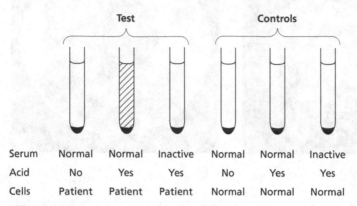

	Test			Controls		
Serum	Normal	Normal	Inactive	Normal	Normal	Inactive
Acid	No	Yes	Yes	No	Yes	Yes
Cells	Patient	Patient	Patient	Normal	Normal	Normal

acquired angio-oedema   angio-oedema which is not inherited or present at birth, usually caused by an acquired deficiency of **C1 inhibitor**; it can be an autoimmune condition or consequent on a low grade B-cell neoplasm

acquired immune deficiency syndrome (AIDS)   an acquired cell-mediated immune deficiency syndrome, consequent on marked reduction of CD4+ T lymphocytes resulting from **HIV** infection

acquired immunity   adaptive immunity that is altered by exposure to antigens, dependent on antigen-presenting cells, T lymphocytes and B lymphocytes

acquired Pelger–Huët anomaly   acquired hypolobulation of neutrophils or other granulocytes, usually indicative of **myelodysplastic syndrome** or **acute myeloid leukaemia**; the cytological features resemble those of the inherited **Pelger–Huët anomaly**

acrocentric   having the **centromere** near one end

ACS2   a gene, <u>A</u>cyl-<u>C</u>oA <u>S</u>ynthetase <u>2</u>, encoding acyl-CoA synthetase 2, gene map locus 5q31 which contributes to an *ETV6-ACS2* fusion gene in myelodys-

plastic syndrome and acute myeloid leukaemia associated with t(5;12)(q31;p13)

actins   an evolutionarily conserved family of intracellular proteins, whose genes exist in multiple copies in all species studied; actin molecules polymerize into intracellular microfilaments that are involved in muscle contraction, cell motility and organelle transport; immunohistochemical demonstration of actin is useful in the diagnosis of rhabdomyosarcoma

activated partial thromboplastin time (aPTT)   a coagulation test in which a contact activator, a **partial thromboplastin** and calcium are added to plasma with the clotting time then being recorded; a test of the **intrinsic pathway** of coagulation (*see* Fig. 17, p. 77)

activated protein C resistance   resistance to the anticoagulant effect of activated **protein C**, often caused by inheritance of a variant of factor V, **factor V Leiden** (*see* **naturally occurring anticoagulants**)

actuarial survival   an estimate of **median survival** made while many patients are still alive

Table 2 WHO criteria for the diagnosis of biphenotypic leukaemia.

Score	B lineage	T lineage	Myeloid
2	cCD79a	CD3 (c or Sm)	MPO
	cIgM	anti-TCR ($\alpha\beta$ or $\gamma\delta$)	
	cCD22		
1	CD19	CD2	CD117
	CD10	CD5	CD13
	CD20	CD8	CD33
		CD10	CD65
0.5	TdT	TdT	CD14
	CD24	CD7	CD15
		CD1a	CD64

If > 2 points is scored for both myeloid and one of the lymphoid lineages the case is classified as biphenotypic; in the original EGIL recommendations CD117 scored 0.5 rather than 1

c, cytoplasmic; CD, cluster of differentiation; Ig, immunoglobulin; MPO, myeloperoxidase; Sm, surface membrane; TdT, terminal deoxynucleotidyl transferase.

Table 3 A simplified explanation of the French-American-British (FAB) classification of acute myeloid leukaemia (AML).

FAB designation	Description
M0	AML with minimal evidence of myeloid differentiation
M1	AML with granulocytic differentiation but little maturation
M2	AML with granulocytic differentiation and maturation
M3 and M3 variant	Acute hypergranular promyelocytic leukaemia and the hypogranular or microgranular variant form
M4	AML with both granulocytic and monocytic differentiation .
M5	AML with monocytic differentiation, either without maturation (M5a or acute monoblastic leukaemia) or with maturation (M5b or acute monocytic leukaemia)
M6	AML with at least half the bone marrow cells being erythroblasts
M7	Acute megakaryoblastic leukaemia

acute basophilic leukaemia an acute myeloid leukaemia with prominent basophilic differentiation

acute biphenotypic leukaemia an acute leukaemia in which there is both myeloid and lymphoid differentiation, defined in the WHO classification as shown in Table 2

acute eosinophilic leukaemia an acute myeloid leukaemia with prominent eosinophilic differentiation

acute erythroleukaemia an acute myeloid leukaemia with prominent erythroid differentiation; the FAB M6 category of AML (Table 3, *see also* Table 4)

acute hypergranular promyelocytic leukaemia an acute myeloid leukaemia characterized by leukaemic cells that are abnormal hypergranular promyelocytes, the FAB M3 category of AML (*see* Tables 3 and 4)

acute leukaemia a leukaemia that, if untreated, leads to death in weeks or months; a leukaemia characterized by continued proliferation with a failure of

Table 4   The WHO classification of acute myeloid leukaemia (AML).

Acute myeloid leukaemia with recurrent genetic abnormalities*
   AML with t(8; 21)(q22;q22)/*AML1-ETO* fusion
   AML with abnormal bone marrow eosinophils and inv(16)(p13q22) or t(16;
      15)(p13;q22)/*CBFB-MYH11* fusion
   Acute promyelocytic leukaemia with t(15; 17)(q22;q12)/*PML-RARA* fusion, and variants
   AML with 11q23 rearrangement and *MLL* abnormality
AML with multilineage dysplasia†
   Following a myelodysplastic syndrome or a myelodysplastic/myeloproliferative syndrome
   Without antecedent myelodysplastic syndrome
Therapy-related AML and myelodysplastic syndrome
   Alkylating agent-related
   Topoisomerase II-inhibitor-related
   Other types
AML not otherwise categorized
   AML, minimally differentiated (resembles FAB M0)
   AML without maturation (resembles FAB M1)
   AML with maturation (resembles FAB M2)
   Acute myelomonocytic leukaemia (resembles FAB M4)
   Acute monoblastic and acute monocytic leukaemia (resembles FAB M5a, M5b)
   Acute erythroid leukaemia
      Erythroleukaemia (resembles FAB M6)
      Pure erythroid leukaemia
   Acute megakaryoblastic leukaemia (resembles FAB M7)
   Acute basophilic leukaemia
   Acute panmyelosis with myelofibrosis
   Myeloid sarcoma (granulocytic or monocytic)

---

* Therapy-related cases may be noted to have one of these abnormalities but are assigned to the category of therapy-related AML.
† Defined as having at least 50% of cells dysplastic in at least 2 lineages.

differentiation so that the dominant cell is a primitive cell referred to as a **blast cell**

acute lymphoblastic leukaemia (ALL) an acute leukaemia in which the predominant cell is a **lymphoblast** of T or B lineage

acute monoblastic leukaemia an **acute myeloid leukaemia** in which the dominant cell is a **monoblast**, the FAB M5a category of AML (*see* Tables 3 and 4)

acute monocytic leukaemia an **acute myeloid leukaemia** in which the leukaemic cells are mainly **promonocytes** and **monocytes** but with at least 20 or 30% of peripheral blood or bone marrow cells being **blast cells**; the FAB M5b category of AML (*see* Tables 3 and 4)

acute myelofibrosis acute myeloid leukaemia with reactive bone marrow fibrosis; the leukaemic cells are com-monly but not always of megakaryocyte lineage

acute myeloid leukaemia (AML) an acute leukaemia in which leukaemic cells belong to any myeloid lineage, i.e. granulocytic, monocytic, erythroid or megakaryocyte lineages, defined in the **WHO classification** as a haematological neoplasm with at least 20% blast cells in the peripheral blood or bone marrow or with a lower percentage of blast cells if there is one of three specified chromosomal rearrangements—t(8;21), inv(16) or t(16;16); AML is further classified as shown in Table 4

acute myelomonocytic leukaemia (AMML) an **acute myeloid leukaemia** in which there is both granulocytic and monocytic differentiation, the FAB M4 category of AML (*see* Tables 3 and 4)

acute non-lymphoblastic leukaemia (ANLL) an alternative designation of **acute myeloid leukaemia**, mainly used in the USA

acute phase reactant one of a number of plasma proteins that rise in concentration in response to acute inflammation or tissue injury, enhancing resistance to infection and promoting tissue repair

acute phase reaction an acute systemic response to infection or inflammation, in which there is a fall in serum albumin, transferrin and iron and a rise in other proteins including C-reactive protein, serum amyloid A protein, factor VIII, fibrinogen and α2 macroglobulin

ADA the gene on 20q that encodes adenosine deaminase, deficiency of which can cause severe combined immunodeficiency

ADAMTS13 a gene at 9q34, encoding a disintegrin-like metalloprotease with thrombospondin type 1 motif, 13, also known as **von Willebrand's factor-cleaving protease**, mutation of which can cause familial **thrombotic thrombocytopenic purpura**

ADCC **antibody-dependent cellular cytotoxicity**

add a cytogenetic abbreviation indicating additional material of unknown origin

Addisonian anaemia *see* **pernicious anaemia**

Addison's disease an illness resulting from chronic failure of the adrenal glands

addresin a tissue-specific **adhesion molecule**

adenine a **purine** base that is a component of both DNA and RNA, pairs with **thymine**

adenocarcinoma carcinoma showing some features of differentiation to glandular structures

adenoma a benign tumour of glandular tissue

adenosine deaminase an enzyme that catalyses the conversion of adenosine to inosine; a deficiency can cause **severe combined immunodeficiency**

adenosine diphosphate (ADP) the nucleotide adenosine, with two attached phosphate moieties; a store of energy; a platelet **agonist**

adenosine triphosphate (ATP) the nucleotide adenosine, with three attached phosphate moieties; an important store of energy

adhesion the process of becoming closely attached to something else

adhesion molecule a molecule that promotes adhesion of cells to each other

adjuvant a substance that non-specifically enhances antigen-specific immune responses

ADP **adenosine diphosphate**

adrenal gland an endocrine gland sited at the upper pole of the kidney

adrenaline *see* **epinephrine**

Adriamycin a trade name for doxorubicin, an anthracycline used in the treatment of lymphomas and carcinomas

adult haemoglobin **haemoglobin A**

adult T-cell leukaemia/lymphoma (ATLL) a subacute neoplasm of T lymphocytes which may have either a leukaemic or a lymphomatous presentation; preceding infection by the **human T-cell lymphotropic virus I** (HTLV-I) is an essential aetiological factor

AE1 a gene, gene map locus 17q21-q22, encoding S̲o̲lute C̲arrier family 4̲, A̲nion exchanger, member 1̲ (*SLC4A1*) also known as the A̲nion E̲xchanger 1̲ and band 3 protein, a component of the red cell membrane (*see* Fig. 64, p. 199); mutation can result in **hereditary spherocytosis, hereditary elliptocytosis** or **Southeast Asian ovalocytosis**; band 3 carries the diego blood group antigens

AF1p a gene, A̲LL1̲ F̲usion gene from chromosome 1̲p̲, also known as *EPS15*— E̲p̲idermal growth factor receptor pathway S̲ubstrate-1̲5̲, gene map locus 1p32; *AF1p* encodes a phosphorylated protein that is a constitutive component of clathrin-coated pits and is required for clathrin-dependent endocytosis; it contributes to the *MLL-AF1p* fusion gene in some cases of M5 acute myeloid leukaemia

AF1q a gene, A̲LL1̲ F̲usion gene from chromosome 1̲q̲, gene map locus 1q21, which contributes to the *MLL-AF1q* fusion gene in some cases of M4 acute myeloid leukaemia; *AF1q* encodes a nuclear protein, the expression of which is usually restricted to the thymus

AF3p21 a gene, *ALL1* Fusion gene from chromosome **3p21**, also known as *SPIN90*—SH3 Protein Interacting with Nck, **90**-KD; gene map locus 3p21, encoding an SH3 adapter protein that is normally expressed in cardiomyocytes; was found to be fused with the *MLL* gene in a patient with therapy-related M5 acute myeloid leukaemia associated with t(3;11)(p21;q23)

AF4 a gene, *ALL1* Fusion gene from chromosome **4**, also known as *MLLT2*—Myeloid/Lymphoid or Mixed Lineage Leukaemia, Translocated to, **2**, gene map locus 4q21, encodes a putative transcription factor widely expressed in normal tissues; *AF4* contributes to the *MLL-AF4* fusion gene in t(4;11)(q21;q23) associated with acute lymphoblastic leukaemia, acute myeloid leukaemia and acute biphenotypic leukaemia

AF5q31 a gene, *ALL1* Fusion gene from chromosome **5q31**, gene map locus 5q31, encodes a homologue of *AF4*, contributed to an *MLL-AF5q31* fusion gene in an infant with pro-B acute lymphoblastic leukaemia and ins(5;11)(q31;q13q23) and an *MLL-AF5q31* fusion in other infants with acute lymphoblastic leukaemia

AF6q21 a gene, *ALL1* Fusion gene from chromosome **6q21**, also known as *FKHRL1*—Forkhead in Rhabdomyosarcoma-Like **1**, gene map locus 6q21; encodes a transcription factor of the *forkhead* family; contributes to the *MLL-AF6q21* fusion gene in acute myeloid leukaemia associated with t(6;11)(q27;q23)

AF6q27 a gene, *ALL1* Fusion gene from chromosome **6q27**, also known as *MLLT4*—Myeloid/Lymphoid or Mixed Lineage Leukaemia, Translocated to, **4**; gene map locus 6q27, encodes a widely expressed normal component of tight and adherens junctions, which has been shown to bind RAS; contributes to the *MLL-AF6q27* fusion gene in M5 acute myeloid leukaemia associated with t(6;11)(q27;q23); the normal gene product is cytoplasmic whereas the fusion gene product is nuclear

AF7p15 a gene, *ALL1* Fusion gene from chromosome **7p15**, gene map locus 7p15, encodes a novel protein with no known homologies located in the intron of 3′ hydroxybutyrate dehydrogenase; contributed to an *ETV6-AF7p15* fusion gene in a patient with acute myeloid leukaemia associated with t(7;12)(p15;p13)

AF9 a gene, *ALL1* Fused gene from chromosome **9**; also known as *MLLT3*—Myeloid/Lymphoid or Mixed Lineage Leukaemia, translocated to, **3**; gene map locus 9p21; encodes a putative nuclear protein; *AF9* contributes to the *MLL-AF9* fusion gene in acute myeloid leukaemia or, less often, acute lymphoblastic leukaemia, associated with t(9;11)(p21-22;q23)

AF9q34 a gene, *ALL1* Fused gene from chromosome **9q34**; gene map locus 9q34, predicted to encode a RAS GTPase-activating protein; *AF9q34* contributed to an *MLL-AF9q34* fusion gene in a case of acute myeloid leukaemia associated with t(9;11)(q34;q23)

AF10 a gene, *ALL1* Fused gene from chromosome **10**, gene map locus 10p12; encodes a widely expressed leucine zipper/zinc finger protein; *AF10* contributes to:
• the *MLL-AF10* fusion gene in t(10;11)(p12;q23) associated with M5 acute myeloid leukaemia and acute lymphoblastic leukaemia;
• a *CALM-AF10* fusion gene in acute myeloid leukaemia

AF15q14 a gene, *ALL1* Fusion gene from chromosome **15q14**, gene map locus 15q14, encoding a protein with no known homologies, that contributed to a *MLL-AF15q14* fusion gene in a patient with acute myeloid leukaemia associated with t(11;15)(q23;q14)

AF17 a gene, *ALL1* Fusion gene from chromosome **17**; also known as *MLLT6*—Myeloid/Lymphoid or Mixed Lineage Leukaemia, Translocated to, **6**; gene map locus 17q21; encodes a zinc finger/leucine zipper protein similar to AF10; contributes to the *MLL-AF17* fusion gene in t(11;17)(q23;q21) associated with M5 acute myeloid leukaemia

AFB   acid-fast bacillus

affinity chromatography separation of proteins by means of differences in affinity for lectins, monoclonal antibodies or other proteins

affinity selection the process by which **germinal centre** B cells that produce high affinity antibodies become **memory cells** or **plasma cells** while other B cells suffer **apoptosis**

afibrinogenaemia an inherited, autosomal recessive, severe reduction or absence of plasma **fibrinogen**

AFX a gene, *ALL1* Fusion gene from chromosome X, also known as *MLLT7*—Myeloid/Lymphoid or Mixed Lineage Leukaemia, Translocated to, 7; gene map locus Xq13; encodes a widely expressed *forkhead* transcription factor; contributes to the *MLL-AFX* fusion gene in T-lineage acute lymphoblastic leukaemia associated with t(X;11)(q13;q23)

agammaglobulinaemia a severe reduction or absence of serum immunoglobulin (*see* **congenital autosomal recessive agammaglobulinaemia** and **X-linked recessive agammaglobulinaemia**)

agar a colloid obtained from certain algae, used for **electrophoresis**, e.g. as citrate agar

agarose a neutral fraction of **agar**, used for **electrophoresis**

agglutination clumping together of cells, particularly erythrocytes

agglutinin an antibody that causes **agglutination** of erythrocytes

aggregation sticking together, particularly of platelets

agnogenic myeloid metaplasia an alternative designation of **idiopathic myelofibrosis**

agonist a molecule having a specific stimulatory effect

agranulocytosis (i) acute drug-induced immune destruction of neutrophils leading to neutropenic sepsis (ii) severe neutropenia of other origin, e.g. congenital

AIDS   acquired immune deficiency syndrome

AILD   angioimmunoblastic lymphadenopathy

AKT1 a gene, *v-akt* murine thymoma viral oncogene homologue 1, also known

as *PKB*—Protein Kinase B, *Rac* serine/threonine protein kinase; gene map locus 14q32.3; encodes a widely expressed serine/threonine kinase, which is activated by a variety of mitogenic signals and which provides a survival signal protecting from apoptosis; the Akt1 protein physically interacts with the product of *TCL1*, which mediates its translocation to the nucleus; akt1 activity is elevated in several human tumours

ALAS1 also known as *ALASn*, a gene, gene map locus 3p21, encoding the ubiquitously expressed δ-amino laevulinate synthase 1

ALAS2 an erythroid-specific gene, gene map locus Xp11.12, also known as *ALASe*, encoding δ-amino laevulinate synthase 2, the enzyme responsible for the first step in **haem synthesis** (*see* Fig. 34, p. 116)

Albers-Schönberg disease *see* **osteopetrosis**

Alder–Reilly anomaly a congenital abnormality of granulocytes characterized by abnormally heavy staining of granules; it may occur as an isolated defect or as a manifestation of a serious inherited metabolic disease

aldolase an enzyme in the erythrocyte **glycolytic pathway** (*see* Fig. 33, p. 113)

aleukaemic leukaemia leukaemia occurring without a rise in the peripheral blood white cell count

algorithm a step by step decision-making process

ALIP abnormal localization of immature precursors

ALK a gene, Anaplastic Lymphoma Kinase; gene map locus 2p23; encodes the transmembrane receptor tyrosine kinase ALK **(CD246)**, a member of the Ltk (Leukocyte Tyrosine Kinase) family, which is normally expressed by scattered cells in the nervous system, gut and testis; *ALK* is involved in a variety of translocations associated with T-lineage anaplastic large cell lymphoma: *ALK*:
• contributes to the *NPM-ALK* fusion gene in the majority of cases of anaplastic large cell lymphoma associated with t(2;5)(p23;q35)

• is cryptically inserted in the region of the *NPM* gene in a minority of cases of anaplastic large cell lymphoma
• contributes to the *TPM3-ALK* fusion gene in the minority of cases of anaplastic large cell lymphoma with t(1;2)(q25;p23)—also described as t(1;2)(q21;p23) and in inflammatory myofibroblastic tumours
• contributes to *ATIC-ALK* fusion gene in the minority of cases of anaplastic large cell lymphoma with a cryptic inv(2)(p23q35)
• contributes to the *RanBP2-ALK* fusion gene in inflammatory myofibroblastic tumours with t(2;2)(p23;q11-13) or inv(2)(p23q11-13)
• contributes to one of two *TFG-ALK* fusion genes (*TFG-ALK$_S$* and *TFG-ALK$_L$*) in occasional cases of anaplastic large cell lymphoma associated with t(2;3)(p23;q21)
• is likely to be rearranged in t(2;13)(p23;q34) associated with anaplastic large cell lymphoma
• contributes to the *CLTC-ALK* fusion gene in a minority of cases of anaplastic large cell lymphoma probably associated with t(2;17)(p23;q23), not t(2;22)(p23;q11.2), and in inflammatory myofibroblastic tumours (note: the designation *CLTCL* for the partner gene is wrong)
• contributed to a *TPM4-ALK* fusion gene in a case of large cell anaplastic lymphoma with NK phenotype associated with t(2;19)(p23;p13) and contributes to the same fusion gene in inflammatory myofibroblastic tumours with t(2;19)(p23;p13.1)
• contributes to a *moesin-ALK* fusion gene, probably resulting from t(X;2)(q11;p23), in large cell anaplastic lymphoma
Full length ALK is expressed in neuroblastomas, rare cases of rhabdomyosarcoma and rare cases of IgA-positive immunoblastic lymphoma

alkaline phosphatase this is a generic term for an enzyme that works optimally at alkaline pH to release phosphate groups from complex molecules; present in the plasma and expressed in various tissues or cells including bone, liver and neutrophils

alkaline phosphatase-anti-alkaline phosphatase (APAAP) technique a technique for identifying **antigens** by means of **antibodies** linked to **alkaline phosphatase**

alkalosis having a blood pH above 7.45

alkylating agent a **cytotoxic drug** which cross-links strands of **DNA** by means of alkyl groups

allele alternative forms of a **DNA** sequence occupying a given chromosomal **locus**, e.g. β^S is an allele of β^A; may refer to a non-coding as well as a coding sequence

allele-specific oligonucleotide an **oligonucleotide** that is specific for one **allele** of a gene, permitting it to be specifically amplified by **PCR**

allele-specific oligonucleotide hybridization (ASO hybridization) a **PCR** technique for identifying specific **alleles** of a **gene** by the use of allele-specific primers

allele-specific polymerase chain reaction *see* **allele-specific oligonucleotide hybridization**

allelic exclusion the process by which further rearrangements of immunoglobulin or T-cell receptor genes are prevented once a functional rearrangement has been made during B- or T-cell development; ensures that B and T cells make only one type of antigen receptor

allergen a **hapten** or **antigen** capable of giving rise to allergic responses

allergy an acquired inappropriate specific immune reactivity to a normally harmless environmental **antigen**, often IgE mediated

alloantibody an antibody recognizing **antigens** on the cells of a genetically different individual

alloantigen an **antigen** expressed on tissues of another genetically different individual

allogeneic genetically different from an individual; relating to any other person except an identical twin

allograft a transplant from a non-identical individual

alloimmune haemolytic anaemia haemolytic anaemia resulting from **alloantibodies**, e.g. caused by transplacental passage of antibodies or transfusion of blood containing alloantibodies

alloimmunization the development of immune responses to **alloantigens**

all-*trans*-retinoic acid (ATRA) a differentiating agent used in the treatment of M3 AML

alopecia loss of hair

Alport's syndrome an inherited syndrome characterized by renal failure and deafness; the classic pattern of inheritance is autosomal dominant but autosomal recessive forms, resulting from mutations in either the basement membrane collagen alpha-3 or alpha-4 genes (*COLA3, COLA4*), and an X-linked form, resulting from mutations in the basement membrane collagen alpha-5 gene (*COLA5*) are known; when there is also **thrombocytopenia** the designation **Epstein's syndrome** is used, this syndrome resulting from a mutation in the non-muscle myosin heavy chain 9 gene (*NMMHC-IIA* or *MYH9*) at 22q11-13 (or 22q12.3-q13.2)

alternative pathway of complement activation complement activation initiated by binding of complement component C3b to bacterial cell walls (*see* **complement system** and Fig. 20, p. 81)

ALX3 a homeobox gene, Aristaless-Like homeobox 3, gene map locus 1p21-p13; expressed by pancreatic beta cells, which is hypermethylated in neuroblastoma

AML acute myeloid leukaemia

AML1 a gene, Acute Myeloid Leukaemia 1, approved name is *RUNX1*—runt-related transcription factor 1; also known as *CBFA2*—Core-Binding Factor, runt domain, Alpha subunit 2; gene map locus 21q22; encodes one of a family of runt-domain-containing proteins which associate with a non-DNA binding protein CBFβ, to form one of the heterodimeric transcription factors, known as the **core binding factors** (CBFs); the AML1/CBFβ complex is required for normal haemo-poiesis and regulates several genes e.g. those encoding myeloperoxidase, CD13, GM-CSF, M-CSF receptor, neutrophil elastase, IL3 and the T-cell receptor enhancer:

• part of *AML1* fuses with part of the *ETO* gene at 8q22 in M2 acute myeloid leukaemia associated with t(8;21)(q22;q22), forming *AML1-ETO*; *AML1-ETO* appear to act as a dominant negative inhibitor of *AML1*

• part of the *EAP, EVI1* and *MDS1* genes at 3q26 in t(3;21)(q26;q22) in association with acute myeloid leukaemia and blast transformation of myeloproliferative disorders, forming *AML1-EAP, AML1-EVI1* and *AML-MDS1*

• part of *ETV6* to form a fusion gene, *ETV6-AML1 (TEL-AML1)*, detected in about 30% of cases of acute lymphoblastic leukaemia, associated with a cryptic t(12;21)(p13;q22)

• part of *MTG16* to form a fusion gene, *AML1-MTG16*, mainly in secondary acute myeloid leukaemia/myelodysplastic syndrome associated with t(16;21)(q24;q22)

• part of *USP25* to form an *AML1-USP25* in myelodysplastic syndrome

• *AML1* has also been found to be rearranged in the following translocations associated mainly with secondary myelodysplastic syndromes (following cytotoxic chemotherapy or irradiation) or acute myeloid leukaemia

t(1;21)(p36;q22) (irradiation associated)
t(5;21)(q13;q22)
t(12;21)(q24;q22)
t(14;21)(q22;q22)
t(15;21)(q22;q22)
t(18;21)(q21)(q22) (irradiation associated)
t(19;21)(q13.4;q22) (irradiation associated)

An autosomal dominant familial disorder characterized by thrombocytopenia and platelet function defects with a propensity to acute myeloid leukaemia has been associated with mis-sense mutations in the *AML1* gene

Point mutations can occur in *AML1* in myelodysplastic syndromes with the mutant gene being a dominant negative inhibitor of wild-type *AML1*

Figure 6   Mitosis.
The process of mitosis, for clarity showing only four of the 46 chromosomes. Cells that are not actively dividing are in **interphase**, interphase having G1, S and G2 phases (*see* Figure 15, p. 71). It is during the S phase that DNA replication occurs, with each chromosome being replicated so that it is composed of two identical daughter chromatids. Mitosis itself has five phases: (a) in **prophase**, the chromosomes condense and become visible although the sister chromatids—joined at the centromere—remain closely associated and are not visible; the nuclear membrane dissolves and the centriole divides, moving towards the two poles of the cell; the polar mitotic spindle starts to form from each centriole; during **prometaphase** (not illustrated) the equatorial spindle develops and the two chromatids become visible; (b) in **metaphase**, the chromosomes—each composed of two chromatids—align, at the equator of the cell, on the mitotic spindle to which they are attached by their centromeres; (c) in **anaphase**, the centromeres divide so that the two chromatids are detached from each other and can be pulled toward the two poles of the cell by contraction of the spindle fibres; (d) in **telophase**, the chromosomes re-condense and the nuclear membrane re-forms around each cluster of chromosomes; the cytoplasm narrows at the equator of the cell and the cell then divides

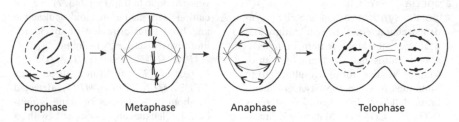

Prophase   Metaphase   Anaphase   Telophase

Biallelic point mutations have been associated with acute myeloid leukaemia with acquired trisomy 21

AML1 may be amplified in acute myeloid leukaemia (by a segmental jumping translocation) and in acute lymphoblastic leukaemia

AMML   acute myelomonocytic leukaemia

amplification   a process of production of multiple copies of DNA sequences *in vitro* (e.g. by **PCR**) or the occurrence of multiple copies of a gene in a cell (e.g. **proto-oncogenes** may be amplified in tumour cells)

amplification-refractory mutation system (ARMS)   a **PCR** method in which primers amplify only a specific mutated **allele**

amyloid   a variety of abnormal proteins derived from different precursor proteins but all characterized by insoluble fibrils with a specific structure—anti-parallel β-pleated sheets with strands arranged perpendicularly to the fibre long axis

amyloidosis   a heterogeneous group of disorders in which there is deposition in the tissues of a waxy starch-like glyco-protein with a distinctive structure (beta pleated sheets); one of the many causes is an overt or occult **plasma cell dyscrasia** giving rise to **light chain-associated amyloidosis**

anabolism   *see* **metabolism**

ANAE   **alpha naphthyl acetate esterase**, one of the **non-specific esterases**

anaemia   a reduction in the haemoglobin concentration in the blood, in comparison with what would be found in a normal individual of the same age and gender

anaphase   the fourth of five phases of **mitosis** in which the **centromere** divides and the two **chromatids** move to either end of the cell (Fig. 6)

anaphylaxis   a life-threatening systemic response to an **allergen**, resulting from the release of histamine and other pharmaco-logical mediators, in which severe hypo-tension and bronchial constriction are prominent elements

anaplastic   a description of cells, the maturation of which shows little re-semblance to that of normal cells of the same lineage

anaplastic large cell lymphoma   a high grade T-cell lymphoma associated with t(2;5) or related translocation (*see* Table 11, p. 153)

ANBE alpha naphthyl butyrate esterase

ANCA anti-neutrophil cytoplasmic antibodies

anergy immunological unresponsiveness to antigenic challenge, particularly of T cells

aneuploid having a chromosome number that is not 46 nor a multiple nor half of 46

aneuploidy presence of a clone of cells with a number of chromosomes which is not 46 nor a multiple nor half of 46

aneurysm a localized dilation of a blood vessel

angiogenesis formation of capillaries and post-capillary venules from pre-existing vessels

angiogram a radiograph of a blood vessel after contrast medium has been injected

angioimmunoblastic lymphadenopathy (AILD) an immune disorder characterized by fever, **lymphadenopathy** and **hypergammaglobulinaemia**; in many if not all cases there is an occult T-cell neoplasm

angioimmunoblastic lymphadenopathy-like (AILD-like) lymphoma a T-cell neoplasm characterized by reactive inflammatory changes in involved lymph nodes and systemic manifestation such as fever and autoimmune disease (*see* Table 11, p. 153)

angio-oedema deep mucocutaneous oedema caused by release of inflammatory cytokines not adequately opposed by **C1 inhibitor**; can occur as an inherited or acquired abnormality

angioplasty reconstruction or dilation of a vessel, usually by minimally invasive methods

angular cheilosis angular **stomatitis**, cracks at the corner of the mouth, a feature of **iron deficiency**

angular stomatitis cracks at the corner of the mouth, a feature of **iron deficiency**

anion a negatively charged ion

anisochromasia increased variation of staining from one erythrocyte to another, reflecting varying haemoglobinization of erythrocytes

anisocytosis increased variation in size from one erythrocyte to another

ANK1 a gene, gene map locus 8p11.2, encoding **ankyrin**, a component of the red cell membrane; mutation can result in **hereditary spherocytosis**

ankyrin a protein of the red cell membrane (*see* Fig. 64, p. 199)

ANLL acute non-lymphoblastic leukaemia

anomaly an abnormality, usually inherited or developmental, affecting a chromosome, cell, tissue, organ or part of the body

anorexia loss of appetite

anorexia nervosa a psychogenic illness in which inadequate intake of calories leads to severe weight loss; can cause **pancytopenia, acanthocytosis** and **gelatinous transformation** of the bone marrow

antagonist a molecule which counteracts the effect of another type of molecule

anthracycline a group of anti-cancer antibiotics including daunorubicin, doxorubicin and epirubicin

antibiotic a molecule synthesized by a living organism, e.g. a fungus, which interferes with the proliferation, growth or differentiation of other organisms or their constituent cells; antibiotics in clinical use include those directed at other micro-organisms and those used for anti-cancer chemotherapy

antibody an **immunoglobulin**, a protein produced by a **plasma cell**, which recognizes and combines with an **antigen**

antibody-dependent cellular cytotoxicity (ADCC) killing that is mediated by a cell, such as a **natural killer cell**, that has **Fc receptors** and thus can bind to an antibody that has already recognized a cellular antigen

anticoagulant a substance that inhibits blood clotting, either *in vitro* or *in vivo*

antifibrinolytic agent a substance which inhibits **fibrinolysis**

antigen a molecule recognized by a specialized structure on the surface membrane of a T or B lymphocyte that has the potential to evoke an immune response; large complex antigens are immunogenic and are therefore designated immunogens; they are capable of eliciting a specific immune response from either B or T lymphocytes, giving rise to humoral and cell-mediated immunity respectively

antigenic drift a slight antigenic change in a micro-organism, which occurs over an extended period of time as a result of a gradual accumulation of mutations

antigenic shift a major, usually sudden, antigenic change in a virus, brought about either by genetic exchanges between related viruses or by exon/whole gene shuffling, both mechanisms representing examples of unequal crossing over between paired chromosomes; the latter mechanism is much more usual (e.g. in the case of the influenza virus)

antigen-presenting cell a specialized cell, e.g. **Langerhans cell, dendritic cell, macrophage** or activated **B cell**, with the function of presenting antigen, in an HLA type II context, to a **helper T cell**

antiglobulin test (Coombs' test) a test for detection of **immunoglobulin** or **complement** components on the surface of erythrocytes (direct antiglobulin test) or for detection of an antibody in the serum capable of binding to erythrocytes (indirect antiglobulin test)

anti-inflammatory agent a drug or other agent which reduces the body's inflammatory responses

antimetabolite a drug which interferes with the participation of normal metabolites such as folic acid, purines or pyrimidines, in metabolic pathways

anti-neutrophil cytoplasmic antibodies (ANCA) autoantibodies characteristic of Wegener's granulomatosis

antiphospholipid syndrome a syndrome including a thrombotic tendency—**thrombophilia**—and recurrent miscarriages associated with the presence of antibodies to phospholipid (*see also* **primary antiphospholipid syndrome**)

antiplasmin an inhibitor of plasmin (*see* Fig. 27, p. 103); mutation of the gene encoding antiplasmin can produce an inactive protein with a resultant haemorrhagic disorder

antisense oligonucleotides short, chemically synthesized, sequence-specific single-stranded DNA molecules that are designed to hybridize to, and block the translation of, their target mRNAs (*see also* **RNA interference**)

antithrombin **a serpin**, an inhibitor of **thrombin** and of activated factors XII, XI, IX and X (see Fig. 27, p. 103); this term now usually refers to the protein that was previously designated antithrombin III, encoded by the *AT3* gene; its anticoagulant effect is greatly increased by the presence of heparin; 1 in 2000–5000 of the Caucasian population have an inherited, **autosomally dominant**, antithrombin deficiency which is associated with significant thrombophilia

anuria failure to produce urine

API2 a gene, **A**poptosis **I**nhibitor **2**, also known as *BIRC3*—**B**aculoviral **I**AP **R**epeat-**C**ontaining protein **3**, gene map locus 11q21; encodes an inhibitor of apoptosis present in normal lymphoid tissue; contributes to the *API2-MLT* fusion gene in MALT lymphoma associated with t(11;18)(q21;q21); in the presence of the fusion gene, there is sequestration of BCL10 protein in the nucleus

APAAP **alkaline phosphatase-anti-alkaline phosphatase technique**, an **immunocytochemistry** technique

APC a gene, **A**denomatous **P**olyposis of the **C**olon, gene map locus 5q21; encodes a large multidomain protein which interacts with the cytoskeleton and components of the wnt/β-catenin signalling system; often regarded as the archetypal **tumour suppressor gene**, somatic mutations are seen in the majority of sporadic colorectal tumours, and germline mutations in *APC* are responsible for familial adenomatous polyposis, an autosomal dominant inherited disease

apheresis the removal of plasma or cellular components, e.g. platelets, from the circulating blood

aplasia failure to develop or acquired absence of a normal tissue or organ

aplastic anaemia **pancytopenia** resulting from chronic bone marrow **aplasia**, either inherited or acquired

apoferritin the protein that binds iron to form **ferritin**; it is an **acute phase reactant**

apoptosis a process of active or programmed cell death; apoptosis is a physiological process but may be exaggerated or suppressed in various disease processes

APT1 previous name for the *TNFRSF6* gene

aPTT activated partial thromboplastin time

AQP1 a gene, gene map locus 7p14, alleles of which encode antigens of the Colton blood group system, carried on an integral membrane water-transport protein, aquaporin 1, also known as Channel-like Integral membrane Protein, 28 RD (*CHIP28*)

ardeparin a low molecular weight heparin

ARF a gene, *see also* Cyclin-Dependent Kinase Inhibitor-2A (*CDKN2A*), gene map locus 9p21; p14^{ARF} is the product of the shorter transcript of the *CDKN2A* gene, the product of the longer transcript being p16^{INK4a}; p14^{ARF} binds to and triggers the degradation of the MDM2 protein (a p53 inhibitor) leading to cell cycle arrest in both the G1 and G2/M phases; deletion of the exon in the *CDKN2A* specifying p14^{ARF} is associated with a worse outcome in aggressive non-Hodgkin's lymphoma

ARG a gene, *ABL*-Related Gene or *ABL2*, gene map locus 1q25, encodes a tyrosine kinase; contributed to a *ETV6-ARG* fusion gene in a cell line with t(1;12)(q25;p13) occurring as a second event in a patient with M3 acute myeloid leukaemia and as a second event in a patient with M4Eo acute myeloid leukaemia

argatroban a thrombin inhibitor, unrelated to heparin

ARMS amplification-refractory mutation system

ARNT a gene, Aryl hydrocarbon Receptor Nuclear Translocator, gene map locus 1q21, encodes a helix–loop–helix transcription factor which heterodimerizes with the dioxin receptor and regulates genes encoding components of the cytochrome P450 system; contributed to an *ETV6-ARNT* fusion gene in a case of M2 acute myeloid leukaemia associated with t(1;12)(q21;p13)

ART4 a gene, gene map locus 12p13.2-p12.1, polymorphism of which lead to expression of the Dombrock blood group antigens

artefact an abnormality that is introduced into a tissue or a peripheral blood sample by some extraneous influence or error in processing

arteriole a small thick walled blood vessel carrying blood away from the heart towards the tissues

arteritis inflammation of an artery

artery a large thick walled blood vessel carrying blood away from the heart towards the tissues

arthritis inflammation of joints

ASH American Society of Hematology

ASO hybridization allele-specific oligonucleotide hybridization

asparaginase an enzyme that destroys the amino acid, asparagine, used in the treatment of acute lymphoblastic leukaemia

aspergillosis disease resulting from infection by a fungus of the Aspergillus genus, e.g. infection by *Aspergillus fumigatus*

aspirate tissue such as bone marrow, obtained by suction applied to a needle

aspiration process of obtaining an aspirate, e.g. of bone marrow

asplenia absence of the spleen

asplenic having no spleen

AT3 the gene at 1q24-q25 that encodes antithrombin, mutation of which can lead to thrombophilia

ataxia telangiectasia a recessively inherited syndrome, resulting from mutation of the *ATM* gene, in which there is cerebellar degeneration, telangiectasiae, defective cell-mediated immunity, increased sensitivity to ionizing radiation and a predisposition to T-lineage prolymphocytic leukaemia and other lymphoid neoplasms

atheroma deposition of lipid in the walls of arteries

ATIC a gene, also known as *AICARFT* (5-Aminoimidazole-4-Carboxamide Ribonucleotide Formyltransferase), gene map locus 2q35; encodes the enzyme that catalyses the penultimate step in the *de novo* purine biosynthetic pathway; contributes to the *ATIC-ALK* fusion gene in the minority of cases of anaplastic large cell lymphoma with a cryptic inv(2)(p23q35)

ATM a gene, Ataxia-Telangiectasia Mutated, gene map locus 11q22-23; a candidate tumour suppressor gene which encodes a serine-threonine kinase with a phosphatidylinositol-3 kinase domain; *ATM* is widely expressed but especially abundant in brain, skeletal muscle and testis; it has a central role in signalling pathways activated by DNA damage; activation of this kinase leads to phosphorylation of **p53**, arresting the cell cycle and permitting DNA repair or apoptosis; *ATM* mutations are the cause of **ataxia-telangiectasia**, a chromosomal instability syndrome; also implicated in T-prolymphocytic leukaemia; *ATM* is often mutated or deleted in mantle cell lymphoma, deleted in cases of chronic lymphocytic leukaemia with del(11)(q23) and mutated in a proportion of other cases of chronic lymphocytic leukaemia

atopy a hereditary predisposition to IgE-mediated disease provoked by common environmental antigens

ATP adenosine triphosphate

ATRA all-*trans* retinoic acid

ATRA syndrome a syndrome of fever, pulmonary infiltrates, weight gain, pleural and pericardial effusions and renal failure that can occur when **acute promyelocytic leukaemia** is treated with all-*trans* retinoic acid (ATRA)

atrophic glossitis inflammation of the tongue with atrophy of the papillae, a feature of **iron deficiency** and **pernicious anaemia**

atrophy regression of an organ or tissue

ATRX a gene, gene map locus Xq13.1-q21.2, that encodes an activator of α globin genes

ATRX syndrome a syndrome of mental retardation and **haemoglobin H disease** resulting from loss or mutation of the *ATRX* gene

atypical chronic myeloid leukaemia (aCML) a chronic myeloid leukaemia that differs clinically, haematologically and at a cytogenetic and molecular genetic level from Philadelphia-positive **chronic granulocytic leukaemia**

atypical lymphocyte a lymphocyte which differs cytologically from a normal lymphocyte; the term is often applied to lymphocytes with features characteristic of **infectious mononucleosis** or other viral infection; also referred to as 'atypical mononuclear cell'

atypical mononuclear cell *see* **atypical lymphocyte**

Auer rod a rod-shaped crystalline structure derived from primary granules, found in the cytoplasm of cells of granulocytic and, less often, monocytic lineage, observed in **acute myeloid leukaemia** and **RAEB-T** category of the **FAB** classification of **myelodysplastic syndromes**

auto- pertaining to self

autoantibody an antibody directed at **antigens** expressed on the body's own cells

autocrine stimulation of a cell by a molecule secreted by the cell itself, creating an 'autocrine loop'

autograft a 'transplant' of autologous tissue; this term is a misnomer since the procedure is not a transplant but merely the storage of **autologous** tissue for subsequent return to the same individual

autohaemolysis test a test for increased destruction of erythrocytes suspended in **autologous** plasma

autoimmune a disease or process in which the body mounts a **humoral** or **cell-mediated** immune response to **autologous** antigens

autoimmune haemolytic anaemia anaemia caused by autoimmune (antibody-mediated) destruction of erythrocytes

autoimmune lymphoproliferative syndrome an inherited condition characterized by hepatosplenomegaly, lymphadenopathy and autoimmune disease (including **autoimmune haemolytic anaemia** and **autoimmune thrombocytopenia**) resulting from mutation in the *TNFRSF6* (fas) gene, previously known as *APT1* (type 1a), the *TNFSFS6* (fas ligand) gene (type Ib) or the *CASP10* (caspase gene) (type II); the disease results from the failure of **apoptosis** of lymphoid cells; diagnostic criteria suggested by the **NIH** are: (i) chronic accumulation of non-malignant lymphocytes; (ii) increased T lymphocytes with the immunophenotype αβ+CD4–CD8– and (iii) defective *in vitro* receptor-mediated lymphocyte apoptosis

Figure 7 Autosomal dominant inheritance—von Willebrand's disease.
A family tree showing the inheritance of von Willebrand's disease (loosely based on an actual family)
showing autosomal dominant inheritance; the disease is passed from parent to child irrespective of gender
with there being a 1 in 2 chance of any child inheriting the condition. Note that only one of non-identical
twins in the second generation is affected. For each individual the factor VIII percentage and the bleeding
time (in minutes) are given.

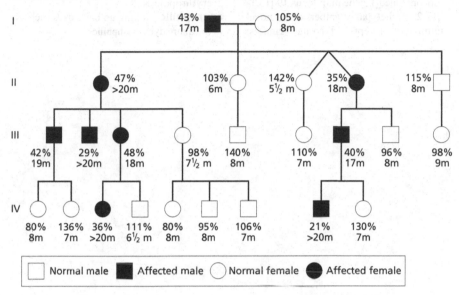

**autoimmune thrombocytopenic pur-
pura** thrombocytopenia caused by autoimmune (antibody-mediated) destruction
of platelets

autologous pertaining to an individual's own cells or tissues

autologous stem cell transplantation
a misnomer, **autologous** cells are re-
infused but this is not a transplant

autophagic vacuole a vacuole in the
cytoplasm of a cell containing material
derived from the cell itself

autosomal pertaining to an **autosome**

autosomal dominant a form of inheritance in which a single copy of an **allele**
on an **autosome** is sufficient to cause an
alteration in phenotype, either an inherited characteristic or an inherited disease
(Fig. 7)

autosomal recessive a form of inheritance in which **homozygosity** (or **compound heterozygosity**) for an **autosomal**
allele is required for a **phenotypic** effect
(Fig. 8)

**Figure 8 Autosomal recessive inheritance—
pyruvate kinase deficiency**.
Pedigree of a hypothetical family in which a boy (IV1)
was found to have severe anaemia resulting from
pyruvate kinase deficiency. His parents, III3 and
III4, were first cousins. They, two of his grandparents
and his great-grandmother were heterozygous
carriers of pyruvate kinase deficiency. This is an
example of autosomal recessive inheritance in a
family in which a consanguineous marriage occurred

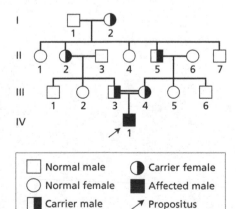

autosome   a chromosome other than X, Y or a mitochondrial chromosome; a diploid cell has two copies of each autosome

AXL   a gene, <u>A</u>ne<u>x</u>e<u>l</u>ekto (Greek for 'uncontrolled'), gene map locus 19q13.1-q13.2, archetypal member of a novel family of receptor tyrosine kinases; over-expressed in chronic granulocytic leukaemia

azathioprine   an antimetabolite used for immune suppression; which can cause **pancytopenia** and **megaloblastic** erythropoiesis

azurophilic   taking up basic dyes such as the azure dyes; **basophilic**

B

2,3-biphosphoglycerate (2,3-BPG) an intermediate in the **glycolytic pathway** that decreases the oxygen affinity of haemoglobin, previously known as 2,3-diphosphoglycerate (*see* Fig. 33, p. 113)

β chain (i) the beta globin chain that forms part of **haemoglobin A** (ii) part of the αβ **T-cell receptor**, a surface membrane structure in T lymphocytes which permits recognition of antigens

β error the lack of a statistically significant difference when a real difference does exist, indicative of inadequate **power** of an experiment or clinical trial

β globin cluster the cluster of genes on chromosome 11 that includes the genes encoding ε, ^Gγ, ^Aγ, δ and β globin chains (*see* Fig. 1)

β globin gene the *HBB* gene, gene map locus 11p15.5, encoding the **β globin chain**

β thalassaemia thalassaemia caused by mutation or, less often, deletion of a **β globin gene** leading to reduced beta globin synthesis

β thalassaemia intermedia a genetically heterogeneous condition intermediate in severity between **thalassaemia trait** and **thalassaemia major**; the severity is very variable but blood transfusions are not essential for the maintenance of life

β thalassaemia major a severe transfusion-dependent thalassaemic condition resulting from **homozygosity** or **compound heterozygosity** for **β thalassaemia**

β thalassaemia trait a clinically mild or inapparent thalassaemic abnormality, resulting from **heterozygosity** for **β thalassaemia**

β₂-glycoprotein I a phospholipid-binding protein, a putative naturally occurring anticoagulant, antibodies to which are strongly associated with thrombophilia and other features of the antiphospholipid syndrome

BAC bacterial artificial chromosome

bacteraemia presence of bacteria in the blood stream

bacterial artificial chromosome (BAC) a bacterial cloning vector capable of maintaining very large fragments of eukaryotic genomic DNA in *E. coli*; essential for genome analysis and mapping

bacterium (plural bacteria) unicellular micro-organisms which may be round, rod-shaped, spiral or comma shaped

babesiosis a disease resulting from infection by protozoan parasites of the genus Babesia

bacillus (plural bacilli) a rod-shaped bacterium

B acute lymphoblastic leukaemia (B-ALL) ALL with cells having a mature B-cell immunophenotype, i.e. expressing surface membrane immunoglobulin

BAD a protein of the BCL2 family that is pro-apoptotic because of its ability to sequester BCL2 and BCLX$_L$; binding of cytokines, such as **interleukin-3**, to their ligands can phosphorylate BAD so that it cannot then sequester these anti-apoptotic proteins

balanced polymorphism the persistence of a polymorphic allele at a stable frequency from generation to generation, usually implies a balance between the beneficial and deleterious effects of the allele

balanced translocation a translocation in which microscopic examination of **metaphase** spreads discloses neither gain nor loss of chromosomal material (Fig. 9, p. 22)

Figure 9   A balanced translocation.
Two diagrammatic representations of a balanced translocation—t(15;17)(q22;q21);
there is exchange of material between two chromosomes with no net gain or loss. The
upper figure shows the two normal and two abnormal chromosomes with their
characteristic banding patterns. The short arm (p), long arm (q), centromere,
telomeres and the two chromatids that make up a chromosome are also indicated. In
the lower diagram chromosome 15 and material derived from it is shown in black and
chromosome 17 and material derived from it in white.

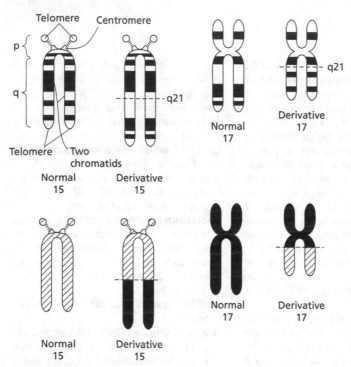

band a chromosomal region that, after staining, can be distinguished from adjoining regions by appearing darker or lighter (*see* Fig. 31, p. 110)

band 3 a red cell membrane protein (**CD233**), also known as anion exchanger 1, encoded by the *AE1* gene at 17q21-q22 (*see* Fig. 64, p. 199)

band cell a late cell of granulocyte lineage with a non-segmented band-shaped nucleus

banding a technique for staining chromosomes so that bands are apparent (*see* **G-banding, Q-banding**)

BARD1 a gene, *BRCA1*-Associated Ring Domain 1, gene map locus 2q, encodes a pro-apoptotic protein bearing a cysteine-rich domain (**RING motif**) which is found in many proteins that regulate cell growth; implicated in familial breast and breast plus ovarian cancer

bare lymphocyte syndrome an immune deficiency syndrome in which lymphocytes are 'bare' of either class I or class II HLA molecules

bare nucleus a nucleus that has lost its cytoplasm, e.g. a mature megakaryocyte that has shed its cytoplasm as platelets, or a cell of any lineage that has lost its cytoplasm during spreading of a blood or bone marrow film

Barr body a clumped area of chromatin representing an inactive X chromosome; a nuclear drumstick in a neutrophil is equivalent to a Barr body in other somatic cells

bartonellosis infection by bacteria of the genus Bartonella, e.g. infection by *Bartonella bacilliformis* which is the cause of Oraya fever

base (i) a proton acceptor (ii) a ring-shaped organic molecule containing nitrogen which is a constituent of DNA and RNA; DNA contains four bases—adenine, guanine, cytosine and thymine; RNA contains four bases—adenine, guanine, cytosine and uracil

base pair (bp) a pair of specific bases, e.g. adenine plus thymine, in the complementary strands of the DNA double helix; bp are the basic units for measuring the length of a DNA sequence

basophil a granulocyte which, on a Romanowsky stain, has large purple granules almost obscuring the nucleus

basophilia (i) increased uptake of basic dyes such as azure blue or methylene blue, conveying a blue colour to cytoplasm (ii) an increased basophil count

basophilic erythroblast an early erythroid precursor, derived from a proerythroblast (*see* Fig. 25, p. 95)

basophilic leukaemia leukaemia with prominent basophilic differentiation

basophilic stippling the presence of evenly dispersed purplish blue dots in the cytoplasm of erythrocytes, representing altered **ribosomes**

BAX a protein that leads to activation of **caspases** and therefore **apoptosis**

B cell a lymphocyte of B lineage, i.e. a cell with the potential to differentiate into an antibody-secreting **plasma cell**, named from the **B**ursa of Fabritius in the chicken

BCL1 a gene, **B**-**C**ell **L**eukaemia/lymphoma **1**, also known as *PRAD1*, *CCND1*; gene map locus 11q13, encodes cyclin D1; cyclins complex with and activate the p34 (**CDC2**) protein kinase, and regulate progress through the cell cycle; dysregulated by proximity to the *IGH* locus as a result of the t(11;14)(q13;q32) translocation in the great majority of patients with mantle cell lymphoma, 20–25% of patients with multiple myeloma and a significant minority of

patients with splenic lymphoma with villous lymphocytes and B-lineage prolymphocytic leukaemia; rearranged in parathyroid adenoma and overexpressed in breast cancer and head and neck cancer

BCL2 a gene, **B**-**C**ell **L**eukaemia/lymphoma **2**; gene map locus 18q21.3; encodes an inner mitochondrial membrane protein which can protect cells in conditions that would otherwise bring about apoptosis; the anti-apoptotic activity of the BCL2 protein is enhanced by phosphorylation, but its precise mechanism of action is not known; the archetypal member of a family of genes encoding proteins with pro- and anti-apoptotic functions; the gene is dysregulated in follicular lymphoma and various other B-lineage lymphomas (10–20% of B-lineage large cell lymphomas) when it is brought into proximity to one of the genes encoding the heavy or light chains of immunoglobulin: the *IGH* locus in t(14;18)(q32;q21), the κ gene in t(2;18)(p12;q21) or the λ gene in t(18;22)(q21;q11); protection from apoptosis may lead to an expanded pool of cells subject to secondary genetic events; *BCL2* is implicated in the majority of cases of follicular lymphoma and in 1–2% of cases of chronic lymphocytic leukaemia, the breakpoints in *BCL2* in follicular lymphoma and in chronic lymphocytic leukaemia being different; *BCL2* rearrangement has also been observed in patients with clonal B-cell proliferation in association with chronic hepatitis C infection

BCL2 a protein, encoded by *BCL2*, that sequesters BAX and is therefore anti-apoptotic

BCL3 a gene, **B**-**C**ell **L**eukaemia/lymphoma **3**, formerly *BCL4*; gene map locus 19q13, belongs to a family of genes that encode inhibitors (IκB proteins) of the transcription factor NFκB$_2$; IκB proteins interact with REL/NFκB proteins in unstimulated cells and sequester them in the cytoplasm by masking nuclear localization signals; on cell stimulation, IκB is degraded, permitting NFκB to translocate to the nucleus and bind to *cis*-acting sequences that induce gene expression; *BCL3* is rearranged, brought into juxtaposition to the *IGH* enhancer and overexpressed in t(14;19)(q32;q13); this translocation is found in less than 1% of cases of chronic lymphocytic leukaemia and is associated with a young age at presentation and poor prognosis

BCL6 a gene, **B**-**C**ell **L**eukaemia/lymphoma **6**, also known as **Z**inc **F**inger protein **51** (*ZNF51*) and **L**ymphoma-**A**ssociated **Z**inc finger gene on chromosome **3** (*LAZ3*); gene map locus 3q27; encodes a zinc finger transcriptional repressor closely related to the Drosophila '*tramtrack*' and '*Broad-complex*' genes; BCL6 protein is expressed by normal germinal centre B cells (and T cells) but not virgin B cells, post-germinal centre B cells (including memory cells) or plasma cells; BCL6 regulates germinal centre formation and T-cell responses; the *BCL6* gene is involved in t(3;14)(q27;q32) and in a great variety of other translocations which have been associated with 30–40% of B-lineage large cell lymphomas; 5' non-coding point mutations in *BCL6* leading to increased expression occur in an even larger proportion of B-lineage large cell lymphomas, in the absence of translocations with a 3q27 breakpoint; high levels of BCL6 expression in diffuse large B-cell lymphoma is associated with a favourable outcome; *BCL6* mutations occur in a proportion of normal B cells (30–50%) that pass through germinal centres and are also associated with germinal centre and post-germinal centre B-cell neoplasms including follicular lymphoma, MALT-type lymphoma, lymphoplasmacytoid lymphoma, diffuse large B-cell lymphoma, Burkitt's lymphoma and a subset of B-chronic lymphocytic leukaemia/small lymphocytic lymphoma and hairy cell leukaemia; *BCL6* mutations are associated with large cell transformation of follicular lymphoma; *BCL6* mutations are found in about a quarter of cases of chronic lymphocytic leukaemia; *BCL6* mutations have been found to be predictive of a worse survival in post-transplant lymphoproliferative disorder; *BCL6* is expressed on the neoplastic cells of nodular lymphocyte predominant Hodgkin's disease and on some cells in a minority of cases of classical Hodgkin's disease; mutations of *BCL6* appear to be common in classical Hodgkin's disease of B-cell origin but in general these diseases are not associated with *BCL6* expression and *BCL6* is therefore unlikely to be relevant in pathogenesis; *BCL6* contributes to:

• a *TTF-BCL6* fusion gene or promoter exchange between *BCL6* and *Rho/TTF* in non-Hodgkin's lymphoma with t(3;4)(q27;p13)

• a *SRP20-BCL6* fusion gene in non-Hodgkin's lymphoma with t(3;6)(q27;p21)

• an *H4-BCL6* fusion gene in non-Hodgkin's lymphoma with t(3;6)(q27;p21)

• an *IKAROS-BCL6* fusion gene in non-Hodgkin's lymphoma with t(3;7)(q27;p12)

• a *BOB1-BCL6* fusion gene in non-Hodgkin's lymphoma with t(3;11)(q27;q23)

• an *LCP1-BCL6* fusion gene in non-Hodgkin's lymphoma with t(3;13)(q27;q14)

BCL7A a gene, **B**-**C**ell **L**eukaemia/lymphoma **7A**, gene map locus 12q24; a widely expressed gene which encodes a predicted protein with no discernible structural or functional motifs; dysregulated by proximity to *IGH* in t(12;14)(q24;q32) associated with B-cell malignancy

BCL7B a gene, **B**-**C**ell **L**eukaemia/lymphoma **7B**, gene map locus 7q11.23, a widely expressed gene which encodes a predicted protein with no discernible structural or functional motifs, closely related to *BCL7A*, not as yet implicated in any haematological malignancy

BCL7C a gene, **B**-**C**ell **L**eukaemia/lymphoma **7C**, gene map locus 16p11, a widely expressed gene which encodes a predicted protein with no discernible structural or functional motifs; closely related to *BCL7A*, not as yet implicated in any haematological malignancy

BCL8 a gene, **B**-**C**ell **L**eukaemia/lymphoma **8**, gene map locus 15q11-13, encodes a predicted protein with no discernible homologies to other known gene products; normally expressed in prostate and testis but not in lymphoid cells; rearranged in 3–4% of diffuse large B-cell lymphomas; probably dysregulated by proximity to *IGH* in t(14;15)(q32;q11-13) which is found in less than 1% of cases of diffuse large B-cell lymphomas

BCL9 a gene, B-Cell Leukaemia/lymphoma **9**, gene map locus 1q21, encodes a predicted protein with no discernible homologies to other known gene products; involved in t(1;14)(q21;q32) in B-lineage acute lymphoblastic leukaemia and other B-cell malignancies in which it is dysregulated by proximity to the *IGH* locus

BCL10 a gene, B-Cell Leukaemia/lymphoma **10**. gene map locus 1p22; *BCL10* is normally ubiquitously expressed at low levels; it encodes a **CARD domain**-containing pro-apoptotic protein; in addition, normal BCL10 protein dimerizes with the product of the *MLT* gene and activates the latter's caspase-like domains; this in turn enhances the activation of the transcription factor NFκB in response to a variety of antigen receptor induced signals; the pro-apoptotic activity of BCL10 requires intact CARD and carboxyl terminal domains, whereas NFκB activation requires an intact CARD but not the full-length carboxyl terminal domain; rearranged in t(1;14)(p22;q32) in some cases of high grade MALT lymphoma, high grade follicle centre cell lymphoma and Hodgkin's disease; t(1;14)(p22;q32) is found in about 5% of MALT lymphomas and in gastric MALT lymphoma mutation is predictive of failure of response to antibiotic therapy; in t(1;14)(p22;q32) *BCL10* is overexpressed following juxtaposition to the *IGH* enhancer; carboxy terminus truncations have been reported in several lymphomas independently of any cytogenetic changes, such truncated proteins can continue to activate NFκB while no longer promoting apoptosis; in the presence of the t(11;18)(q21;q21) translocation in gastric MALT lymphoma, which results in the AP12-MLT fusion protein, there is sequestration of BCL10 protein in the nucleus; mutations

within the *BCL10* gene have been reported to occur in a variety of cancers but this may be a cloning artefact

BCL11A a gene, B-Cell Leukaemia/lymphoma **11A**, mouse, homologue of; also known as *evi9*; gene map locus 2p13; *evi9* is a common site for retroviral integration in murine myeloid leukaemias; encodes an evolutionarily conserved zinc-finger protein with highest expression in brain, spleen, and testis; it is brought into proximity to the *IGH* enhancer in 'childhood chronic lymphocytic leukaemia' associated with t(2;14)(p13;q32); the same translocation with dysregulation of *BCL11A* is also observed in atypical chronic lymphocytic leukaemia/non-Hodgkin's lymphoma

BCL11B a gene, B-Cell Leukaemia/lymphoma **11B**, also known as *CTIP2*, gene map locus 14q32.1, encodes a protein structurally similar to BCL11A; highly expressed during normal T-cell differentiation and is probably responsible for the transcriptional activation of *HOX11L2* in a quite common t(5;14)(q35;q32) cryptic translocation in T-lineage acute lymphoblastic leukaemia; it is expressed in cell lines derived from patients with adult T-cell leukaemia/lymphoma

BCLX$_L$ a protein that sequesters BAX and is therefore anti-apoptotic

BCR Breakpoint Cluster Region, gene map locus 22q11.21, encodes a widely expressed cytoplasmic protein which has serine/threonine kinase activity, at least two SH-2 domains and enhances GTPase activity of p21^{rac} (*see* **RAC1**); in addition, normal BCR protein is known to interact with the DNA repair protein, XPB; *BCR* contributes to:

• a *BCR-ABL* fusion gene, encoding a tyrosine kinase, as a result of the t(9;22)(q34;q11) translocation in chronic granulocytic leukaemia, a significant proportion of cases (particularly adults) with acute lymphoblastic leukaemia and a small minority of cases of acute myeloid leukaemia

• a *FGFR1-BCR* fusion gene in chronic myeloid leukaemia associated with t(8;22)(p11;q11)

Figure 10   Bence Jones protein.
Demonstration of Bence Jones protein in the urine of a patient with IgG multiple
myeloma. Electrophoresis of the urine (lane 5) shows an albumin band and a discrete
heavy band early in the gamma region (top). Lanes 1 and 10 are control serum
samples. Lanes 2 and 3 show albumin only whereas lanes 6–9 are negative.
Immunofixation (bottom) shows that the band is identified with anti-lambda but
not anti-gamma antiserum. It is therefore a lambda Bence Jones protein.

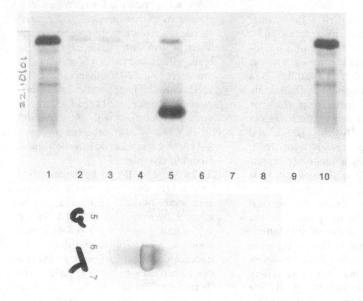

BCR-ABL   the fusion gene on chromosome
22 formed as a result of t(9;22)(q34;q11),
encoding BCR-ABL protein

BCR-ABL   a non-receptor tyrosine kinase
encoded by the *BCR-ABL* fusion gene

BCSH   British Committee for Standards in
Haematology

Bence Jones myeloma multiple
myeloma in which the **paraprotein** synthesized is a monoclonal light chain
rather than a complete immunoglobulin

Bence Jones protein a monoclonal
light chain (kappa or lambda) synthesized in multiple myeloma, either as the
only paraprotein present or together with
a monoclonal immunoglobulin; Bence
Jones protein, as initially described by
Henry Bence Jones, was a protein that
coagulated at 45°C to 55°C but redis-
solved on heating to a higher temperature; it is now usually demonstrated
by electrophoresis and immunofixation
(Fig. 10)

benign 'not harmful', a description of
a non-aggressive neoplasm

benign lymphoid aggregate an
aggregate of lymphocytes present in the
bone marrow as a reactive phenomenon,
better referred to as a 'reactive lymphoid
aggregate'

benign monoclonal gammopathy a
very low grade B-lineage lymphoid neoplasm with cells secreting small amounts
of a **paraprotein**; the designation '**monoclonal gammopathy of undetermined significance**' is now preferred

Bernard–Soulier syndrome an inherited, autosomal recessive, platelet abnormality characterized by giant platelets
that do not aggregate normally with ristocetin; it can result from mutations in
the *GPIBA*, *GP1BB*, *GPV* or *GPIX* genes

BFU-E   **burst forming unit-erythroid**

bHLH basic helix loop helix; a protein
motif found in certain transcription
factors which allows binding to a DNA

sequence known as the E box, which is found in the regulatory regions of many genes; HLH proteins fall into two classes—Class I HLH proteins, e.g. E2A, are widely expressed and are capable of homodimerization and/or heterodimerization, Class II HLH proteins, e.g. TAL1, are expressed in a tissue-specific manner and bind DNA only as heterodimers with class I proteins

BHLHB1 a gene, **B**asic **H**elix–**L**oop–**H**elix protein, class **B**, **1**, gene map locus 21q22, encodes a transcription factor normally only expressed in neural tissues; overexpressed when brought into proximity to the *TCRAD* (αδ) locus in a patient with T-lineage acute lymphoblastic leukaemia associated with t(14;21)(q11.2;q22)

bias in the statistical sense, a systematic factor resulting in **inaccuracy**

bile the fluid containing bilirubin and bile salts secreted by the liver and concentrated in the gall bladder

bilirubin a pigmented breakdown product of haemoglobin, produced by macrophages and by liver parenchymal cells; in the liver it is conjugated with glucuronic acid prior to excretion in the bile (Fig. 11)

bioinformatics the study of information content and information flow in biological systems and processes

biopsy the removal of tissue from a living person for diagnostic purposes

biphenotypic a leukaemia with a single leukaemic cell population having features of two lineages—haemopoietic or B or T lymphoid, e.g. myeloid and B-lymphoid

Birbeck granules granules characteristic of **Langerhans cells**

bite cell an erythrocyte from which a **Heinz body** has been removed by a **macrophage** of the **reticuloendothelial system**, leading to the formation of a cell from which a bite appears to have been taken, a **keratocyte**

bivalirudin a hirudin derivative, a **thrombin** inhibitor

Blackfan–Diamond syndrome see **Diamond–Blackfan syndrome**

black water fever acute intravascular haemolysis occurring in falciparum malaria

blast cell a primitive cell or haemopoietic or lymphoid lineage, e.g. a myeloblast or a lymphoblast (Fig. 12)

blast crisis **blast transformation** of **chronic granulocytic leukaemia**

blast transformation the transformation of a low grade leukaemia to an acute leukaemia, e.g. blast transformation of chronic granulocytic leukaemia

bleeding time the time for which bleeding continues from a standardized skin puncture or incision, determined by platelet number and function

B lineage a lineage of lymphoid cells that differentiate into antibody-synthesizing **plasma cells**

blood component constituents of blood separated from whole blood with minimal manipulation, mainly red cells, platelets or plasma but also leucocytes, cryoprecipitate and 'cryosupernatant'

blood product a biological product prepared by fractionation or processing of a blood component, e.g. immunoglobulin, albumin

blood tap jargon used to describe an attempt at bone marrow aspiration that yields only blood

Bloom's syndrome a rare recessively inherited condition, most common among Ashkenazi Jews, characterized by growth retardation, telangiectatic erythema, photosensitivity, immune deficiency, subfertility and an increased risk of cancer, including leukaemia; Bloom's syndrome results from a mutation in the *BLM* gene leading to a deficiency of the BLM protein, a member of the RecQ family of DNA helicases, which associates with chromosomes during **meiosis**; Bloom's syndrome cells show genomic instability with an increased frequency of sister **chromatid** exchange and an increased rate of **somatic mutation**

B lymphocyte a lymphocyte, also known as a B cell, with the potential to mature into an antibody-secreting **plasma cell** (Fig. 13)

BMT **bone marrow transplantation**

boat-shaped cell a cell the shape of which resembles a boat viewed from

Figure 11   The results of red cell breakdown.

Normal red cell breakdown and intravascular and extravascular haemolysis (not to scale). Red cells at the end of their life span and abnormal or antibody-coated red cells are phagocytosed by macrophages of the reticulo–endothelial system. The haemoglobin of the red cells is degraded to globin, iron and protoporphyrin, the latter then being converted to bilirubin. Unconjugated bilirubin is transported to the liver. In intravascular haemolysis, haemoglobin is released from red cells and binds to plasma haptoglobin. The complexes thus formed are cleared by the parenchymal cells of the liver which degrade haemoglobin and convert protoporphyrin to bilirubin. Bilirubin, whether produced in the liver or transported there, is conjugated to form bilirubin glucuronide. Conjugated bilirubin is excreted in the bile and enters the intestine. Within the intestine, bacteria convert bilirubin to urobilinogen, which is either reabsorbed and excreted in the urine or passes further down the intestinal tract where it is known as stercobilinogen. Extravascular haemolysis, if marked, leads to release of more haemoglobin than can be bound by haptoglobin with the result that free haemoglobin is filtered from the plasma by the kidneys, leading to haemoglobinuria. Some haemoglobin is resorbed by renal tubules and converted to haemosiderin, which later appears in the urine as the renal tubular cells are shed.

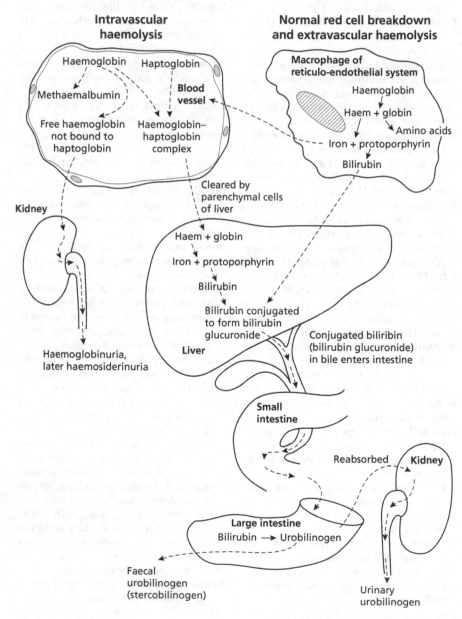

Figure 12   A lymphoblast.
A transmission electron micrograph of a lymphoblast from a patient with acute lymphoblastic leukaemia. There is a high nucleocytoplasmic ratio and the nucleus shows little chromatin condensation.

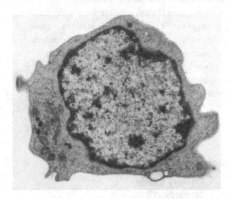

above, suggestive of the presence of haemoglobin S but not pathognomonic

BOB1 a gene, **B**-cell specific **O**ctomer-**B**inding transcription factor, also known as *POU2AF1*—**POU** domain, class **2**, **A**ssociating **F**actor **1**, gene map locus 11q23.1; encodes a B-cell specific coactivator of octamer-binding transcription factors, Oct1 and Oct2; the gene contributes to the *BOB1-BCL6* fusion gene in B-lineage non-Hodgkin's lymphoma associated with t(3;11)(q27;q23); *BOB1* is expressed in the neoplastic cells of nodular lymphocyte predominant Hodgkin's disease but not those of classical Hodgkin's disease

BOB-1 a co-activator of the transcription factors, Oct1 and **Oct2**

Bombay blood group the hh O blood group in which there is inability to express A and B antigens as a result of a lack of the precursor H substance which, in turn, results from the lack of a specific glycosyltransferase that is encoded by the *H* allele at the *FUT1* locus (*see* Fig. 3, p. 4)

bone marrow the tissue present in the cavity of bones that has the potential to produce blood cells; yellow marrow is predominantly fat whereas red marrow has a high percentage of haemopoietic cells

bone marrow fibrosis the deposition of increased amounts of **reticulin** (reticulin fibrosis) or reticulin plus **collagen** (collagen fibrosis) in the bone marrow

bone marrow necrosis the non-selective death of bone marrow cells, e.g. due to an inadequate blood supply for the metabolic needs of the tissue

bone marrow transplantation (BMT) the engraftment of haemopoietic stem cells by means of the intravenous infusion of bone marrow cells, either derived from the individual himself (**autologous transplantation**) or from another individual (**allogeneic transplantation**)

bone scan an imaging technique using a radioactive isotope; increased isotope uptake in areas of increased **osteoblast** activity causes 'hot spots' on the scan; it should be noted that this is not a recommended test for detection of the **osteolytic** lesions of **multiple myeloma** since these often do not give rise to any abnormality on a bone scan

borreliosis a disease resulting from infection by micro-organisms of the genus Borrelia; relapsing fever

bp base pair

2,3-BPG 2,3-biphosphoglycerate, also known as 2,3-DPG

B prolymphocytic leukaemia a leukaemia of relatively large mature B-lineage cells with plentiful cytoplasm and a large prominent nucleolus (Fig. 14)

BRCA1 a gene, **Br**east **Ca**ncer, type **1**, gene map locus 17q21; encodes a widely expressed nuclear phosphoprotein which may be involved in DNA repair; implicated in familial breast and breast plus ovarian cancer

BRCA2 a gene, **Br**east **Ca**ncer 2, early-onset, gene map locus 13q12.3; encodes a DNA repair protein that functions in conjunction with the RAD51 recombinase; implicated in familial breast and breast plus ovarian cancer

breakpoint the point in a gene or on a chromosome where a breakage occurs, leading to rearrangement of a gene or a chromosome

bromodomain an evolutionarily conserved motif found in proteins associated with chromatin and in nearly all nuclear

Figure 13   Production and maturation of the B lymphocyte.
Precursor B lymphoblasts are produced in the bone marrow from the common lymphoid progenitor. They rearrange first an immunoglobulin heavy chain gene and then one or more light chain genes. The naïve B cell passes into the blood stream and thus to a primary follicle of the lymph node. If the naïve B cell recognizes antigen presented by a specialized antigen-presenting cell, further development occurs, to either an immunoblast, giving rise to a medullary plasmacytoid lymphocyte, or to a B blast, which remains in the follicle. The follicle also contains follicular dendritic cells which, by means of their Fc and complement receptors, can trap antigen in the form of immune complexes. If the B blast is presented with antigen by a follicular dendritic cell and is aided by helper T cells, it becomes a centroblast and undergoes somatic hypermutation, affinity maturation and isotype switching; by this stage the primary follicle has become a secondary follicle. The centroblast becomes a centrocyte and, on leaving the follicle, the mature B cell ultimately becomes either a memory B cell or an antibody-secreting plasma cell in bone marrow or other tissues.

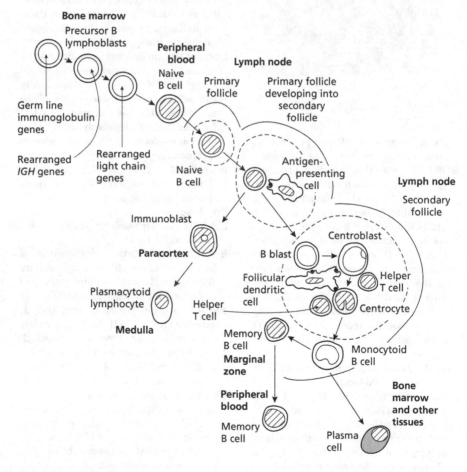

histone; bromodomains have been shown to bind to acetylated histones

bronchi   intermediate sized air passages

bronchioles   small air passages

bronchitis   acute or chronic inflammation of the **bronchi**

bronchoconstriction   reversible narrowing of the airways

brucellosis   disease resulting from infection by organisms of the genus Brucella

BSH   British Society for Haematology

Figure 14 A prolymphocyte.
Transmission electron micrograph of a prolymphocyte in B-lineage prolymphocytic leukaemia. The very large nucleolus and abundant cytoplasmic mitochondria are apparent.

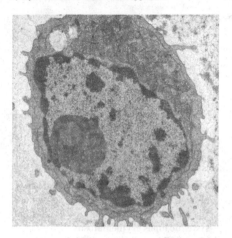

BTK a gene, **B**ruton agammaglobuli-naemia **T**yrosine **K**inase, also known as **B**-cell **P**rogenitor **K**inase, *BPK*, gene map locus Xq21.3-q22, encodes a nonreceptor tyrosine kinase that is essential for B-cell development; germline mutations in this gene lead to X-linked agammaglobulinaemia, characterized by a failure of B-cell development and agammaglobulinaemia, but with normal T and NK cells

***BTL**   see CHIC2*

buffer a substance that tends to control the hydrogen ion concentration in a solution so that pH change on adding an acid or an alkali is lessened

buffy coat the beige-coloured layer of white cells that appears above the red cells when blood is centrifuged or allowed to sediment

Burkitt's lymphoma a highly aggressive B-cell lymphoma with distinctive cytological, histological, cytogenetic and molecular genetic features

burr cell an unsatisfactory term which is sometimes used to describe a variety of types of **spiculated cell**

burst forming unit-erythroid (BFU-E) an erythroid **progenitor** which gives rise to a number of erythroid colonies (CFU-E) (*see* Fig. 41, p. 122)

busulphan an alkylating agent occasionally used in the treatment of chronic myeloid leukaemias and other myeloproliferative disorders

C

c   (i) a cytogenetic abbreviation indicating a **constitutional** abnormality (ii) expressed in the cytoplasm (iii) an indication that a gene is a human cellular gene, homologous to a viral gene, e.g. *c-ABL* cf. *v-abl*

C   one of the **complement** components or an abbreviation for the pyrimidine, cytosine

C1   also known as C1 esterase, the first component of the **complement** pathway, composed of one molecule of C1q, two molecules of C1s and two molecules of C1r (*see* **complement system**)

C1 esterase inhibitor   C1 inhibitor, the inhibitor of the activated form of the first component of **complement**

C1 esterase inhibitor deficiency   an inherited or acquired deficiency of **C1 esterase inhibitor**

C1 inhibitor   *see* **C1 esterase inhibitor**

C1q deficiency   an inherited deficiency of C1q, when homozygous associated with high probability of developing **systemic lupus erythematosus**

C1r and C1s deficiency   an inherited deficiency of C1r and C1s, when homozygous associated with high probability of developing **systemic lupus erythematosus**

C2   a component of the classical and mannose-binding lectin complement pathways (*see* **complement system**)

C2 deficiency   an inherited deficiency of C2, when homozygous associated with high probability of developing **systemic lupus erythematosus**

C3   a component of the classical, alternative and mannose-binding lectin complement pathways (*see* **complement system**)

C3 deficiency   an inherited deficiency of C3, when homozygous associated with susceptibility to pyogenic infections, membranoproliferative glomerulonephritis and rash

C4   a component of the classical and mannose-binding lectin complement pathways (*see* **complement system**)

C4 deficiency   an inherited deficiency of C4, when homozygous associated with increased probability of developing **systemic lupus erythematosus**

C4A, C4B   genes at 6p21.3 encoding complement component 4, which carries antigens of the Chido/Rodgers blood group system

C4ST   a gene, Chondroiton 4-O-Sulphotransferase 1, gene map locus 12q23, which is rearranged and dysregulated in t(12;14)(q23;q32) in chronic lymphocytic leukaemia

C5, C6, C7, C8 and C9   components of the classical, alternative and mannose-binding lectin complement pathways (*see* **complement system**)

Cabot's rings   thread-like rings or loops within red cells, mainly described on films stained with a **Wright's stain** and very uncommon in **May–Grünwald–Giemsa** stained films

cachectic   suffering from **cachexia**

cachexia   marked wasting, e.g. due to severe malnutrition or malignant disease

cadherin   a member of the family of calcium-dependent cell adhesion molecules which mediate **homotypic** cell-cell adhesion; they include N-cadherin (neuronal cadherin), P-cadherin (placental cadherin) and E-cadherin (epithelial cadherin); 'classical' cadherins have a highly conserved cytoplasmic domain that associates with intra-cellular actin microfilaments via catenins; 'non-classical' cadherins are more diverse and have cytoplasmic domains that connect to intermediate filaments, e.g. desmin (see also **protocadherin**)

caisson disease decompression illness occurring in deep-sea divers, consequent on too rapid decompression leading bubbles of nitrogen to appear in the blood stream, can cause **bone marrow necrosis**

Calabar swellings subcutaneous swelling of the shins as a consequence of loiasis

CALM a gene, Clathrin Assembly Lymphoid Myeloid leukaemia, gene map locus 11q14, also known as Phosphatidylinositol-binding Clathrin Assembly Lymphoid Myeloid leukaemia protein—*PICALM* and Assembly Protein, **180** kD—*AP180*; encodes a phosphoinositide-binding protein which promotes the assembly of and restricts the size of clathrin-coated vesicles; *CALM* contributes to
• a *MLL-CALM* fusion gene in acute myeloid leukaemia associated with inv(11)(q14.2q23.1)
• a *CALM-AF10* fusion gene in acute myeloid leukaemia

CAN Cain gene, also known as *NUP214*—Nucleoporin, **214** kD; gene map locus 9q34.1; *CAN* is so named because of its proximity to the *ABL* gene at 9q34 (Cain and Abel, the sons of Adam) also indicating Cancer gene intron on Nine; encodes a protein which forms part of the nuclear pore complex; *CAN* contributes to
• the *DEK-CAN* (*DEK-NUP214*) fusion gene in t(6;9)(p23;q34) associated with acute myeloid leukaemia in which the fusion protein localizes to the nucleus and may function as a transcription factor
• the *SET-CAN* (*SET-NUP214*) fusion gene, formed by fusion of two genes at 9q34, associated with acute myeloid leukaemia

cancellous bone trabecular bone, bone composed of anastomosing spicules

cancer a general term usually used to indicate any malignant neoplasm

cancer suppressor gene *see* **tumour suppressor gene**

Candida a genus of fungi capable of causing superficial or deep infections, the latter particularly in patients with immune deficiency or other illnesses

candidiasis disease resulting from infection by micro-organisms of the genus Candida

CAPD continuous ambulatory peritoneal dialysis

capillary (i) a small thin walled blood vessel connecting arterioles to venules (ii) a very fine tube

carbonic anhydrase an erythrocyte enzyme which catalyses the conversion of CO_2 and H_2O into carbonic acid, H_2CO_3; the most abundant protein in an erythrocyte after haemoglobin, being present in sufficient quantities to produce a visible band if a protein stain is used for staining haemoglobin electrophoresis membranes

carboxyhaemoglobin haemoglobin that has been chemically altered by combination with carbon monoxide

carcinocythaemia circulation of carcinoma cells in the peripheral blood

carcinogen a substance capable of giving rise to cancer

carcinogenesis the process by which an external influence or substance, e.g. a chemical or a radioactive isotope, gives rise to cancer

carcinogenic able to cause cancer

carcinoid tumour a neuroendocrine tumour that secretes serotonin

CARD domain Caspase Recruitment Domain; a homotypic interaction motif present in proteins that regulate apoptosis e.g. **BCL10, caspase** 2, ApaF1

carrier a person who has one copy of a mutant gene that causes a significant phenotypic abnormality in **homozygotes**, a **heterozygote** for a mutant gene

cascade a sequence of reactions, e.g. the coagulation cascade

caseating granuloma a granuloma with central **caseation** necrosis, typical of tuberculosis but not pathognomonic

caseation a form of tissue necrosis when a crumbly cheese-like material is produced

CASP10 a caspase gene, gene map locus 2q23-q34, mutations of which underlie type II **autoimmune lymphoproliferative syndrome**, also known as *FLICE*, FAD-Like Ice

caspase   a family of cysteine proteases that mediate **apoptosis**

Castleman's disease   an inflammatory condition of lymph nodes, also known as angiofollicular lymph node hyperplasia and giant lymph node hyperplasia; **human herpesvirus 8 (HHV8)** infection is one aetiological factor

CAT scan   **computerized axial tomography scan**

catabolism   the breakdown or degradation of large energy-rich molecules within cells (*see also* **metabolism**)

catalyse   to increase the rate of a chemical reaction

cathepsin G   a protease which is one of the constituents of azurophilic granules of neutrophils

cation   positively charged ion

cat scratch disease   a disease resulting from infection by micro-organisms of the genus Afipia or the genus Rochalimaea, transmitted by the bite or scratch of a cat and causing fever and lymphadenopathy

CBC   **complete blood count**

CBFB   a gene, **C**ore **B**inding **F**actor **B**eta, gene map locus 16q22; encodes a transcription factor that does not bind DNA directly but interacts with one of three *runt* domain containing proteins encoded by either *RUNX1* (*AML1*), *RUNX2* (*AML3*) or *RUNX3* (*AML2*) to form one of three possible heterodimeric active transcription factors; each transcription factor has a distinct normal pattern of expression and function (see also *AML1* and Fig. 29, p. 107); *CBFB* contributes to the fusion gene *CBFB-MYH11* in M4Eo acute myeloid leukaemia associated with inv(16)(p13q22) and t(16;16)(p13;q22); the fusion gene probably has a dominant negative effect on *AML1* function

CBP   CREB (**C**yclic adenosine monophosphate **R**esponsive **E**lement **B**inding protein) binding protein, *CREBBP*; gene map locus 16p13; encodes a widely expressed bromodomain protein which binds to and coactivates CREB—a transcription factor activated by signals that lead to elevated cAMP levels; in addition CBP has inherent acetylase activity; CBP coactivates several tissue-specific transcription factors including the haemopoietic transcription factors, AML1 and GATA1, and the muscle-specific transcription factor, MyoD; mutations in *CBP* result in the Rubinstein–Taybi syndrome (RTS), characterized by mental retardation, skeletal abnormalities, and an increased propensity for neoplasms, including leukaemia; part of *CBP* fuses with:

• part of the *MOZ* gene to form *MOZ-CBP* in M5 acute myeloid leukaemia associated with t(8;16)(p11;p13)

• part of the *MLL* gene to form *MLL-CBP* in M2 acute myeloid leukaemia and therapy-associated myelodysplastic syndrome associated with t(11;16)(q23;p13)

• part of the *MORF* gene at 10q22 to form both *MORF-CBP* and *CBP-MORF* genes in M5 acute myeloid leukaemia associated with t(10;16)(q22;p13)

CCAAT/Enhancer-Binding Protein ε   a basic leucine zipper motif, myeloid-specific transcription factor encoded by *C/EBPε*

CCNA1   the gene encoding cyclin A1, gene map locus 13q12.3-q13, normally expressed in testes and brain, it is overexpressed in about a quarter of patients with acute myeloid leukaemia

CCNA2   the gene encoding cyclin A2, gene map locus 4q27, a widely expressed cyclin which promotes both G1/S and G2/M transitions (*see* **cell cycle**); repressed by **PLZF**; it is overexpressed in breast cancer

CCNB1   the gene encoding cyclin B1, gene map locus 5q12, widely expressed, predominantly in the G2/M phase of the **cell cycle** when it is phosphorylated and translocated into the nucleus; with **CDK1** and **cyclin F**, is a component of M-phase promoting factor; degraded by **ubiquitin**-mediated proteolysis at the end of metaphase; it is overexpressed in malignant and some benign breast disorders, and in squamous metaplasia of the oesophagus

CCNC   the gene encoding cyclin C, gene map locus 6q21; along with **CDK8**, cyclin

C forms an inhibitory component of the RNA polymerase II holoenzyme complex; it is hemizygously deleted in some cases of acute lymphoblastic leukaemia

CCND1 *see BCL1*

CCND2 the gene encoding cyclin D2, gene map locus 12p13, normally expressed during the G1 phase of the **cell cycle**; brought into proximity to the λ gene enhancer in t(12;22)(p13;q11) associated with a case of Richter's transformation; there was also loss of a negative regulatory element; it is overexpressed in colorectal cancer, gastric cancer (indicates poor prognosis) and male germ cell tumours

CCND3 the gene encoding cyclin D3, gene map locus 6p21.1, normally expressed late in the G1 phase of the **cell cycle**; it is:
• dysregulated by proximity to the *IGH* locus in 2–4% of patients with multiple myeloma and in some patients with splenic lymphoma with villous lymphocytes and transformed marginal zone lymphoma associated with t(6;14)(p21;q32)
• dysregulated by proximity to the λ gene in one patient with multiple myeloma associated with t(6;22)(p21;q11)

CCNE the gene encoding cyclin E, gene map locus 19q13.1, overexpressed in several types of cancer including bladder and gastric cancer, overexpressed in chronic lymphocytic leukaemia

CCNF the gene encoding cyclin F, also known as **F-Box** only protein **1**, *FBX1*; gene map locus 16p13.3, encodes a protein containing a novel domain, the F-box which is present in proteins involved in **ubiquitin**-mediated proteolysis; a component of M-phase promoting factor

CCNG1 the gene encoding cyclin G, gene map locus 5q32-q34, encodes a protein induced by DNA-damaging agents via a **p53**-dependent mechanism; normally expressed in lymphocytes, skeletal muscle, ovary and kidney; unusual amongst cyclins in that its mRNA level does not vary during the **cell cycle**

CCNG2 the gene encoding cyclin G2, a protein closely related to **cyclin A**, normally expressed in spleen, thymus and prostate, reaches its highest levels of expression in late G2 phase of the **cell cycle**

CCNH the gene encoding cyclin H, gene map locus 5q13.3-q14; encodes a protein which, along with **CDK7** comprises **C**dk-**A**ctivating **K**inase (CAK)

CCNT1 the gene encoding cyclin T1, gene map locus chromosome 12, *see CDK9*

CD cluster of differentiation, a system for classifying monoclonal antibodies according to their antigenic specificity; antibodies within the same cluster recognize the same antigen, as determined by immunoprecipitation, binding inhibition experiments or both; antibodies of the same CD category have similar, but not necessarily identical, patterns of tissue reactivity

CD1 a cell surface glycoprotein, a family of transmembrane proteins (CD1a, CD1b, CD1c, CD1d and CD1e) noncovalently linked with β2 microglobulin; CD1a, CD1b and CD1c function in T-cell responses to glycolipid antigens; expressed on cortical thymocytes (CD1a strongly, CD1b moderately and CD1c weakly) and thought to have a role in thymic T-cell development; expressed on about a third of normal B cells (CD1b and c), mature and some immature dendritic cells, interdigitating reticulum cells (CD1b and c), Langerhans cells and intestinal epithelium (CD1d only); not expressed on mature T cells; has a role in antigen presentation. CD1a is expressed on Langerhans cells, but not on interdigitating dendritic cells, follicular dendritic cells or macrophages

CD1 is expressed on blast cells of some T-lineage acute lymphoblastic leukaemia, the cells of some B-cell neoplasms and the cells of Langerhans cell histiocytosis; it is less often expressed in chronic lymphocytic leukaemia than on normal B cells, although in other B-cell neoplasms expression is often increased

CD2 receptor for sheep red blood cells, (previous designations LFA-2 and leucocyte function-associated antigen 1), binds to **CD58** on antigen presenting cells and is costimulatory for B cells, expressed on cortical and late thymocytes, mature T cells, most NK cells; expression in T cells increases with repeated antigen stimulation; expressed on cells of systemic mastocytosis but not on normal mast cells; a recombinant protein bearing the CD2-binding moiety of CD58 (alefacept) has been used to target memory T cells in the therapy of psoriasis

CD2 is expressed on blast cells of many cases of T-lineage acute lymphoblastic leukaemia and cells of many leukaemias/lymphomas of mature T cells; may be expressed on the leukaemic cells in M3 and M4Eo acute myeloid leukaemia

CD3   a complex of at least five membrane-bound polypeptides (CD3γ, CD3δ, CD3ϵ, CD3zeta and CD3eta) that are non-covalently associated with each other and with the T-cell receptor; expressed on late thymocytes and mature T cells, the complex is essential for antigen recognition and binding by T cells and subsequent signal transduction; monoclonal antibodies to CD3 (muromonab) have been used for the treatment of renal and cardiac allograft rejection and acute graft-versus-host disease; a bi-specific CD3, CD19 antibody has therapeutic potential in non-Hodgkin's lymphoma

CD3 is expressed on blast cells of many cases of T-lineage acute lymphoblastic leukaemia and neoplastic cells of many leukaemias/lymphomas of mature T cells

CD4   a cell surface glycoprotein, co-receptor for MHC class-II restricted antigen-induced T-cell activation (*see* Fig. 42, p. 123); co-expressed with CD8 on cortical thymocytes and expressed on a major subset of late thymocytes and mature T cells (helper/inducer) without co-expression of CD8; expressed on immature myeloid cells, eosinophils, monocytes, macrophages and Langerhans cells but not interdigitating dendritic cells or follicular dendritic cells, receptor for human herpesvirus 7; receptor for **HIV**, binding to the envelope protein gp120; the number of CD4+ lymphocytes is greatly reduced in advanced HIV infection and overt **AIDS**; a chimaeric anti-CD4 monoclonal anti-body (keliximab) has been used in therapy of severe asthma and anti-CD4 monoclonal antibodies have also been used in psoriasis

CD4 is expressed on blast cells of many cases of T-lineage acute lymphoblastic leukaemia and on cells of many leukaemias/lymphomas of mature T cells; sometimes expressed on blast cells in acute myeloid leukaemia, particularly in M4 and M5 acute myeloid leukaemia; expressed in Langerhans cell histiocytosis

CD5   a cell surface glycoprotein, a signal transducing molecule that modulates signalling through the T- and B-cell receptor complexes: ligand of the B-cell antigen **CD72**; expressed on cortical and late thymocytes and some early thymocytes, on mature T cells, on a subset of normal B cells (found in the mantle zone of germinal centres and in small numbers in the blood); CD5+ lymphocytes are expanded in various autoimmune diseases, e.g. rheumatoid arthritis and high circulating levels of soluble CD5 are seen in Sjogren's Syndrome; ricin-conjugated-CD5 monoclonal antibodies (XomaZyme-CD5 Plus) have been used for the treatment of acute graft-versus-host disease

CD5 is expressed on blast cells of many cases of T-lineage acute lymphoblastic leukaemia, and cells of many T-lineage leukaemias/lymphomas and on cells of chronic lymphocytic leukaemia and mantle cell lymphoma; expression of CD5 in diffuse large B-cell lymphoma is associated with adverse prognostic features and worse survival

CD6   an adhesion molecule mediating binding of developing thymocytes to thymic epithelium, expressed on thymocytes at all stages of development but may be weakly expressed on the most immature cells; expressed on the majority of peripheral blood T cells and a subset of normal B cells (involved in the production of autoreactive antibodies); CD6+ T cells are thought to be involved in graft-versus-host disease; expressed at low levels on a subset of CD34+ haemopoietic stem cells and may mediate their attachment to stromal cells by binding to **CD166**

CD6 is expressed on the cells of chronic lymphocytic leukaemia; it is expressed fairly consistently on the blast cells of T-lineage acute lymphoblastic leukaemia

CD7 a cell surface glycoprotein, a member of the immunoglobulin superfamily of cell surface glycoproteins, expressed on thymocytes, the majority of mature T cells and NK cells; expressed on some **common lymphoid progenitor cells**; expressed a subset of immature myeloid cells; ricin-conjugated monoclonal antibodies to CD7 have been used for the treatment of T-cell leukaemias and lymphomas and, together with anti-CD3, for the treatment of acute graft-versus-host disease

CD7 is expressed on blast cells of T-lineage acute lymphoblastic leukaemia, leukaemic cells of T-lineage prolymphocytic leukaemia and, less often, the cells of other T-lineage leukaemias/lymphomas; it is expressed on blast cells of a significant minority (c. 15%) of cases of acute myeloid leukaemia—this expression may be useful in monitoring minimal residual disease

CD8 a heterodimeric glycoprotein, having an α and a β chain encoded by closely linked genes on chromosome 2; a co-receptor for MHC class I molecules; the α chain gene also gives rise to an alternatively spliced transcript that encodes a small secreted polypeptide which is thought to have an immunoregulatory role; expressed on cortical thymocytes together with **CD4**; expressed on a subset of late thymocytes and mature T cells without co-expression of CD4, these being cytotoxic/suppressor T cells that recognize antigen in the context of class I major histocompatibility antigens; expressed on macrophages but not osteoclasts; expressed on NK cells

CD8 is expressed on cells of most cases of large granular lymphocyte leukaemia and on cells of a smaller proportion of cases of other T-lineage leukaemias/lymphomas

CD8 lymphopenia a congenital immune deficiency syndrome resulting from mutation in the *ZAP-70* gene, gene map locus 2q12, which encodes a **tyrosine kinase** important in T-cell signalling

CD9 MRP-1, a cell surface glycoprotein, a member of the transmembrane 4 or tetraspanin superfamily of proteins, expressed on haemopoietic stem cells, megakaryocyte progenitors, platelets, early B cells, activated B and T cells, eosinophils, basophils, normal and neoplastic mast cells, endothelial cells, neural and glial cells of the brain and peripheral nerves, vascular and cardiac smooth muscle and epithelial cells; expressed on bone marrow stromal cells; in platelets is associated with **CD36**; expression in melanoma and breast cancer may be indicative of a better prognosis; however, has a role in transendothelial migration of melanoma cells

CD9 is expressed by B-lineage acute lymphoblastic leukaemia cells, the leukaemic cells of hypergranular promyelocytic leukaemia and less often the leukaemic cells in other types of acute myeloid leukaemia

CD10 a cell surface glycoprotein, neutral endopeptidase or neprilysin, a cell surface metalloproteinase, the common ALL antigen, expressed on a subset of normal B-cell progenitors including B cells in germinal centres and '**haematogones**'—non-neoplastic immature B-lineage lymphoid cells that are seen particularly in the bone marrow of children; expressed on a minority (less than 10%) of circulating B cell in neonates, on neutrophils, on bone marrow stromal cells, on renal, bronchial and intestinal epithelium and on breast myoepithelium; expressed on a significant proportion of many non-haemopoietic tumours including: renal cell, transitional cell and prostatic carcinoma, pancreatic and hepatocellular carcinoma, melanoma and various sarcomas

CD10 is expressed on blast cells of the majority of cases of B-lineage acute lymphoblastic leukaemia, more weakly on the blast cells of some cases of T-lineage acute lymphoblastic leukaemia, on the cells of many cases of follicle centre cell lymphoma and a lower proportion of cases of other B-lineage non-Hodgkin's lymphomas; expressed on some myeloma cells

CD11a a cell surface glycoprotein, LFA1α (α chain of leucocyte function associated antigen 1) or $α_L$ integrin, shares a beta subunit (**CD18**) with other members of a family of leukocyte surface membrane antigens; CD11a is expressed as a heterodimer with CD18; CD11a/CD18 is an adhesion molecule of the $β_2$ integrin family ($α_Lβ_2$ integrin) which is expressed on all leucocytes and is important in many inflammatory and immune responses; expressed on macrophages but not osteoclasts; CD11a/CD18 is necessary for lymphocyte recirculation through lymph nodes; CD11a/CD18 binds to ICAM-1 (**CD54**), ICAM-2 (**CD102**) and ICAM-3 (**CD50**); expression is absent in **leucocyte adhesion deficiency** type I, a congenital disorder characterized by neutrophilia and recurrent bacterial infections due to deficiency of the beta-2 integrin subunit (CD18) of the leukocyte cell adhesion molecule; anti-CD11a antibodies have been used experimentally in the treatment of psoriasis

CD11a is expressed (with CD18) in some cases of multiple myeloma; CD11a/CD18 may be expressed in follicular lymphoma and strong expression is indicative of a better prognosis; not expressed on chronic lymphocytic leukaemia cells; expression in acute myeloid leukaemia correlates with a worse prognosis

CD11b a cell surface glycoprotein, $α_M$ integrin chain, also known as mac1 or MO1, it shares a beta subunit (**CD18**) with other members of a family of leukocyte surface membrane antigens; CD11b/CD18 is $α_Mβ_2$; it is a C3bi receptor (CR3 complement receptor); also binds to **CD54** and extracellular matrix proteins; expressed on mature monocytes and macrophages but not osteoclasts; expressed on NK cells; expressed more weakly on mature neutrophils but expression is increased when neutrophils are activated; sometimes expressed on basophils and variably expressed on mast cells; expressed on a subset of B cells (CD5+ activated B cells) and a subset of T cells (cytotoxic CD8+ T cells); expressed, together with high levels of **CD11c**, on a subset of

mature thymic dendritic cells; CD11b/CD18 promotes binding and phagocytosis of complement coated particles and has a role in interactions of neutrophils and monocytes with stimulated endothelium; expression is absent in **leucocyte adhesion deficiency** type I, a congenital disorder characterized by neutrophilia and recurrent bacterial infections due to deficiency of the beta-2 integrin subunit (CD18) of the leukocyte cell adhesion molecule; administration of **G-CSF** increases expression of CD11b/CD18 on neutrophils; on monocytes CD11b is expressed more strongly than CD15 whereas on neutrophils the reverse is true; used by *Mycobacterium tuberculosis*, the human immunodeficiency virus and flaviviruses, such as the West Nile virus, to enter cells

CD11b is expressed on hairy cells; expressed on cells of many cases of acute myeloid leukaemia, particularly those with monocytic differentiation; occasionally expressed on chronic lymphocytic leukaemia cells

CD11c a cell surface glycoprotein, $α_X$ integrin chain, also known as p150 (p150, 95); it shares a beta subunit (**CD18**) with other members of a family of leukocyte surface membrane antigens; it is expressed as a heterodimer with CD18 (CD11c/CD18 or $α_Xβ_2$ integrin); expressed on monocytes, macrophages, NK cells and neutrophils (more weakly than on monocytes); not expressed on osteoclasts; expressed on normal and neoplastic mast cells but not basophils; expressed on some but not all dendritic cells—specifically, on peripheral blood dendritic cells of myeloid origin but not on those of lymphoid origin; expressed on some but not all mature lymph node dendritic cells; expressed, together with CD11b, on a subset of mature thymic dendritic cells; expressed on activated T and B cells; CD11c is a ligand for iC3b and fibrinogen; expression is absent in **leucocyte adhesion deficiency** type I, a congenital disorder characterized by neutrophilia and recurrent bacterial infections due to deficiency of the beta-2 integrin subunit

(CD18) of the leukocyte cell adhesion molecule

CD11c is expressed on hairy cells and cells of some cases of hairy cell variant leukaemia and splenic lymphoma with villous lymphocytes and occasionally on chronic lymphocytic leukaemia and small lymphocytic lymphoma cells but not usually on cells of other lymphoproliferative disorders

CDw12 the gene encoding this antigenic determinant has not yet been cloned; expressed on monocytes, neutrophils, natural killer cells and platelets

CD13 a membrane-bound zinc-binding metalloproteinase, also known as aminopeptidase N; expressed as a homodimer, that degrades regulatory peptides and may modify peptides bound to MHC class II molecules; expressed on early committed progenitors of granulocytes and monocytes and on maturing cells of these lineages; expressed on dendritic cells; expressed on macrophages and osteoclasts; expressed on mast cells and their precursors; expressed on endothelial cells when there is angiogenesis but not expressed on normal endothelial cells; expressed on bone marrow stromal cells, osteoclasts, bile duct canalicular cells, proximal tubule cells of the kidney and the intestinal brush border (where CD13 is thought to function as a coronavirus receptor)

CD13 is expressed on the blast cells of the majority of cases of acute myeloid leukaemia, being more often negative in M6 and M7 acute myeloid leukaemia; expressed on some myeloma cells

CD14 a glycosylphosphatidylinositol (GPI)-anchored cell surface glycoprotein, receptor for endotoxin (lipopolysaccharide–lipopolysaccharide binding protein complex); expressed on monocytes and macrophages and more weakly on neutrophils; not expressed on basophils or mast cells; expressed on circulating dendritic cells and some immature tissue dendritic cells; expressed on macrophages but not osteoclasts; when endotoxin is bound to CD14 of neutrophils and monocytes there is release of tumour necrosis factor and upregulation of cellular adhesion molecules; soluble CD14 is required for endotoxin signalling to endothelial and epithelial cells

CD14 is expressed on the blast cells of many cases of acute myeloid leukaemia, particularly those showing monocytic differentiation—it is a fairly specific but not very sensitive marker of M4 and M5 acute myeloid leukaemia; aberrant expression of CD14 in chronic lymphocytic leukaemia has been associated with a worse prognosis; expressed in the majority of cases of Langerhans cell histiocytosis

CD15 a fucose-containing, cell surface glycoprotein, also known as alpha-3 fucosyltransferase, which is the ligand of E and P selectins (**CD62E** and **CD62P**); expressed on maturing cells of monocyte lineage and more weakly on maturing cells of neutrophil and eosinophil lineages, from the promyelocyte stage onwards; not expressed on basophils or mast cells; CD15s is the sialylated form; monoclonal antibodies detect either the sialylated form, CD15s (e.g. McAb FH6 or CSLEX1) or non-sialylated form of CD15 (LeuM1 and 80H5); the sialylated form is the ligand for CD62E; Rambam–Hasharon syndrome is an autosomal recessive inborn error of fucose metabolism associated with neutrophilia and recurrent infections; the immune defect, designated **leucocyte adhesion deficiency type II**, results from lack of sialylated CD15 (CD15s) which is a ligand for selectins—as a result, neutrophils which fail to express CD15s cannot bind normally to endothelial E and P selectins and cannot migrate normally into tissues; in addition, the patient's red blood cells lack H substance, a fucosylated glycoprotein, which is the precursor molecule of the A, B and O blood groups and consequently patients manifest the **Bombay** blood type

CD15 is expressed on the blast cells of many cases of acute myeloid leukaemia particularly those with monocytic differentiation; it is expressed on Reed–Sternberg cells and mononuclear Hodgkin's cells (except in nodular lymphocyte predominant Hodgkin's disease), a worse prognosis in Hodgkin's disease having been related to expression of non-sialylated rather than sialylated CD15; expressed on cells of a small proportion of cases of non-Hodgkin's lymphoma

CD15u   sulphated CD15

CD16   a glycosylphosphatidylinositol (GPI)-anchored integral membrane protein, part of the low affinity Fcγ receptor, FcRIII which mediates phagocytosis and antibody-dependent cytotoxicity; expressed on NK cells (mature NK cells but not NK precursors or immature NK cells), some T cells, neutrophils and macrophages but not eosinophils or osteoclasts; not expressed on basophils or mast cells constitutive expression in neutrophils is cytoplasmic with transient surface membrane expression occurring when they are exposed to complement; includes CD16a and CD16b, which differ somewhat in structure but are expressed on the same range of cells

Polymorphisms in FcγRIIIa correlate with responsiveness to rituximab (anti-CD20) therapy

CD16 is expressed on the cells of a significant minority of cases of acute myeloid leukaemia—a fairly specific but not very sensitive marker of M4 and M5 acute myeloid leukaemia; expressed by some NK-cell neoplasms, specifically aggressive NK cell leukaemia/lymphoma and some cases of nasal-type NK-cell leukaemia lymphoma but not blastic NK-cell lymphoma

CDw17   an antigenic determinant defined by the lactosyl disaccharide group of the glycosphingolipid lactosyl ceramide; the protein carrying this antigenic determinant is not known; expressed on monocytes, neutrophils, basophils (but not mast cells), platelets, a subset of B cells and tonsillar dendritic cells

CD18   an integral membrane protein, the β chain of the β$_2$ integrins CD11a/CD18, CD11b/CD18 and CD11c/CD18; mutations in the CD18 gene are responsible for **leucocyte adhesion deficiency type I**, a congenital disorder characterized by neutrophilia and recurrent bacterial infec-

tions; CD18 binds unopsonized bacteria and fungi, thus promoting phagocytosis; CD18 is expressed on all leucocytes; a proteolytically truncated form of CD18 is a marker of activation of neutrophils and monocytes; β2 integrins are expressed on activated eosinophils, permitting their adhesion to ICAM-1 on endothelial cells; expressed on basophils; variably expressed on mast cells; not expressed on normal plasma cells; administration of **G-CSF** increases expression of CD11b/CD18 on neutrophils

CD18 may be expressed on myeloma cells; CD11a/CD18 may be expressed in follicular lymphoma and strong expression is indicative of a better prognosis; not expressed on chronic lymphocytic leukaemia cells

CD19   a cell surface glycoprotein, a signal transduction molecule, regulating B-cell development, activation and proliferation; part of a large signal transduction complex that also involves **CD21** and **CD81**, expressed on B lymphocytes and their precursors; it is one of the earliest of the B-lineage restricted antigens to be expressed; expressed on follicular dendritic cells; may be expressed on normal plasma cells and their precursors

CD19 is expressed on the cells of the majority of cases of B-lineage acute lymphoblastic leukaemia and leukaemia/lymphoma of B-lineage; not usually expressed on myeloma cells; an anti-CD19 immunotoxin conjugated to the tyrosine kinase inhibitor, Genistein, has been employed in therapy of acute lymphoblastic leukaemia and B-lineage non-Hodgkin's lymphoma; a bi-specific CD3, CD19 antibody has therapeutic potential in non-Hodgkin's lymphoma

CD20   a cell surface glycoprotein, expressed on B lymphocytes and their precursors but not the earliest identifiable precursors; weakly expressed on a T-cell subset; expressed on follicular dendritic cells; humanized murine monoclonal antibodies to CD20, rituximab (Mabthera, Rituxan), have been used in severe autoimmune disease including pure red cell aplasia, autoimmune haemolytic anaemia, immune thrombocytopenia in the context of graft-versus-host disease and polyneuropathy caused by IgM antibodies; anti-CD20 antibodies may also be useful in Epstein–Barr virus related post-transplant lymphoproliferative disease and in human herpesvirus 8-related multicentric Castleman's disease

CD20 is expressed on blast cells of some cases of B-lineage acute lymphoblastic leukaemia but not on the most immature B lymphoblasts; expressed on cells of the majority of cases of B-lineage leukaemia/lymphoma but more weakly expressed in chronic lymphocytic leukaemia than in other mature B-cell neoplasms; expressed in a minority of cases of multiple myeloma but more often expressed in plasma cell leukaemia; expressed on neoplastic cells in nodular lymphocyte predominant Hodgkin's disease and expressed, more weakly on the neoplastic cells of 30–40% of classical Hodgkin's disease; the murine monoclonal antibodies to CD20, including some linked to a radionucleide (e.g. Yttrium-90 (90Y)-ibritumomab and Iodine-131(^{131}I)-tositumomab), are used in treatment of B-cell neoplasms, such as follicular lymphoma, chronic lymphocytic leukaemia and cold haemagglutinin disease; the monoclonal antibody FMC7, widely used in diagnosis, appears to bind to a particular conformation of CD20, probably a multimeric CD20 complex

CD21 a cell surface glycoprotein, forms part of a large signal transduction complex that also involves **CD19** and **CD81**; a **complement** receptor, CR2 or C3dR, that binds C3d, C3dg and iC3b; complement may activate B cells through CD21 binding with activated B cells no longer expressing CD21; a receptor for **EBV**; expressed on a subset of normal B cells including follicular mantle zone and marginal zone lymphocytes; not expressed on B-cell precursors; expressed on follicular dendritic cells, helping to distinguish them from interdigitating dendritic cells, Langherhans cells and macrophages; CD21 monoclonal antibodies, used in conjunction with CD24 mono-

clonal antibodies, have been found useful in controlling post-transplant lymphoproliferative disorder

CD21 is expressed on cells of most cases of chronic lymphocytic leukaemia and on cells of about 50% of cases of B-lineage non-Hodgkin's lymphoma but expression on chronic lymphocytic leukaemia cells is weaker than on normal B cells and does not support EBV transformation; weakly expressed on hairy cells; expressed on cells of some cases of T-lineage acute lymphoblastic leukaemia; expressed by neoplastic cells of a minority of cases of Hodgkin's disease; when linked to a radionucleide, monoclonal CD21 antibodies have been used in therapy of B-cell neoplasms

CD22 <u>S</u>ialic acid-binding <u>I</u>mmunoglobulin-like <u>Lec</u>tin <u>2</u>, siglec-2, an adhesion and signalling cell surface glycoprotein, which is a member of the sialoadhesion subclass of the Ig superfamily; CD22 modulates the effect of antigen signalling in B cells; expressed on B lymphocytes and in the cytoplasm of their precursors; variably expressed on mast cells; expression on basophils is detected with some but not all monoclonal antibodies

CD22 is expressed in the cytoplasm of the blast cells of most cases of B-lineage acute lymphoblastic leukaemia but less frequently on the surface membrane; expressed on the surface membrane of cells of most cases of B-lineage leukaemia/lymphoma, including hairy cell leukaemia but with the exception of the cells of chronic lymphocytic leukaemia in which expression is weak or absent; anti-CD22 monoclonal antibodies, e.g. epratuzumab, including murine and humanized antibodies linked to a radionucleide, have been used for the treatment of B-lineage non-Hodgkin's lymphoma; an anti-CD22 recombinant immunotoxin has been used in the treatment of hairy cell leukaemia

CD23 a cell surface glycoprotein, low affinity Fcε receptor (FcεRII); a negative feedback regulator of IgE synthesis; expressed on B cells in the follicular mantle but not by proliferating germinal centre B cells; expressed on 30–40% of peripheral blood B cells, on activated B cells, a subset of T cells, eosinophils, monocytes, macrophages, Langerhans cells, follicular dendritic cells, platelets and some stromal cells; mediates cytokine release by monocytes; soluble CD23 is a B-cell growth factor; expressed less often on the cells of polyclonal B-cell lymphocytosis than on normal B cells; expressed on epithelial cells, e.g. of stomach. intestine and lung

CD23 is expressed on cells of most cases of chronic lymphocytic leukaemia and small lymphocytic lymphoma but in only a minority of cases of prolymphocytic leukaemia and other categories of non-Hodgkin's lymphoma; expressed more often in low grade lymphoma than in high grade; soluble CD23 is of prognostic significance in chronic lymphocytic leukaemia

CD24 a heavily glycosylated **glycosylphosphatidylinositol** (GPI)-anchored cell surface glycoprotein, expressed on B lymphocytes and their precursors, on activated T lymphocytes, on neutrophils, on eosinophils, on some epithelial cells and on carcinoma cells including cells of small cell carcinoma of the lung; CD24 has been reported to be a ligand for P-selectin (**CD62**), a lectin expressed on platelets and vascular endothelium; CD24/CD62 binding could represent a mechanism for tumour dissemination; CD24 monoclonal antibodies, used in conjunction with CD21 monoclonal antibodies, have been found to be useful in controlling post-transplant lymphoproliferative disorder

CD24 is expressed on the blast cells of the majority of cases of B-lineage acute lymphoblastic leukaemia but not those associated with a cytogenetic rearrangement with an 11q23 breakpoint; expressed on the cells of the majority of cases of B-lineage leukaemia/lymphoma and on blast cells of some cases of acute myeloid leukaemia, particularly M4 and M5 acute myeloid leukaemia for which it is a fairly specific but not very sensitive marker; weakly expressed on hairy cells

CD25 a cell surface glycoprotein, the α chain of **interleukin 2 receptor** (IL2Rα); high affinity IL2R is a complex of CD25 with **CD122** and **CD132**; expressed on activated B cells and T cells and on a subset of regulatory T cells, on monocytes and on the cells of polyclonal B-cell lymphocytosis; sometimes expressed on basophils but not expressed on normal mast cells; a humanized anti-CD25 monoclonal antibody, dacluzumab (Zenapax), has been used for prevention of cardiac allograft rejection and acute renal allograft rejection; anti-CD25 antibodies have been used experimentally in the treatment of psoriasis; a first exon deletion mutation in the CD25 gene has been described, leading to a severe immunodeficiency syndrome

CD25 is expressed on hairy cells, on the cells of the great majority of cases of adult T-cell leukaemia/lymphoma and sometimes on other high grade lymphomas including anaplastic large cell lymphoma; expressed on mononuclear Hodgkin's cells and Reed–Sternberg cells; in non-Hodgkin's lymphoma, serum CD25 correlates with tumour burden; may be expressed on neoplastic mast cells, both in systemic mastocytosis and acute mast cell leukaemia; an immunotoxin directed at CD25 (LMB-2) has been used in therapy of hairy cell leukaemia, Hodgkin's disease, cutaneous T-cell lymphoma and adult T-cell leukaemia lymphoma

CD26 a membrane bound serine exopeptidase—dipeptidyl peptidase IV; adenosine deaminase binding protein; interacts with **CD45** and is a costimulatory molecule for T-cell activation; cleaves an essential cofactor for the entry of HIV into CD4+ Th1 T cells; up-regulated on Th1 T cells by γ-interferon; cleaves peptides from several chemokines, reducing their ability to mediate chemotaxis without affecting their angiostatic potential; expressed on mature thymocytes, activated T cells, B cells, NK cells, macrophages, renal proximal tubule cells, fibroblasts, some epithelial cells (including those of small intestinal epithelium, prostatic cells and biliary canalicular cells), brain, heart, skeletal muscle, endothelial cells and splenic sinus lining cells; lack of expression of CD26 has been found useful in the identification of circulating neoplastic cells in mycosis fungoides/Sézary syndrome; lymphoma cells in other types of T-cell lymphoma may also fail to express CD26

CD27 a member of the tumour necrosis factor receptor superfamily which exists as a homodimer; expressed on some T cells, memory B cells (but not immature or mature but naïve B cells) and NK cells; an early activation marker on T cells; the ligand for CD27 is **CD70** which belongs to the tumour necrosis family; binding of CD70 to its ligand, in the presence of **interleukin-2**, increases differentiation of memory B cell to plasma cells; the cytoplasmic tail of CD27 can bind to a fas-like molecule, Siva, which in turn induces apoptosis; expressed on the cells of polyclonal B-cell lymphocytosis, which may be an expansion of memory B cells; expressed by normal plasma cells

CD27 is often expressed on neoplastic B cells, e.g. in most cases of chronic lymphocytic leukaemia, three-quarters of cases of follicular lymphoma and two-thirds of cases of diffuse large B-cell lymphoma; more likely to be expressed by plasma cells in monoclonal gammopathy of undetermined significance than by myeloma cells; when expressed on neoplastic B cells, is often co-expressed with its ligand

CD28 a member of the immunoglobulin superfamily of cell surface molecules which allows T cells to proliferate in the presence of phorbol esters; exists as a homodimer, which binds to co-stimulatory receptors such as **CD80** and **CD86** on antigen-presenting cells; expressed on mature thymocytes, most T cells, activated B cells and plasma cells

CD29 a glycoprotein, platelet GpIIa; β_1 integrin chain; the β chain of VLAs (very late activation antigens) including VLA-1 (CD49a/CD29), VLA-2 (CD49b/CD29), VLA-3 (CD49c/CD29) and VLA-4 (CD49d/CD29); VLA-2 is platelet glycoprotein IaIIa, a platelet collagen receptor; VLA-4, $\alpha_4\beta_1$ integrin is expressed on

haemopoietic progenitor cells and is the ligand of VCAM-1 on bone marrow stromal endothelium, permitting transendothelial migration of haemopoietic progenitors; VLA-4 is expressed on T cell and permits their adhesion to VCAM-1 on activated endothelium and subsequent transmigration; β_1 integrins ($\alpha_2\beta_1$ and $\alpha_3\beta_1$) are expressed on thymic epithelial cells and mediate adhesion of thymocytes; expressed on basophils; expressed on normal mast cells

Expressed on neoplastic mast cells; VLA-4 is expressed in follicular lymphoma. VLA-3 is expressed at high levels in chronic lymphocytic leukaemia

CD30 a cell surface antigen (initially recognized by the Ki-1 monoclonal antibody), a member of the nerve growth receptor superfamily expressed on activated B cells and T cells; on T cells is a late activation marker; binds to **CD153** on neutrophils, activated T cells, monocytes and macrophages; weakly expressed on late erythroid cells and late cells of granulocyte lineage, expressed on plasma cells

CD30 is strongly expressed on Hodgkin's cells and Reed–Sternberg cells (except in nodular lymphocyte predominant Hodgkin's disease), elevated levels of serum CD30 correlating with poor prognosis; strongly expressed on the lymphoma cells of systemic anaplastic large cell lymphoma (but not cutaneous anaplastic large cell lymphoma) and may be weakly expressed on the cells of other types of large cell non-Hodgkin's lymphoma; expressed on cells of about a third of cases of transformed mycosis fungoides; expressed by some carcinomas and some germ cell tumours; CD30 monoclonal antibodies linked to magnetic microbeads have been used experimentally for the isolation of mononuclear Hodgkin's cells and Reed–Sternberg cells

CD31 a cell surface glycoprotein, Platelet/Endothelial Cell Adhesion Molecule (PECAM-1); an adhesion molecule of the immunoglobulin gene superfamily involved in homophilic and heterophilic cell adhesion; activation of integrins occurs following CD31 cross-linking;

expressed on endothelial cells, platelets, megakaryocytes, haemopoietic progenitors, monocytes, macrophages, neutrophils, eosinophils, NK cells, a subset of T cells and plasma cells; mediates binding of CD34-positive haemopoietic precursors cells to stroma; on platelets, it is a negative regulator of aggregation induced by collagen; expressed on endothelial cells including those of the bone marrow; has a role in the transendothelial migration of neutrophils and monocytes; CD31 on high endothelial cells is a ligand for **CD38** on T cells; interacts with αvβ3 integrin on endothelial cells and a subset of T cells; CD31 on endothelial cells is up-regulated by verotoxin, promoting adhesion of platelets; increased phosphorylation of PECAM-1 on endothelial cells following interaction with erythrocytes of sickle cell anaemia leads to increased transendothelial migration of monocytes; thought to be a minor histocompatibility antigen, well defined polymorphism of which increase the risk of acute graft-versus-host disease following bone marrow transplantation

CD31 is expressed on plasma cells in monoclonal gammopathy of undetermined significance and on plasma cells of plasmacytic multiple myeloma but much less often expressed in plasmablastic multiple myeloma and plasma cell leukaemia; expressed in benign and malignant tumours of vascular origin, in histiocytic sarcoma and occasionally in other tumours

CD32   a cell surface glycoprotein, a low affinity IgG receptor—FcγRII; expressed on monocytes, macrophages, Langerhans cells, neutrophils, eosinophils, platelets, mast cells, B cells and placental endothelial cells; expressed on NK cells of some individuals; there are two different receptors detected by antibodies of this cluster, FcγRIIA (expressed on neutrophils, eosinophils, macrophages and platelets) and FcγRIIB (expressed on neutrophils, macrophages, mast cells and B cells); the cytoplasmic tail of the molecule is essential for the formation of phagolysosomes; allelic variants of the Fcγ receptor confer differing phagocytic capacities, providing a mechanism for heritable susceptibility to immune complex disease; certain polymorphisms in FcγRII are associated with an increased incidence of lupus nephritis

CD32 is often expressed in acute myeloid leukaemia, more often in M4 and M5 categories but not with sufficient specificity for this to be diagnostically useful

CD33   Sialic acid-binding Immunoglobulin-like Lectin 3, siglec-3; a sialic acid-dependent adhesion molecule expressed on myeloblasts, promyelocytes and myelocytes and expressed weakly on mature neutrophils; expressed more strongly on monocytes than neutrophils; expressed on some dendritic cells, which are viewed as being of myeloid origin, but not on others viewed as being of lymphoid origin; sometimes expressed on basophils and usually expressed on mast cells; expressed on some NK cells

CD33 is expressed on the blast cells of the majority of cases of acute myeloid leukaemia, being particularly strongly expressed on cells of M3 and M5 acute myeloid leukaemia; may be weakly expressed in acute lymphoblastic leukaemia; anti-CD33 monoclonal antibodies, some coupled to an antitumour antibiotic or a radionucleide, e.g. gentuzumab ozogamicin (Myelotarg), are of potential therapeutic value in acute myeloid leukaemia and myelodysplastic syndromes

CD34   a monomeric cell surface glycoprotein, a cell adhesion molecule expressed on lymphoid and haemopoietic stem cells, and used for selection of haemopoietic stem cells; expressed on the earliest identifiable mast cell precursors; expressed on endothelial cells including those of the bone marrow; expression on high endothelial cells of lymph node veins permits binding to endothelium by lymphocytes expressing L-selectin (**CD62L**), the lymphocyte homing receptor

CD34 is expressed on the blast cells of most cases of acute myeloid leukaemia, many cases of B-lineage acute lymphoblastic leukaemia (pro-B and common but not pre-B or mature B) and some

cases of T-lineage acute lymphoblastic
leukaemia

CD35 a single chain cell surface glycoprotein existing in four allotypic forms
(A,B,C,D): C3b/C4b **complement** receptor (CR1); expressed by erythroid
cells, neutrophils, eosinophils, basophils,
monocytes, B cells and 10–15% of T cells;
not expressed on normal mast cells;
expressed on follicular dendritic cells but
not Langerhans cells or interdigitating
dendritic cells; mediates phagocytosis;
has a role in splenic clearance of complement coated erythrocytes; binds to C3b
and C4b in immune complexes and promotes their clearance; mediates adhesion
to and phagocytosis of complement-
coated particles; makes C3b and C4b
more susceptible to cleavage; expressed
on glomerular podocytes; CD35 carries
the Knops blood group antigens; permits
entry of HIV into cells

CD35 is often expressed in acute
myeloid leukaemia, more often in M4
and M5 categories but not with sufficient
specificity for this to be diagnostically
useful; may be expressed on neoplastic
mast cells both in systemic mastocytosis
and in acute mast cell leukaemia;
expressed in non-Hodgkin's lymphoma
but not usually expressed by chronic lymphocytic leukaemia cells

CD36 a trans-membrane protein, platelet
glycoprotein IV, thrombospondin receptor, fatty acid translocase; expressed on
megakaryocytes and platelets; expressed
on erythroblasts, fetal red cells, monocytes, macrophages, microvascular endothelium, retinal pigment epithelial cells
and adipocytes; has a role in platelet
aggregation, cell adhesion, inhibition
of angiogenesis and recognition and
removal of apoptotic cells; mediates scav-
enging of oxidized low density lipoprotein by macrophages; involved in creation
of foam cells in early atherosclerosis;
CD36 binds erythrocytes parasitized by
P. falciparum thus contributing to their
sequestration and survival and to the
pathology of the disease (e.g. cerebral
malaria); some polymorphisms in the
CD36 gene enhance susceptibility to cere-

bral malaria whilst others confer protection against malaria; CD36 deficiency is
present in at least 2 to 3% of Japanese,
Thais and Africans but in less than 0.3%
of Caucasians and can be involved in
some cases of isoimmune neonatal
thrombocytopenia and refractoriness to
transfusion of HLA-matched platelets;
antibodies to CD36 are detected in the
majority of cases of thrombotic thrombocytopenic purpura and in a significant
proportion of cases of autoimmune
thrombocytopenic purpura and heparin-
induced thrombocytopenia; they may
also contribute to thrombosis in patients
with the lupus anticoagulant

CD36 is expressed on megakaryoblasts
in M7 acute myeloid leukaemia and some
cases of M4, M5 and M6 acute myeloid
leukaemia

CD37 MB-1, a member of the transmembrane 4 or tetraspanin superfamily of proteins, involved in signal transduction; forms
complexes with **CD53**, **CD81**, **CD82** and
MHC class II molecules on the surface of
B cells; strongly expressed on mature B
cells but expressed weakly on T cells, neutrophils and monocytes so that strong
expression can be used a B-cell marker

CD37 may be expressed on late B lymphoblasts that also express cytoplasmic μ
chain but not on more immature B lymphoblasts; monoclonal antibodies linked
to a radionucleide have been used in the
therapy of B-cell neoplasms

CD38 a transmembrane glycoprotein,
NAD+ glycohydrolase/ADP-ribosyl
cyclase which has ectoenzymatic activity
but also functions as a receptor with a
role in cell adhesion and signalling;
expressed on thymic cells, early B and T
cells, germinal centre B cells, some T
cells (most tissue T cells but a minority
of peripheral blood T cells; expressed
by naïve CD45RA+ T cells but not
CD45RO+ memory T cells), activated
NK cells, a subset of monocytes (but not
tissue macrophages), osteoclasts, plasma
cells, haemopoietic progenitors, basophils but not mast cells, red cells and
platelets; pancreatic β cells—where
expression is essential for insulin secre-

tion, neurones, Purkinje cells, astrocytes and neurofibrillary tangles in Alzheimer's disease, retinal cells, renal tubular cells, prostatic epithelium and sarcolemma of smooth and striated muscles; binds to extracellular matrix; binds to CD38 ligand (**CD31**) on high endothelial cells, T-cell subsets, NK cells, monocytes and platelets; in HIV infection, the number of CD8+CD38+ T cells increases with progression to AIDS with the expression of CD38 on CD8+ T cells being of independent prognostic significance

CD31 binding to CD38 leads to apoptosis of bone marrow B cells but protects tonsillar B cells from apoptosis and leads to proliferation of splenic B cells

CD38 is expressed on myeloma cells, on cells of primary effusion lymphoma, on cells of some cases of splenic lymphoma with villous lymphocytes and some cases of chronic lymphocytic leukaemia; in multiple myeloma, expression correlates with a worse prognosis; in chronic lymphocytic leukaemia, expression correlates with clonal origin from a less mature cell and with worse prognosis; expressed in acute myeloid leukaemia and acute lymphoblastic leukaemia, strong expression in acute myeloid leukaemia correlating with better prognosis

Expression of CD38 on myeloid cells is up-regulated by **all-*trans*-retinoic acid** (ATRA) and is likely to lead to binding of leukaemic cells to CD31 on endothelial cells in the ATRA syndrome and in the similar syndrome induced by arsenic in patients with acute promyelocytic leukaemia

CD39 ATP diphosphohydrolase, expressed on the surface of vascular endothelium and essential for the hydrolysis of extracellular ATP to ADP and AMP in platelet recruitment and adhesion; expressed on activated B cells, activated NK cells, some macrophages, some dendritic cells and some plasma cells;

CD39 is expressed on chronic lymphocytic leukaemia cells

CD40 a cell surface glycoprotein, a member of the tumour necrosis factor receptor superfamily; interacts with CD40 ligand

on T cells (CD40L, **CD154**) and this drives B-cell proliferation; expressed on B cells and precursors, but not on the most immature B lymphoblasts, and is involved in growth, differentiation and isotype switching of B cells, T-cell-dependent B-cell responses and rescue of germinal centre B cells from apoptosis; expressed weakly on plasma cells; also expressed on T cells, activation leading to increased expression of its ligand and secretion of cytokines and chemokines including IL1, IL6, IL8, IL12, IL15; expressed on CD34+ haemopoietic progenitors, monocytes, (but not those in cord blood), macrophages, platelets, endothelial cells, fibroblasts and some epithelial cells; variably expressed on normal and neoplastic mast cells; expressed weakly on immature dendritic cells, such as those in skin and other peripheral tissues, but expressed strongly on mature follicular dendritic cells in lymph nodes; has a role in cytokine production by macrophages and dendritic cells

Expressed in B-cell tumours including acute lymphoblastic leukaemia; expressed on Reed–Sternberg cells and Hodgkin's cells in lymphocyte predominant and classical Hodgkin's disease; expressed, together with CD40 ligand, on cells of some cases of non-Hodgkin's lymphoma (mantle cell lymphoma and follicular lymphoma) so that an autocrine cytokine loop could occur; similarly co-expressed, with its ligand, in cells of some cases of chronic lymphocytic leukaemia; expressed in the majority of cases of Langerhans cell histiocytosis; may be expressed in acute myeloid leukaemia and expression correlates with worse prognosis; expressed on carcinoma cells

CD41a platelet glycoprotein IIb/IIIa complex (αIIbβ3 integrin); the genes encoding both αIIb and β3 integrins are at 17q21.32 but are not closely linked; expressed on megakaryocytes and platelets; involved in the increased interaction of platelets with endothelium on exposure to verotoxin; has a role in megakaryocyte-dependent fibroblast growth; receptor for von Willebrand's factor, fibronectin, fibrinogen and throm-bospondin; mutations in the genes for both platelet glycoprotein IIb and IIIa have been shown to be associated with different types of **Glanzmann's thrombas-thenia**; not expressed on normal mast cells; monoclonal antibodies to glyco-protein IIb/IIIa are used therapeutically as potent antithrombotic agents, e.g. in patients having coronary angioplasty

Expressed on megakaryoblasts of M7 acute myeloid leukaemia; may be ex-pressed on neoplastic mast cells

CD41b platelet glycoprotein IIb; forms a heterodimer with β_3 integrin (**CD61**) with the heterodimer ($\alpha_{IIb}\beta_3$) being expressed on multipotent myeloid stem cells (**CFU-GM**), bipotent erythroid–megakaryocyte stem cells, megakaryocyte colony-forming cells (**CFU-MK**), megakaryo-cytes and platelets; mediates binding of haemopoietic stem cells to stromal fib-ronectin; mediates platelet adhesion to subendothelial matrix and platelet aggregation induced by fibrinogen, von Willebrand's factor, thrombin, collagen, ADP and adrenaline; polymorphisms in CD41b are responsible for the HPA3 platelet alloantigen system

CD41b is expressed on megakary-oblasts of M7 acute myeloid leukaemia

CD42a platelet glycoprotein IX; ex-pressed on megakaryocytes and platelets; the CD42a-d (or GpIb-IX-V) complex is the platelet receptor for **von Willebrand's factor** and **thrombin**; it mediates adhesion to the subendothelium which in turn causes platelet activation and converts $\alpha_{IIb}\beta_3$ (*see* **CD41b**) from a low affinity to a high affinity state; the response to thrombin and other agonists is thereby enhanced; mutations of the CD42a gene can cause **Bernard–Soulier syndrome**

CD42a is expressed on megakary-oblasts of M7 acute myeloid leukaemia

CD42b platelet glycoprotein Ibα; ex-pressed on megakaryocytes and platelets; CD42a-d complex is the platelet receptor for **von Willebrand's factor** and **thrombin**, the actual binding site being on the CD42b molecule; CD42b forms a heterodimer with CD42c with the heterodimer also being associated with CD42a and CD42d; mutations of the CD42b gene can cause **Bernard–Soulier syndrome** and **platelet-type von Willebrand's disease** in which the platelets have increased affinity for von Willebrand's factor, as a result of a gain of function mutation; polymorphisms of CD42b have been related to arterial thrombosis; has a role in megakaryocyte-dependent fibroblast growth; not expressed on normal mast cells

CD42b may be expressed, but usually only weakly, by megakaryoblasts of M7 acute myeloid leukaemia; positivity in acute myeloid leukaemia is usually the result of adherent platelets; may be expressed on neoplastic mast cells

CD42d platelet glycoprotein Ibβ; forms a heterodimer with CD42b and binds non-covalently with CD42a and CD42d to form the CD42a-d receptor complex; mutation of the CD42c gene can lead to **Bernard–Soulier syndrome**

CD42e platelet glycoprotein V, part of the CD42a-d complex; although the actual binding site is on CD42b, the presence of CD42e is necessary in order for the complex to provide a strong thrombin-binding site

CD43 a mucin-like, heavily glycosyl-ated and heavily sialylated glycoprotein, sialophorin or leukosialin, expressed on T lymphocytes, occasionally on activated B cells; expressed on myeloid cells includ-ing haemopoietic progenitors; expressed on basophils and mast cells; in some circumstances inhibits adhesion and in other circumstances may promote it; CD43 is an anti-adhesive molecule in resting leucocytes and is down-regulated on activation; has a role in neutrophil locomotion; CD43 has a role in activa-tion of T cells, B cells, NK cells and monocytes; it is aberrantly glycosylated in **Wiskott–Aldrich syndrome**; **CD54** is a ligand for CD43

CD43 is expressed in T-lineage acute lymphoblastic leukaemia and T-lineage non-Hodgkin's lymphoma, chronic lym-phocytic leukaemia, small lymphocytic lymphoma, mantle cell lymphoma and Burkitt's lymphoma but rarely in follicular lymphoma; expressed in a proportion of lymphoplasmacytoid lymphomas and marginal zone lymphomas; may be expressed by neoplastic mast cells

CD44   a transmembrane protein expressed as a family of multiple isoforms generated by alternative RNA splicing; it is an adhesion molecule (CD44H, H-CAM); expressed on all blood cells, except platelets, and in non-haemopoietic tissues; expressed on haemopoietic stem cells and may mediate binding to hyaluronate; expressed on mast cells as well as basophils; expressed on macrophages and osteoclasts; expressed on plasma cells, expressed on fibroblasts and some epithelial cells; CD44 has a role in neutrophil attachment to endothelial cells, development of cytotoxicity and generation of IL6 and in lymphocyte homing and development of lymphocyte cytotoxicity; it may have a role in the attachment of haemopoietic stem cells to stroma; expressed on white matter of brain; CD44 is not expressed in normal liver but is expressed in bile duct epithelium in some bile duct diseases; it probably has a role in autoimmune biliary disease, by promoting lymphoepithelial interactions; CD44 carries the Indian blood group antigens

CD44 is expressed on multiple myeloma cells; it is expressed on most lymphoma cells, particularly those of low grade lymphoma and increased levels of serum CD44 have been found of prognostic significance; expressed normally on chronic lymphocytic leukaemia cells; expressed by neoplastic mast cells; certain splice variants of the CD44 gene are over-represented in several human carcinomas, where they may indicate increased likelihood of tumour progression

CD45   the leucocyte common antigen—a protein-tyrosine phosphatase, receptor-type, c-ptprc, that removes phosphate groups from tyrosine residues of target proteins, expressed on all haemopoietic cells except mature red cells and their immediate precursors; expressed on early cells of neutrophil lineage but expression diminishes with maturation; more strongly expressed on monocytes than neutrophils but eosinophils show similar expression to monocytes; strongly expressed on T and B lineage lymphocytes; necessary for receptor-mediated activation of T and B cells; augments signalling through antigen receptors on T and B cells; different isoforms exist formed by differential splicing of exons 4, 5 and 6 to give CD45RA, CD45RB and CD45RC respectively as well as CD45RO (lacking any of exons 4, 5 or 6); CD45 is the common epitope; expressed on tonsillar plasma cells and on reactive plasma cells produced in response to increased IL6 secretion, but weakly expressed if at all on normal bone marrow plasma cells; expressed by mast cells; follicular dendritic cells are CD45–

CD45 is strongly expressed on T and B lineage lymphoblasts in most cases of acute lymphoblastic leukaemia; more strongly expressed in T-lineage acute lymphoblastic leukaemia than B-lineage acute lymphoblastic leukaemia and about 20% of cases of B-lineage acute lymphoblastic leukaemia are negative; weakly expressed on blast cells of acute myeloid leukaemia; expressed by neoplastic mast cells; Hodgkin's cells and Reed–Sternberg cells of classical Hodgkin's disease are CD45– but neoplastic cells of nodular lymphocyte predominant Hodgkin's disease are positive; sometimes expressed by myeloma cells; radiolabelled CD45 antibodies may be useful in eliminated neoplastic cells prior to stem cell transplantation

CD45RA   a high molecular weight isoform of the leucocyte common antigen, expressed on haemopoietic progenitors, B cells, naïve T cells and monocytes; expressed in most B-lineage neoplasms

CD45RB   an isoform of the common leucocyte antigen, expressed on B cells, a T-cell subset, monocytes, macrophages and neutrophils

CD45RC   a high molecular weight isoform of the leucocyte common antigen, expressed on B cells and a T-cell subset; monoclonal antibodies may recognize a sialylated form of the sequence encoded by the C exon

CD45RO a low molecular weight isoform of the leucocyte common antigen, expressed on neutrophils, a B-cell subset, T-cell subsets (memory T cells), monocytes, macrophages; expressed weakly and strongly, respectively, on two subsets of thymic dendritic cells

CD45RO is expressed in T-cell lymphomas but also in some B-cell lymphomas

CD46 a dimeric cell surface membrane protein, **M**embrane **C**ofactor **P**rotein (MCP) acting as a cofactor for proteolytic cleavage of C3b and C4b; ubiquitous—expressed on all nucleated cells (not erythrocytes); receptor for the measles virus; CD46 is incorporated into the HIV envelope and protects the virus and HIV-infected cells against complement deposition

CD47 an adhesion molecule, integrin-associated protein; thrombospondin receptor and receptor for transmembrane **S**ignal **R**egulatory **P**rotein alpha (hence SIRP ligand)—an inhibitory receptor expressed on myeloid cells; CD47 is expressed on many cell types including haemopoietic cells; it is a glycoprotein component of the Rh protein complex; knockout studies in mice have shown CD47 to be important in neutrophil migration in response to bacterial infection; thrombospondin forms a bridge between apoptotic cells and phagocytes by binding of CD47 to **CD36**

Binding of either thrombospondin or CD47 antibodies to CD47 in chronic lymphocytic leukaemia can induce cell death

CD47R redesignation of CDw149, MEM-133; expressed on lymphocytes and monocytes

CD48 a surface membrane glycoprotein closely related to the activation protein, Blast-1; a member of the Ig supergene family, expressed on monocytes and almost all T cells and B cells; expressed on EBV-induced B-lineage blasts; ligand of **CD244**; a weak binder of **CD2** and therefore acts as an adhesion molecule and as a costimulatory molecule for T cells; has a role in graft-versus-host disease; is bound

to **glycosylphosphatidylinositol** (GPI) and is therefore reduced in paroxysmal nocturnal haemoglobinuria

CD49a a membrane glycoprotein, $\alpha 1$ integrin chain

CD49b a membrane glycoprotein, $\alpha 2$ integrin; integrin $\alpha_2\beta_1$ (very late antigen-2, VLA-2) is platelet glycoprotein Ia/IIa (CD49b/CD29) which mediates adhesion of mature megakaryocytes and platelets to collagen; $\alpha_2\beta_1$ integrins are also expressed on thymic epithelial cells, B cells, activated T cells, monocytes, endothelial cells and fibroblasts; the $\alpha 2$ gene is polymorphic, leading to lesser or greater expression of IaIIb on platelets; VLA-2 is a principal vector used by neutrophils for locomotion in extravascular tissues; permits coxsackie and adenoviruses to enter cells

CD49c a membrane glycoprotein, $\alpha 3$ integrin chain; $\alpha_3\beta_1$ integrin (very late antigen-3, VLA-3) is expressed on thymic epithelial cells and mediates adhesion of thymocytes to thymic epithelium; expressed on B cells, monocytes, platelets and kidney glomerular cells; usually expressed on chronic lymphocytic leukaemia cells although they fail to express CD29

CD49d a membrane glycoprotein, $\alpha 4$ integrin chain; $\alpha_4\beta_1$ integrin (very late activation antigen-4, VLA-4) permits adhesion of megakaryocyte-colony forming units and immature megakaryocytes to fibronectin, adhesion of bone marrow progenitor cells to fibronectin of basement membrane and adhesion of haemopoietic progenitor cells to VCAM-1 on bone marrow stromal cells and activated endothelial cells; VLA-4-mediated adhesion of progenitor cells to basement membrane and bone marrow endothelial cells may permit transendothelial and trans-basement membrane migration of progenitor cells; $\alpha_4\beta_1$ integrin (VLA-4) permits adhesion of eosinophils to VCAM-1 (**CD106**) of endothelial cells; expressed on basophils; expressed on normal and neoplastic mast cells; $\alpha_4\beta_1$ and $\alpha_4\beta_7$ integrins mediate adhesion of normal B cells and B-lineage lymphoma cells to fibronectin and may promote their proliferation; VLA-4 is expressed on plasma cells

CD49d/CD29 (VLA-4) is expressed on myeloma cells, follicular lymphoma cells and neoplastic mast cells

CD49e   a membrane glycoprotein, $\alpha 5$ integrin chain; $\alpha_5\beta_1$ integrin (very late antigen-5, VLA-5) is expressed on mature megakaryocytes and strongly promotes their adhesion to fibronectin; promotes adhesion of thrombin stimulated megakaryocytes to fibrinogen; VLA-5 is expressed on neutrophils and mediates their binding to fibronectin of connective tissue and their locomotion; VLA-5 is expressed on haemopoietic progenitor cells and, since it binds to fibronectin, may permit their migration through basement membrane; expressed on plasma cells; expressed on mast cells

VLA-5 is expressed on neoplastic mast cells; it is usually expressed by chronic lymphocytic leukaemia cells although they fail to express CD29; expressed on myeloma cells

CD49f   a membrane glycoprotein, $\alpha 6$ integrin chain; $\alpha_6\beta_1$ integrin (very late antigen-6, VLA-6) is expressed on megakaryocytes, platelets, most epithelial cells, monocytes and T lymphocytes; expression on thymic epithelial cells mediates adhesion of thymocytes; expression on megakaryocytes mediates their binding to laminin; $\alpha_6\beta_1$ integrin is expressed on the Th1 subset of helper T lymphocytes, expression being upregulated by IL-12

CD50   ICAM-3 (**I**nter**c**ellular **A**dhesion **M**olecule-**3**), an adhesion and co-stimulatory molecule, a member of he immunoglobulin superfamily of adhesion receptors, expressed on immature and mature leucocytes and dendritic cells; a ligand for the β_2 integrin CD11a/CD18 and for α_d/CD18; plays a role in the interaction of T lymphocytes with antigen-presenting cells

CD50 is expressed on cells of acute and chronic myeloid leukaemias, chronic lymphocytic leukaemia, hairy cell leukaemia, multiple myeloma and non-Hodgkin's lymphoma

CD51 α_v integrin chain, the α chain of the vitronectin receptor, $\alpha_v\beta_3$ integrin (CD51/CD61); the vitronectin receptor is expressed on platelets, macrophages, osteoclasts and endothelial cells; upregulated on endothelial cells after exposure to verotoxin; expressed on mast cells; $\alpha_v\beta_3$ integrin is also expressed on late megakaryocytes and may aid their adhesion to vitronectin; $\alpha_v\beta_3$ is expressed on neutrophils, permitting their binding to vitronectin and their locomotion; α_v can also pair with β_5, β_6 and β_8

CD51 is expressed by neoplastic mast cells

CD52   a **g**lycosyl**p**hosphatidy**l**inositol (GPI)-anchored protein, reduced in paroxysmal nocturnal haemoglobinuria; expressed on thymocytes, lymphocytes, eosinophils, monocytes and macrophages (but not neutrophils), and epithelial cells of the epididymus and seminal vesicles; expression by chronic lymphocytic leukaemia cells is similar to that of normal lymphocytes; antibodies to CD52, e.g. alemtuzumab (CAMPATH-1), can give long-term depletion of T lymphocytes when used *in vivo* and can be used for purging T lymphocytes *in vitro*; a combination of CAMPATH-1M for *in vitro* purging and CAMPATH-1G administered to the recipient has been used to reduce graft-versus-host disease without a concomitant increase in failure of engraftment

Alemtuzumab is useful in T-prolymphocytic leukaemia, may be useful in eliminating minimal residual disease in B-lineage chronic lymphocytic leukaemia and can be used for *in vivo* purging for autologous stem cell transplantation in chronic lymphocytic leukaemia

CD53   OX44, a member of the transmembrane 4 or tetraspanin superfamily of proteins, expressed on leucocytes, has a role in signal transduction; structurally similar to and forms complexes with **CD37**

CD54   a cell surface glycoprotein, ICAM-1 (**I**nter**c**ellular **A**dhesion **M**olecule-**1**), an adhesion molecule that is a ligand for β_2 integrins, CD11a/CD18 and CD11b/

CD18; expressed on activated endothelial cells including those of the bone marrow, activated B lymphocytes and activated T lymphocytes; expressed on dendritic cells, permitting their binding to CD11a on T cells; up-regulated on microvascular endothelial cells following exposure to verotoxin, promoting neutrophil adhesion; expressed on macrophages and osteoclasts; functions as a rhinovirus receptor; permits adhesion and transendothelial migration of VLA-4-expressing haemopoietic progenitors; activated eosinophils express β2 integrins, permitting their adhesion to ICAM-1 on endothelial cells; expression of ICAM-1 is increased when the erythrocytes of sickle cell anaemia adhere to endothelium; binds erythrocytes parasitised by *P. falciparum* thus contributing to their sequestration and survival and to the pathology of the disease (e.g. cerebral malaria); polymorphisms in the CD54 gene may predispose to cerebral malaria; expressed on basophils and mast cells; expressed on circulating dendritic cells; expressed on plasma cells

CD54 is expressed on neoplastic mast cells; expressed on myeloma cells; expressed on the blast cells of about three-quarters of patients with acute myeloid leukaemia; serum CD54 is of prognostic significance in non-Hodgkin's lymphoma and in high grade lymphoma correlates with tumour burden; soluble CD54 is increased in chronic lymphocytic leukaemia although it is not expressed on the leukaemic cells

CD55 a **glycosylphosphatidylinositol** (GPI)-linked cell surface glycoprotein, decay accelerating factor (DAF), binds C3b, C4b, C3bBb, C4b2a and protects against inappropriate **complement activation**; widely expressed including expression on erythroid cells; reduced expression in paroxysmal nocturnal haemoglobinuria (PNH); ligand for **CD97**; CD55 antibodies can be used to identify cells of the PNH clone; CD55-deficient red cells have also been detected in a proportion of patients with lymphoproliferative disorders; receptor for echovirus, coxsackie virus, picornaviruses and enterovirus

The Cromer blood group system consists of antigens carried on the DAF molecule: in the rare Inab phenotype, all Cromer system antigens are lacking; this has been associated with mutations in the DAF gene resulting in a complete absence of DAF; such individuals are not known to have any associated abnormalities

CD56 an isoform of N-CAM, **N**eural **C**ell **A**dhesion **M**olecule, a member of the immunoglobulin superfamily, expressed on cells in the cerebellum and cerebral cortex (neurones, astrocytes and Schwann cells), mediates homophilic adhesion of neural cells; expressed on NK cells (mature and immature but not pre-NK cells), a subset of CD4+ T cells and a subset of CD8+ T cells; expressed on activated lymphocytes; expressed on a subset of peripheral blood monocytes and bone marrow macrophages and osteoclasts; not expressed on normal plasma cells

CD56 is usually expressed in large granular lymphocyte leukaemia of NK lineage and sometimes in large granular lymphocyte leukaemia of T-cell lineage; expressed on blastic NK cell leukaemia/lymphoma, aggressive NK cell leukaemia/lymphoma and nasal-type NK cell lymphoma; expressed on the cells of many patients with acute myeloid leukaemia; expressed in many cases of multiple myeloma and somewhat less often in plasma cell leukaemia; may promote homotypic adhesion of myeloma cells to bone marrow macrophages; down-regulated on extramedullary myeloma cells in comparison with bone marrow myeloma cells; according to some studies, not expressed on the plasma cells of monoclonal gammopathy of undetermined significance; expressed on the cells of small cell carcinoma of the lung and neural-derived tumours such as neuroblastoma and astrocytoma; CD56 expression has been linked to a worse prognosis in acute myeloid leukaemia associated with t(8;21) and t(15;17)

CD57 a carbohydrate determinant found on a number of polypeptides and lipids; expressed on NK cells, subsets of T cells,

B cells, monocytes and a subset of Schwann cells

CD57 is usually expressed on large granular lymphocyte leukaemia of T-cell lineage and sometimes in large granular lymphocyte leukaemia of NK lineage

CD58   a glycoprotein that occurs as a transmembrane protein with a cytoplasmic domain and as a **glycosylphosphatidylinositol** (GPI)-anchored membrane protein; Leucocyte Function Associated antigen-3 (LFA-3), the ligand of **CD2**, expressed on leucocytes, dendritic cells, erythrocytes, endothelial cells, epithelial cells and fibroblasts; expressed on a proportion of lymphoid stem cells; not expressed on normal plasma cells; mediates adhesion between killer cells and their targets, between antigen-presenting cells and T cells and between thymocytes and thymic epithelium; provides costimulatory signals in immune responses; expressed by mast cells; reduced expression in paroxysmal nocturnal haemoglobinuria (PNH)

CD58 is expressed on blast cells in the majority of cases of acute myeloid leukaemia and B-lineage acute lymphoblastic leukaemia; expressed by neoplastic mast cells and may permit adhesion of neoplastic mast cells showing aberrant expression of CD2 to each other; expressed on myeloma cells

CD59   a   **glycosylphosphatidylinositol** (GPI)-linked cell surface glycoprotein, MIC11, which associates with the final component of the complement pathway, C9, inhibiting incorporation of C5b-8 to form a membrane attack complex (hence 'protectin'); reduced in paroxysmal nocturnal haemoglobinuria, a disease which is characterized by abnormal complement sensitivity; CD59 antibodies can be used to identify cells of the PNH clone; CD59-deficient red cells have also been identified in a proportion of patients with lymphoproliferative disorders; a patient doubly heterozygous for different nonsense mutations in the CD59 gene leading to CD59 deficiency has been reported to have haemolytic anaemia and thrombosis causing cerebral infarction, but none of the other features of PNH; widely expressed including expression in erythrocytes, neutrophils, lymphocytes, monocytes, platelets and mast cells; has a signalling role in T-cell activation; is incorporated into the HIV envelope and protects the virus and HIV-infected cells against complement deposition

CD59 is expressed on neoplastic mast cells

CD60   a glycolipid which provides costimulatory signals for T cells; expressed on a subset of CD8+ T cells, platelets, thymic epithelium, glomeruli, smooth muscle cells and astrocytes; revised classification as **CD60a, CD60b** and **CD60c**

CD60a   a glycolipid, GD3

CD60b   a glycolipid, 9-O-acetyl-GD3

CD60c   a glycoclipid, 7-O-acetyl-GD3

CD61   a surface membrane glycoprotein, the β3 integrin chain, GpIIIa; part of the GpIIb/IIIa complex, $\alpha_{IIb}\beta_3$ integrin; expressed on platelets and megakaryocytes (in association with CD41) and on monocytes, macrophages, osteoclasts, endothelial cells and platelets (in association with CD51, forming the vitronectin receptor, CD51/CD61); expressed on mast cells; GpIIb/IIIa is a receptor for fibrinogen, fibronectin, vitronectin and **von Willebrand's factor**; a point mutation in the CD61 gene results in **Glanzmann's thrombasthenia** type B; polymorphisms in CD61 are responsible for the HPA1 and HPA4 platelet alloantigen systems

Expressed on blast cells of M7 acute myeloid leukaemia and may be expressed weakly by leukaemic cells of other subtypes of acute myeloid leukaemia; CD61 is expressed on neoplastic mast cells

CD62E   E selectin, Endothelium Leucocyte Adhesion Molecule (ELAM-1, LECAM-2), expressed on activated endothelium and mediates rolling of neutrophils, monocytes and lymphocytes at sites of inflammation; expression of E selectin occurs after stimulation by lipopolysaccharide and inflammatory cytokines such as IL1 and tumour necrosis factor; up-regulated by exposure to verotoxin, promoting neutrophil adhesion; a lack of expression of E-selectin on endothelial cells has been linked to recurrent infections in a child, probably caused by impaired adhesion of neutrophils to endothelium; certain polymorphisms in CD62E are associated with early onset coronary artery disease; also expressed on proliferating endothelial cells; a ligand for **CD162** (cutaneous leucocyte antigen) which is expressed on lymphocytes; mediates eosinophil adhesion to endothelial cells but is less efficient at this than P selectin; polymorphisms in E selectin have been associated with premature atherosclerosis; expression of E-selectin is increased when the erythrocytes of sickle cell anaemia adhere to endothelium

CD62L L selectin (LECAM-1/LAM-1). Expressed on B and T lymphocytes, some NK cells, thymocytes, haemopoietic progenitors, monocytes and neutrophils; mediates homing of lymphocytes to high endothelial venules of peripheral lymphoid tissues and rolling of leucocytes (neutrophils, monocytes and lymphocytes) on activated endothelium at sites of inflammation; a ligand of **CD34** and **CD162**; the expression of CD62L on neutrophils is up-regulated by inflammatory stimuli and down-regulated by corticosteroids; expressed on megakaryocytes and mediates adhesion to fibroblasts; the number of cells co-expressing CD34 and L-selectin is predictive of rapid engraftment following autologous stem cell transplantation

CD62L is expressed on the majority of leukaemic cells and in acute myeloid leukaemia high levels of soluble CD62L in the serum correlate with a worse prognosis; expressed normally on chronic lymphocytic leukaemia cells

CD62P P selectin (LECAM-3), platelet alpha-granule membrane protein, located in the storage granules of platelets and endothelial cells (Weibel–Palade bodies) and translocated to the surface when endothelial cells are activated; mobilized to the cell surface on platelet activation and enriched in platelet microvesicles; surface CD62P expression on CD41a+ or CD42b+ platelets can be used as a measure of platelet activation; mediates adhesion of platelets to endothelium and

rolling of neutrophils and eosinophils on activated endothelium; mediates adherence of lymphocytes and monocytes to a lesser extent; upregulated on microvascular endothelial cells by exposure to verotoxin, promoting adhesion of platelets; expressed on megakaryocytes and mediates adhesion to fibroblasts; binds to **CD162** on lymphocytes and **CD24** on neutrophils and B lymphocytes; P-selectin expression is reduced on the endothelial cells of premature babies, a factor that may delay transendothelial migration of neutrophils; soluble P selectin is increased in autoimmune thrombocytopenic purpura and following deep vein thrombosis; certain polymorphisms in CD62E are associated with reduced incidence of myocardial infarction; mediates adhesion of sickle cells to endothelium; binds to a protein that is exported to the surface of red cells infected by *Plasmodium falciparum*

CD63 melanoma associated antigen 1, ME491, a member of the transmembrane 4 or tetraspanin superfamily of proteins, stored in cytoplasmic granules or lysosomes of platelets, endothelial cells, neutrophils, monocytes and macrophages and is exported to the cell surface on activation; expressed on fibroblasts, osteoblasts, smooth muscle cells, neural tissue and melanoma cells; expressed on mast cells; deficient in the platelets of **Hermansky–Pudlak syndrome**

CD63 is expressed more strongly on neoplastic mast cells than on normal mast cells

CD64 FcγRI—high affinity receptor for IgG, expressed on monocytes, CD34+ monocyte progenitors, macrophages and activated neutrophils and eosinophils, a subset of circulating dendritic cells, germinal centre dendritic cells and promyelocytes; expression is up-regulated by interferon gamma and IL10 and down-regulated by IL4; has a role in antigen capture for presentation to T cells, antibody-dependent cellular cytotoxicity, endocytosis of immune complexes and removal of abnormal cells, such as the erythrocytes in thalassaemia; a non-coding mutation in the CD64 transcript which reduces mRNA stability and hence phagocytic expression of CD64 has been reported; individuals with this CD64 deficiency have no known abnormalities

CD64 expression has a high degree of both sensitivity and specificity for the diagnosis of M4 and M5 acute myeloid leukaemia (although it is also expressed, more weakly, in M3 acute myeloid leukaemia)

CD65 a carbohydrate ceramide dodecasaccharide, expressed on cells of granulocyte lineage from the promyelocyte stage onwards and, more weakly, on monocytes; a ligand for E-selectin

CD65 is expressed on blast cells of many cases of acute myeloid leukaemia; expression may be critical for extravascular infiltration by leukaemic cells

CD65s is the sialylated form; CD65s is expressed on granulocytes and monocytes

CD65s is expressed on cells of myeloid leukaemias; its expression appears as CD34 expression disappears; aberrantly expressed on cells of some patients with pro-B acute lymphoblastic leukaemia

CD66a member of the carcinoembryonic antigen family, also known as biliary glycoprotein I; expressed on neutrophils and epithelial cells; has a role in cell adhesion and signalling in neutrophils; a receptor for *Neisseria* spp; radiolabelled monoclonal antibodies to CD66a, b, c and e have been used for conditioning prior to stem cell transplantation

CD66b (previously CD67), biliary glycoprotein, member of the carcinoembryonic antigen family, product of the *CGM6* gene; a **glycosylphosphatidylinositol** (GPI)-anchored protein, expressed in neutrophils and metamyelocytes and weakly by myelocytes, has a role in cell adhesion and signalling

CD66c member of the carcinoembryonic antigen family, a **glycosylphosphatidylinositol** (GPI)-linked expressed in neutrophils and epithelial cells, has a role in cell adhesion and signalling, expressed in colonic carcinoma

Expressed by cells of a subset of B-lineage acute lymphoblastic leukaemia but not normal B-cell precursors so can be used for monitoring minimal residual disease

CD66d member of the carcinoembryonic antigen family, expressed on neutrophils, function uncertain

CD66e a glycoprotein which is a constituent of embryonic endodermal epithelium, carcinoembryonic antigen, **glycosylphosphatidylinositol** (GPI)-linked, expressed (weakly) by epithelial cells and strongly by carcinoma cells of gastrointestinal origin; has a role in cell adhesion and possibly in metastasis of tumour cells; found in the serum where is referred to as carcinoembryonic antigen (CEA) and is used as a tumour marker

CD66f pregnancy-specific glycoprotein, expressed in the placenta and fetal liver; may protect the fetus from the maternal immune system

CD67   *see* CD66b

CD68 macrosialin, a member of the family of haemopoietic mucin-like molecules that includes CD34 and CD43; expressed within the cytoplasm of monocytes, macrophages and osteoclasts and more weakly on neutrophils and basophils; expressed early in the neutrophil lineage, possibly before chloroacetate esterase, but expression is lost with maturation whereas in the monocyte lineage it is retained; expressed on mast cells; expressed on some B lymphocytes

CD68 is expressed on blast cells of many patients with acute myeloid leukaemia and is useful for the immunohistochemical demonstration of myeloid differentiation; expressed by megakaryocytes and in M7 acute myeloid leukaemia; expressed in systemic mastocytosis; expressed weakly on cells of B-lineage acute lymphoblastic leukaemia; occasionally expressed on hairy cells and chronic lymphocytic leukaemia cells; expressed in the majority of cases of Langerhans cell histiocytosis

CD69 a transmembrane protein that functions as a signal transmitting receptor in the early stages of cellular activation; not expressed on resting peripheral blood lymphocytes but following activation can be expressed on B cells, T cells (particularly) and NK cells; activated T cells which express CD69 are mainly CD8+CD45RO+; expression on T cells is induced by **IL15** and by contact with activated endothelium expressing ICAM-1; expression on activated T cells rapidly declines in the absence of exogenous stimuli; detection of lymphocytes expressing CD69 after exposure to a specific antigen can be used to demonstrate response to that antigen; expressed on some thymocytes; constitutively expressed on monocytes, epidermal Langherhans cells, mast cells, platelets and bone marrow myeloid precursors; expressed on activated neutrophils and eosinophils; expressed on mantle zone B cells and some germinal centre B cells and has a role in B-cell development; expressed on mast cells and overexpressed in reactive mast cells in monoclonal gammopathy of undetermined significance and myelodysplastic syndromes (but less strongly expressed in these reactive cells than in systemic mastocytosis); CD69 is expressed on cells of 80% of cases of low grade B-lineage lymphoproliferative disorders (non-Hodgkin's lymphoma and chronic lymphocytic leukaemia) and 53% of high grade non-Hodgkin's lymphoma; expressed on lymphoma cells of nasal-type NK cell lymphoma and sometime on cells of aggressive NK-cell leukaemia/lymphoma but not those of blastic NK cell lymphoma; overexpressed on the mast cells of indolent systemic mastocytosis

CD70 a member of the tumour necrosis factor receptor family, ligand for **CD27**; the interaction of CD70 with its ligand is probably functionally important early after antigenic stimulation; expressed on 10% of peripheral blood B cells and B cells in about 10% of germinal centres; expressed on activated B cells and T cells

CD70 is expressed more often on neoplastic than on normal B cells, being expressed in about a third of cases of follicular lymphoma, about three-quarters of cases of large B-cell lymphoma and in some cases of chronic lymphocytic leukaemia; expressed by Reed–Sternberg

cells; when expressed on malignant cells there is often co-expression of the ligand, CD27; can function as a receptor and facilitate proliferation of neoplastic cells; expressed by nasopharyngeal carcinoma and some thymic carcinomas

CD71 **transferrin** receptor; mediates iron uptake; expressed on early and late erythroid precursors and on activated B and T lymphocytes and proliferating cells in general; expressed on early cells of neutrophil lineage but lost on maturation; expressed on mast cells

CD71 is expressed on immature erythroid cells in M6 acute myeloid leukaemia; often expressed in T-lineage acute lymphoblastic leukaemia and may be expressed in aggressive lymphomas; expressed on neoplastic mast cells; expressed on Reed–Sternberg cells

CD72 an antigen expressed on B cells and B-cell precursors; ligand for **CD5** and **CD100**; CD72 is a negative regulator of B-cell responses with these negative signals being turned off by binding of CD100 on T cells to CD72 on B cells

CD72 is expressed on lymphoblasts in many cases of B-lineage acute lymphoblastic leukaemia; co-expressed with its ligand, CD5, on chronic lymphocytic leukaemia cells; strongly expressed on hairy cells

CD73 a **glycosylphosphatidylinositol** (GPI)-anchored protein, ecto 5′ nucleotidase, expressed on subsets of B and T cells, follicular dendritic cells, epithelial cells and endothelial cells; a costimulatory molecule for T cells; catalyses dephosphorylation of purine and pyrimidine ribo- and deoxyribonucleoside monophosphates to nucleosides: the preferred substrate is AMP

CD73 is expressed on some B lymphoblasts but not the most immature

CD74 invariant (γ) chain of the MHC class II complex, expressed on B cells but not B-cell precursors, activated T cells, monocytes, macrophages, activated endothelial and activated epithelial cells

CD75 carbohydrate determinants—nonsialylated/masked lactosamine epitopes

CD75s alpha-2,6-sialylated lactosamines (formerly CDw75 and CDw76); CDw75 is a **CD22** ligand; expressed on circulating

B cells and germinal centre B cells of secondary follicles but not B-cell precursors, a small subset of T cells, erythrocytes and some epithelial cells; expressed on B cells including mantle zone B cells of secondary follicles, a subset of T cells and subsets of endothelial and epithelial cells

CD75s is expressed on immature B lymphoblasts and cells of mature B-lineage neoplasms

CDw76   a deleted CD designation (*see* CD75s)

CD77   a carbohydrate, Pk blood group antigen, expressed on germinal centre B cells; in endothelial cells, CD77 functions as a receptor for verotoxin with resultant apoptosis of the cells

CD77 is expressed by the cells of Burkitt's lymphoma and post-transplant lymphoproliferative disorder; weakly expressed on the cells of follicular centre cell lymphoma; expressed by cells of a minority of patients with multiple myeloma but in a majority of patients with plasma cell leukaemia

CDw78   a deleted CD designation

CD79a   part of the immunoglobulin-associated heterodimeric B-cell antigen receptor complex; expressed on B cells and their precursors, and on plasma cells; a useful 'pan-B' marker applicable in immunocytochemistry and immunohistochemistry—monoclonal antibodies available detect an intracellular epitope

CD79a is expressed on blasts cells of B-lineage acute lymphoblastic leukaemia and on mature B-lineage leukaemias and lymphomas; expressed on neoplastic cells in nodular lymphocyte predominant Hodgkin's disease and expressed, more weakly on the neoplastic cells of a significant minority of cases of classical Hodgkin's disease

CD79b   part of the B-cell antigen receptor complex; crucial for the correct intracellular assembly and transport of the complex; expressed on mature B cells and late B-cell precursors (pre-B cell)

CD79b is expressed on most neoplasms of mature B cells but weakly or not at all on the cells of chronic lymphocytic leukaemia and in only about a half of cases of lymphoplasmacytoid lymphoma and a quarter of cases of hairy cell leukaemia; the lack of expression in chronic lymphocytic leukaemia is useful in helping to differentiate this condition from non-Hodgkin's lymphoma; expressed on the blast cells of some cases of acute lymphoblastic leukaemia

CD80   ligand of **CD28** and **CD152**; co-regulator, with **CD86**, of T-cell activation; engagement of the T-cell receptor without co-stimulation may lead to anergy rather than clonal expansion; expressed on T cells, activated B cells and some dendritic cells; expressed weakly on immature dendritic cells, such as those in skin and other peripheral tissues, but expressed strongly on mature dendritic cells in lymph nodes; expressed in the majority of cases of Langerhans cell histiocytosis

CD81   a tetraspanin; part of a large signal transduction complex, together with **CD19** and **CD21**; broadly expressed on haemopoietic cells but not on erythrocytes, platelets or neutrophils; expressed on lymphocytes, endothelial cells, epithelial cells and hepatocytes; on lymphocytes and hepatocytes is a receptor for the hepatitis C virus

CD82   Kangai 1, a member of the transmembrane 4 or tetraspanin superfamily of proteins, which functions in signal transduction; almost ubiquitous tissue expression; strongly expressed on early haemopoietic progenitor cells; moderately expressed on neutrophils and monocytes but expressed weakly on only about a third of peripheral blood lymphocytes (T and B cells); a tumour metastasis suppressor gene whose transcription is down regulated during the tumour progression of several human adenocarcinomas (prostate, pancreas and breast); the enhancer of the CD82 gene is positively regulated by **p53** and loss of p53 function during tumour progression is associated with a loss of CD82 expression

CD82 is expressed in chronic lymphocytic leukaemia, acute myeloid leukaemia and blast crisis of chronic myeloid leukaemia

CD83 a transmembrane protein, which is expressed weakly on activated B cells and activated T cells; expressed on interdigitating dendritic cells and Langerhans cells; may not be expressed on circulating or bone marrow dendritic cells but is up-regulated on culture of circulating dendritic cells; usually expressed weakly or not at all in Langerhans cell histiocytosis; expressed on activated neutrophils

CD84 a cell surface glycoprotein, expressed on mature B cells, thymocytes, a subset of T cells, monocytes, macrophages and platelets; a receptor for the product of the *SAP* gene

CD85 Leukocyte Immunoglobulin-like Receptor 1, LIR1; expressed on circulating B cells, a minority of circulating T cells and a subpopulation of circulating NK cells; expressed on monocytes and macrophages; strongly expressed on plasma cells, hairy cells, mantle zone B cells and germinal centre cells

CD86 a cell surface protein, expressed weakly on immature dendritic cells, such as those in skin (Langerhans cells) and other peripheral tissues, but expressed strongly on mature dendritic cells in lymph nodes, e.g. interdigitating reticulum cells; usually expressed weakly or not at all on the cells of Langerhans cell histiocytosis; expressed on monocytes, activated B cells, memory B cells and germinal centre B cells; a ligand of **CD28**, **CD80** and **CD152**; co-regulator, with CD80, of T-cell activation; plays a critical role in induction and regulation of the immune response

CD86 is expressed by Hodgkin's cells and Reed–Sternberg cells; expressed on some acute myeloid leukaemia myeloblasts and has been found to correlate with worse prognosis; is more often expressed in M4 and M5 categories of acute myeloid leukaemia but not with sufficient specificity for this to be diagnostically useful; expressed on neoplastic cells in about half of patient with multiple myeloma, expression correlating with a worse prognosis

CD87 plasminogen activator receptor uPAR, u-PAR, a **glycosylphosphatidyl-inositol** (GPI)-anchored protein, receptor for urokinase and pro-urokinase and also for vitronectin; expressed on activated T cells, NK cells, monocytes, neutrophils, platelets and many non-haemopoietic cells; has a possible role in the migration of leucocytes into tissues

CD88 a cell surface glycoprotein, C5a receptor, expressed on neutrophils and monocytes and has a role in their activation; sometimes expressed on basophils but not on mast cells (with the exception of skin mast cells); expressed on smooth muscle cells, pulmonary epithelial and endothelial cells and alveolar macrophages

CD89 Fcα receptor, expressed on myeloid cells from the promyelocyte to the neutrophil stage, promonocytes, monocytes, splenic and alveolar macrophages and activated eosinophils; induces phagocytosis, the respiratory burst, bacterial killing and degranulation; eosinophils of atopic individuals show up-regulation of CD89

CD90 Thy-1, a **glycosylphosphatidylinositol** (GPI)-anchored glycoprotein expressed on lymphocytes and co-expressed with CD34 on a proportion of haemopoietic stem cells and prothymocytes; also expressed on neurones and in secreted form by neuronal accessory cells; following autologous stem cell transplantation, the number of CD34+CD90+ cells infused correlates with durability of engraftment

Expressed on the leukaemic cells in 5% of patients with acute myeloid or acute lymphoblastic leukaemia

CD91 α_2 macroglobulin receptor, also known as low density lipoprotein receptor-related protein and heat shock protein receptor; expressed on monocytes and macrophages, including Kupffer cells and alveolar macrophages, neurones, astrocytes, smooth muscle cells, testicular Leydig cells and ovarian granulosa cells; binds protease–inhibitor complexes such as protease–α_2 macroglobulin complexes and processes and presents heat shock proteins

CD92 an antigen expressed on neutrophils, monocytes, platelets and endothelium

CDw93   expressed on neutrophils, monocytes and endothelial cells

CD94   Killer cell Lectin-like Receptor,
subfamily D, member 1, KLRD1; an
MHC Class I-specific NK receptor
molecule, expressed on mature NK cells
but not pre-NK cells or immature NK
cells; binding of cells expressing CD94 to
cells expressing **MHC Class I** alleles leads
to inhibition of cytotoxicity whereas
binding to virus-infected cells failing to
express MHC Class I permits cytotoxicity; expressed on a subset of T cells;
expressed on cells of nasal T/NK lymphoma, aggressive NK-cell leukaemia
lymphoma and a minority of extranodal
cytotoxic T-cell lymphomas but not cells
of blastic NK-cell leukaemia/lymphoma

CD95   Fas/APO-1, a transmembrane
protein belonging to the TNF family
that mediates programmed cell death
(apoptosis) when trimerized by cross-
linking to Fas ligand; cross linking leads
to activation of caspases, a family of proteases that mediate apoptotic cell death;
expressed on activated (non-cytotoxic)
T and B lymphocytes; responsible for
eliminating autoreactive T cells during
ontogenesis and for maintaining lymphocyte homeostasis; inherited Fas mutations are responsible for an autoimmune
lymphoproliferative syndrome; CD95/Fas
is expressed on thymic medullary epithelial
cells; Fas is expressed on early erythroblasts whereas Fas ligand is expressed
on late erythroblasts, permitting negative
feedback control which can be abrogated
by high concentrations of erythropoietin;
Fas is expressed on dendritic cells; expressed on reactive plasma cells and
normal tonsillar plasma cells so that
they are susceptible to apoptosis but not
expressed on normal bone marrow
plasma cells; an HIV protein, type 1 nef,
upregulates Fas on CD4+ lymphocytes,
leading to apoptosis and T-cell depletion;
the Fas/FasL pathway may specifically
kill virally infected or transformed cells

The Fas gene is mutated in a significant proportion (about 10%) of cases of
multiple myeloma and non-Hodgkin's
lymphoma, particularly MALT-type
lymphoma and extra-nodal B-lineage diffuse large cell lymphoma; not expressed
on chronic lymphocytic leukaemia cells
and this may contribute to the prolonged
survival of chronic lymphocytic leukaemia cells; not expressed in acute lymphoblastic leukaemia and expressed in
only a half of cases of diffuse large cell
lymphoma and Burkitt's lymphoma; Fas
is expressed on Reed–Sternberg cells of
most cases of Hodgkin's disease; Fas is
often overexpressed in the myelodysplastic
syndromes and Fas ligand may be inap-
propriately expressed on CD34+ stem
cells so that Fas-Fas ligand interactions
contribute to increased apoptosis

Fas ligand is expressed on activated
lymphocytes, monocytes, neutrophils and
thymocytes but not on normal CD34+
stem cells. Fas ligand is expressed in the
anterior chamber of the eye so that lymphocytes entering the anterior chamber
bind to Fas ligand and undergo apoptosis.
Fas ligand is upregulated on macrophages
by HIV infection so that lymphocytes
that come in contact with macrophages
undergo apoptosis

Expression of Fas ligand is increased
in chronic lymphocytic leukaemia/small
lymphocytic lymphoma and marginal
zone lymphoma; fas ligand is expressed
on myeloma cells and may induce apoptosis in T cells; Fas ligand is expressed on
Reed–Sternberg cells of about a third of
cases of Hodgkin's disease but although
Fas may be coexpressed apoptosis does
not appear to occur

CD96   a protein, a member of the immunoglobulin gene superfamily expressed on
activated T cells and activated NK cells,
peaking 6 to 9 days after the activating
stimulus

CD97   a glycoprotein expressed strongly
by monocytes and macrophages and less
strongly by neutrophils; not expressed by
resting lymphocytes but upregulated on
activation; a member of the EGF-TM7
family of cell surface proteins; alternative
exon splicing leads to several isoforms
which have varying numbers of extracellular EGF repeats; related to the secretin
and calcitonin receptors; interacts with

the human complement regulator, CD55 —the physiological role of this is not known

CD98 a protein, Solute Carrier family 3, member 2, SLC3A2; an L-phenylalanine transporter; expressed on activated monocytes, T lymphocytes and B lymphocytes

Expressed on neoplastic cells in most patients with multiple myeloma—failure of expression appears to correlate with resistance to melphalan therapy

CD99 MIC2, a transmembrane sialoglycoprotein encoded by the first identified Y chromosomal structural gene; located on the pseudo-autosomal region of the Y chromosome; the corresponding X chromosomal gene, *MIC2X* escapes X inactivation; broadly expressed on haemopoietic and lymphoid cells (including thymocytes, T cells and B cells); involved in cell-cell adhesion during haemopoietic cell differentiation and apoptosis of immature thymocytes; expressed on a subset of pancreatic islet cells

CD99 is not expressed on Reed–Sternberg or Hodgkin's cells; expressed on the blast cells in the majority of cases of acute myeloid leukaemia and acute lymphoblastic leukaemia and on cells of Ewing's tumour, primitive neuroectodermal tumours and peripheral neuroepitheliomas; useful in the diagnosis of atypical fibroxanthoma; expressed more weakly in Burkitt-type acute lymphoblastic leukaemia than precursor-B acute lymphoblastic leukaemia; Epstein–Barr virus LMP down-regulates CD99 expression on B cells, possibly contributing to viral oncogenesis in EBV-positive Hodgkin's disease

CD100 a transmembrane semaphorin expressed on late haemopoietic cells, T cells, germinal centre B cells, NK cells, neutrophils and monocytes; more strongly expressed on activated T cells and B cells; has a role in cell adhesion; ligand of **CD45**; induces B-cell aggregation and down-regulates B-cell expression of **CD23**; can be cleaved from the cell surface to give a functional soluble semaphorin, which inhibits monocyte migration;

interaction with **CD72** on B lymphocytes is essential for production of T-cell dependent antibodies

CD101 a protein, Immunoglobulin Superfamily, member 2, IGSF2; expressed on monocytes, neutrophils, cutaneous dendritic cells and activated T cells

CD101 is a marker of Langerhans cell histiocytosis cells

CD102 Intercellular adhesion molecule 2 (ICAM-2); an adhesion molecule that is the ligand of the β_2 integrin **CD11a/ CD18**; expressed on endothelial cells, platelets, monocytes and some lymphocytes; acts as a costimulatory molecule in the immune response and has a role in lymphocyte recirculation

CD103 human mucosal lymphocyte antigen 1, alpha subunit; a cell surface antigen, αE integrin, which forms a heterodimer with $\beta7$ integrin; expressed on mucosa-associated T lymphocytes, other intra-epithelial lymphocytes and a small subset of peripheral blood lymphocytes (2–6%); expressed on monocytes

CD103 is expressed by hairy cells and in adult T-cell leukaemia/lymphoma and enteropathy-associated T-cell non-Hodgkin's lymphoma

CD104 a cell surface antigen, $\beta4$ integrin chain, expressed as α_6/β_4 integrin in keratinocytes; expressed on Schwann cells and some tumour cells; mutations in the $\beta4$ integrin gene have been found in children with the non-lethal form of junctional epidermolysis bullosa and pyloric atresia; these cases have all been compound heterozygotes for a nonsense and a mis-sense mutation; compound heterozygosity for two nonsense mutations or homozygosity for a single nonsense allele results in stillbirth; $\alpha_6\beta_4$ integrin is also expressed on thymic epithelial cells, permitting the adhesion of thymocytes

CD105 endoglin, a homodimeric membrane glycoprotein that is a high-affinity receptor for transforming growth factor $\beta1$ and $\beta3$; expressed on endothelial cells, activated monocytes, macrophages, early B-cell precursors, stromal cells of the bone marrow, erythroid precursors and some haemopoietic stem cells; in the embryo, CD105 expression is essential for myeloid and erythroid differentiation; encoded by the target gene that is mutated in hereditary haemorrhagic telangiectasia

CD106 a cell surface antigen, VCAM-1, **V**ascular **C**ell **A**dhesion **M**olecule; a member of the immunoglobulin gene superfamily; expressed on activated endothelium, some tissue macrophages, dendritic cells and bone marrow fibroblasts; expression of VCAM-1 is increased by IL1α, TNFα, IL4 and lipopolysaccharide; upregulated by exposure to verotoxin, promoting neutrophil adhesion to endothelium; mediates the adhesion of monocytes, lymphocytes and eosinophils to activated endothelial cells; to a lesser extent, mediates adhesion of neutrophils, probably by means of binding to an α_4 integrin; expression of VCAM-1 is increased when the erythrocytes of sickle cell anaemia (SS) adhere to endothelium, which further increases adhesion of SS reticulocytes, expressing $\alpha_4\beta_1$ integrin, to activated endothelium; expressed at a low level on bone marrow stromal cells, expression being upregulated by TNFα, IL1, IL4 and IL13; administration of G-CSF leads to release of neutrophil proteases in the bone marrow with cleavage of VCAM-1 on bone marrow stromal cells, which may lead to release of haemopoietic stem cells

Soluble VCAM-1 is increased in chronic lymphocytic leukaemia and, although it is not expressed on the leukaemic cells, correlates with tumour burden; soluble VCAM-1 is increased in acute leukaemia, Hodgkin's disease and advanced-stage non-Hodgkin's lymphoma; increased serum levels in non-Hodgkin's lymphoma correlate with a worse prognosis

CD107a **L**ysosomal **M**embrane **P**rotein **1** (LAMP-1), expressed by degranulated platelets, activated T cells, neutrophils and activated endothelium; mediates mononuclear cell adhesion to vascular endothelium

CD107b **L**ysosomal **M**embrane **P**rotein **2** (LAMP-2), expressed on activated platelets and weakly on activated endothelium and neutrophils; mediates mononuclear cell adhesion to vascular endothelium

CD108 a protein expressed on red cells and lymphoblasts and more weakly on lymphocytes; expressed on erythrocytes; the JMH blood group antigen

CD109 a **glycosylphosphatidylinositol** (GPI)-linked glycoprotein, $\alpha_v\beta_3$ integrin, expressed on activated T cells, platelets, megakaryocytes, endothelial cells and haemopoietic stem cells

CD110 thrombopoietin receptor, a member of the cytokine receptor superfamily, expressed on a stem cell subset, megakaryocytes and, weakly, on platelets; encoded by the *MPL* gene at 1p34; homologue of the murine viral oncogene, *v-mpl* (**M**yeloproliferative **L**eukaemia **V**irus); mutations in *MPL* are found in patients with congenital amegakaryocytic thrombocytopenia; expressed by common myeloid but not common lymphoid progenitor cells

CD111 a protein, nectin-1/**P**olio**v**irus **R**eceptor-**L**ike, PVRL1; a component of adherens junctions; expressed on a stem cell subset, macrophages, neutrophils and neurones; an adhesion molecule and receptor for *Herpes simplex* viruses; two isoforms are known with differing intracellular domains; mutations in the *PVRL1* gene have been found in kindreds with the cleft lip/palate–ectodermal dysplasia syndrome (CLPED1)

CD112 a protein, nectin-2/PRR2, expressed on neurones, endothelial cells epithelial cells, monocytes, megakaryocytes, neutrophils and a stem cell subset; a component of adherens junctions; two isoforms are known with differing intracellular domains

CD113 an unassigned CD number

CD114 the receptor for granulocyte colony-stimulating factor (G-CSFR); CSF3R; expressed at all stages of neutrophil differentiation and on monocytes, platelets and endothelial cells; has a major role in regulation of proliferation and differentiation of cells of neutrophil lineage; mutations of this gene are responsible for some cases of severe congenital neutropenia; binding to G-CSF down-regulates CD114 and induces gelatinase B release

CD115 a glycoprotein, M-CSF receptor (Macrophage Colony Stimulating Factor Receptor) or CSF1, a receptor tyrosine kinase which is encoded by the *FMS* (*CSF1R*) gene; expressed on monocytes and macrophages, placental cells and some choriocarcinoma cells;

CD115 is expressed by some acute myeloid leukaemia cells; mis-sense point mutations in codons 301 or 969 of the *FMS* gene have been found in chronic myelomonocytic leukaemia and M4 acute myeloid leukaemia; in one series, 1/51 haematologically normal subjects were shown to have the mutation in codon 969; this may represent a marker of predisposition to myeloid malignancy

CD116 the α chain of the Granulocyte-Macrophage Colony Stimulating Factor Receptor (GM-CSFR), the β chain being **CDw131**; expressed on monocytes, macrophages, neutrophils, eosinophils and dendritic cells; sometimes expressed on basophils but not on mast cells; the gene for this protein is located in the pseudoautosomal region of the short arm of the X and Y chromosomes, distal to the CD99 locus

CD117 *c-KIT*, the receptor for stem cell factor (SCF-R), a receptor tyrosine kinase; expressed on haemopoietic precursors, myeloblasts, primitive erythroid cells, mast cells, a subset of NK cells and a range of non-haemopoietic cells including the interstitial cells of Cajal Auerbach's plexus, melanocytes, testis, vascular endothelium, stromal fibroblasts, astrocytes, renal tubules, breast glandular epithelium and sweat glands; not expressed on basophils; expressed on early B lymphoid cells and immature thymic T cells; point mutations in *c-KIT* have been found in familial piebaldism and megacolon and in gastrointestinal stromal tumours which are thought to be derived from interstitial cells of Cajal, express CD117, and respond to therapy with imanitib mesylate, a c-KIT inhibitor

CD117 is expressed by the blast cells of most cases of acute myeloid leukaemia

with megakaryoblasts as well as myeloblasts expressing the antigen; expressed in systemic mastocytosis; expressed on some myeloma cells but not on the cells of plasma cell leukaemia; rarely expressed in T-lineage acute lymphoblastic leukaemia

CD118 interferon α.β receptor; a broadly expressed protein

CDw119 an interferon receptor, IFNγR1; expressed on monocytes, macrophages, B cells and endothelium; a mutation in the gene encoding this protein causes susceptibility to atypical mycobacterial infections

CD120a a receptor for tumour necrosis factor α; Tumor Necrosis Factor Receptor subfamily, member 1A, TNFRI; expressed on haemopoietic and non-haemopoietic cells, most strongly on epithelial cells; mutations in the *TNFR1* gene have been linked with familial autosomal dominant periodic fever syndromes

CD120b a receptor for tumour necrosis factor α; Tumour Necrosis Factor Receptor subfamily, member 1B, TNFRII; expressed on haemopoietic and non-haemopoietic cells, most strongly on myeloid cells, activated T cells and activated B cells; polymorphisms in the *TNFR2* gene have been linked with familial combined hyperlipidaemia

CD121a a receptor for IL1α and IL1β; IL1R type 1, IL1RI, expressed on T cells

CD121b a receptor for IL1, IL1R type II, IL1RII; possibly inhibits IL1 activity by binding IL1 that would otherwise bind to IL1RI; expressed on B cells, monocytes and macrophages

CD122 Interleukin 2 Receptor **beta** chain (IL2Rβ); together with **CD25** and **CD132**, forms a high affinity IL2R which is expressed on T cells, B cells, NK cells, monocytes and macrophages; CD122 is also a subunit of IL15R which is expressed on activated monocytes and on various non-haemopoietic cells; not expressed by basophils or mast cells; targeted disruption of the murine gene leads to uncontrolled B-cell proliferation with hypergammaglobulinaemia and an autoimmune haemolytic anaemia; KIT-ligand (SCF) and flt-3 ligand induce expression of CD122 on CD34^{bright} haemopoietic progenitor cells which can then be induced to differentiate to NK cells by the action of IL15

CD123 Interleukin 3 Receptor alpha chain (IL3Rα); the α subunit is ligand specific whereas the β subunit, **CD133**, is shared with GM-CSFR and IL5R; the gene is located in the pseudoautosomal region at the end of the short arm of the X and Y chromosomes expressed on haemopoietic stem cells, granulocytes, monocytes and megakaryocytes; expressed on basophils but not mast cells; expressed on lymphoid dendritic cells

Expressed on blast cells of the majority of patients with acute myeloid leukaemia but not expressed on normal CD34+CD38− bone marrow stem cells

CD124 Interleukin 4 Receptor alpha chain (IL4Rα), combines with the IL4Rβ chain, **CD132**, to form the receptor; expressed on T cells, B cells and haemopoietic cells; also contributes the α chain of IL13R, combining with IL13Rβ chain to form the receptor; susceptibility to atopy and increased levels of expression of CD23 have been associated with a mis-sense mutation in codon 576 of the IL4Rα gene; several mis-sense mutations at codon 50 have been associated with susceptibility to asthma, atopy and elevated IgE levels

CDw125 Interleukin 5 Receptor alpha chain (IL5Rα), which combines with **CDw131**, the β chain, to form a high affinity IL5 receptor; expressed on eosinophils, activated B cells and basophils; soluble isoforms of the IL5R α chain occur normally because of alternative splicing

CD126 Interleukin 6 Receptor alpha chain (IL6Rα); expressed on T cells, activated B cells and monocytes; in reactive conditions, expressed on plasmablasts and immature plasma cells but not mature plasma cells

CD126 is expressed on plasma cells in about 50% of patients with monoclonal gammopathy of undetermined significance and 90% of patients with multiple myeloma; may have a role in maintaining growth and survival of neoplastic plasma cells since IL6 binds to CD126 triggering association with the signal transducing molecule, **CD130**

CD127 Interleukin 7 Receptor alpha chain (IL7Rα), combines with the β chain, **CD132**, to form a high affinity receptor; expressed on most T cells, being down-regulated on T-cell activation; expressed on B-cell precursors and monocytes

CDw128a Interleukin 8 Receptor Alpha (IL8RA, IL8Rα); a high affinity receptor for IL8

CDw128b Interleukin 8 Receptor Beta (IL8RB, IL8Rβ), a low affinity receptor for IL8

CD130 a widely expressed molecule that associates with **CD126** after CD126 has bound to its ligand, IL6, and similarly associates with the IL11R after it has bound IL11; receptor for oncostatin M; part of the signalling system after cells have bound IL6 or IL11; expressed on activated B cells and plasma cells

CD130 is expressed on plasma cells in about 40% of patients with multiple myeloma at diagnosis and a similar proportion of cases of monoclonal gammopathy of undetermined significance; may have a role in maintaining growth and survival of neoplastic plasma cells; expressed on about 90% of cases of relapsed multiple myeloma and in about half of these is co-expressed with CD126

CDw131 the β subunit of GM-CSFR (combining with CD116), of the IL3R (combining with CD123) and of the IL5R (combining with CDw125); expressed on most myeloid cells

CD132 the common γ chain of a number of cytokine receptors:
• Combining with CD122 and CD25 to form the high affinity IL2R
• Combining with CD124 to form the high affinity IL4R
• Combining with CD127 to form the high affinity IL7R
• Combining with IL15Rα and CD122 to form the IL15R
• Also part of the receptor for IL9
Expressed on T cells, B cells, NK cells, monocytes, macrophages and neutrophils; mutation leads to sex-linked **severe combined immunodeficiency**

CD133 a protein, AC133, expressed on stem cell/progenitor cell subsets which can give rise to endothelial cells as well as haemopoietic cells

Expressed on blast cells of the majority of patients with acute myeloid leukaemia and acute lymphoblastic leukaemia but not expressed on normal CD34+CD38– bone marrow stem cells. In patients with acute myeloid leukaemia, expression correlates with other markers of immaturity, with M0 subtype being most often positive and with M3/M3 subtype not showing expression. Expression is more frequent in B-lineage than T-lineage acute lymphoblastic leukaemia and is characteristic of acute lymphoblastic leukaemia with t(4;11) and rearrangement of the *MLL* gene

CD134 a protein, OX40, a member of the TNF receptor superfamily; expressed on activated lymphocytes; an early activation marker on germinal centre T cells; interacts with its ligand expressed on antigen-presenting cells; interaction of CD134 with its ligand has an important role in acute graft-versus-host disease and numbers of CD134+ T lymphocytes correlate with chronic-graft-versus host disease

CD134 is expressed in many T-cell lymphomas including angioimmunoblastic, angiocentric and histiocyte-rich T-cell lymphoma but not in anaplastic large cell lymphoma

CD135 flt3, a receptor tyrosine kinase, a growth factor receptor that binds to FLT3 ligand; expressed on multipotent stem cells, myelomonocytic precursors and early B-cell progenitors; has a role in the proliferation and differentiation of haemopoietic progenitors

CD135 is expressed on blast cells in acute lymphoblastic leukaemia, acute myeloid leukaemia and the blast crisis of chronic granulocytic leukaemia; acquired mutations in *FLT3* have been found in acute myeloid leukaemia and indicate a poor prognosis

CDw136 a receptor tyrosine kinase, receptor for macrophage stimulating protein; expressed on macrophages and ciliated epithelial cells; has a role in induction of macrophage migration

CDw137 a protein, a member of the tumour necrosis receptor family, encoded by a gene at 1p36; expressed by activated T and B cells and monocytes; a costimulatory molecule in T-cell proliferation; B cells, activated T cells and monocytes express CD137 ligand; soluble CD137 stimulates proliferation of peripheral blood monocytes; expressed by endothelial cells and vascular smooth muscle cells in abnormal tissues, particularly malignant tumours, but not in normal tissues

CD138 a heavily glycosylated transmembrane molecule (heparan sulphate proteoglycan), an adhesion molecule, LFA-3 or Syndecan-1, that mediates the interaction between cells and the extracellular environment—mediating adhesion and regulating growth factor activities; expressed on post-germinal centre B cells but not germinal centre B cells; expressed on epithelial cells; expressed by plasma cells including early plasma cells but not expressed by reactive plasmablasts

CD138 is expressed by multiple myeloma cells and in some lymphomas including lymphoplasmacytoid lymphoma; serum CD138 is of prognostic significance in multiple myeloma; expressed on neoplastic cells of some cases of classical Hodgkin's disease but not on the cells of nodular lymphocyte predominant Hodgkin's disease; cells of chronic lymphocytic leukaemia show weak or moderate cytoplasmic and membrane expression; expressed on HIV-associated primary effusion lymphoma; CD138-coated beads can be used for purifying myeloma cells; has been used, together with pan-B monoclonal antibodies, for purging peripheral blood stem cell harvests for autologous transplantation in multiple myeloma

CD139 a protein, expressed on B cells, monocytes, neutrophils and follicular dendritic cells

CD139 is expressed on cells of some but not all cases of chronic lymphocytic leukaemia

CD140a   Platelet-Derived Growth Factor Receptor Alpha (PDGFRα), a receptor tyrosine kinase

CD140b   Platelet-Derived Growth Factor Receptor Beta (PDGFRβ), a receptor tyrosine kinase; expressed on endothelial cells, smooth muscle cells, fibroblasts, glial cells, chondrocytes, B and T lymphocytes and myeloid cells including megakaryocytes and platelets

The gene encoding CD140b, which is on chromosome 5, is often deleted in the 5q– syndrome and is rearranged in several uncommon chronic myeloid leukaemias (*see PDGFRB*)

CD141   a cell surface glycoprotein, **thrombomodulin**, expressed on endothelial cells; the cofactor for thrombin-mediated expression of activated protein C; heterozygosity for a mis-sense mutation in the thrombomodulin gene has been associated with familial thrombophilia

CD142   **tissue factor**; CD142 plus factor VIIa initiates the **coagulation cascade** through factors X and IX; VIIa is the catalytic subunit while CD142 is the regulatory subunit; induced on monocytes and endothelial cells by inflammatory mediators

CD143   Angiotensin-Converting Enzyme (ACE); expressed on some endothelial cells, and some epithelial and neuronal cells, monocytes, activated macrophages, a small number of T cells and spermatozoa; metabolizes angiotensin II and bradykinin; increased expression of CD143 on endothelial cells may be relevant to the development of atherosclerosis; has a role in binding spermatazoa to the ovum

CD144   VE-cadherin, a protein expressed on endothelium that mediates homotypic adhesion

CDw145   a protein that is expressed constitutively on endothelial cells and some bone marrow stromal cells

CD146   a protein, a member of the immunoglobulin gene superfamily, also known as MUC18 and S-endo; expressed on endothelium and activated T cells; a component of the endothelial junction, involved in cell–cell cohesion; monoclonal CD146 antibodies can be used to identify and select circulating endothelial cells; a marker for melanoma, associated with tumour progression and metastasis

CD147   a protein known as neurothelin, basigin, EMMPRIN (Exracellular Matrix Metalloproteinase Inducer); a member of the immunoglobulin gene superfamily, an adhesion molecule; expressed on leucocytes (neutrophils, monocytes and lymphocytes) and erythrocytes and their precursors, macrophages, dendritic cells, platelets and endothelial cells; possibly an adhesion molecule. CD147 is upregulated when T and B lymphocyte are activated; receptor for cyclophilin A (a cyclosporin binding protein); anti-CD147 has some efficacy in graft-versus-host disease

CD148   a protein, HPTP-eta, p260 phosphatase; expressed on neutrophils, eosinophils, monocytes, T cells, some B cells, NK cells, dendritic cells, platelets and epithelial cells; expressed on memory B cells and on the cells of polyclonal B-cell lymphocytosis, which may represent an expansion of memory B cells; a membrane tyrosine phosphatase, which acts as a transducing molecule but also modulates signalling, e.g. through the T-cell receptor/CD3 complex

CDw149   an antigen that has been redesignated **CD47R**

CD150   a protein, Signalling Lymphocyte Activation Molecule (SLAM), IPO-3; a member of the immunoglobulin gene superfamily; expressed on thymocytes, B cells, some T cells and dendritic cells; a costimulatory molecule on B cells and dendritic cells; a mutation in the *SAP* (SLAM-Associated Protein) gene, which encodes a ligand of SLAM, is the cause of **X-linked lymphoproliferative disease**

CD151   Platelet-Endothelial Tetraspan Antigen 3 (PETA3), a member of the transmembrane 4 or tetraspanin superfamily of proteins, expressed on endothelial cells, platelets, monocytes and immature haemopoietic cells

CD152   a protein, Cytotoxic T associated Lymphocyte Antigen 4 (CTLA4), expressed on activated T cells; shows partial homology with **CD28**; like CD28, binds **CD80** and **CD86** and is probably mainly a negative regulator of T-cell activation; mis-sense mutations in codon 17 have been reported to be associated with autoimmune endocrinopathies; a CD152-immunoglobulin fusion protein has been used experimentally in the treatment of psoriasis

CD153 a cytokine, **CD30** ligand or CD30L, shows homology with tumour necrosis factor; expressed on neutrophils, activated T cells, monocytes and macrophages

CD153 (CD30 ligand) is expressed, together with CD30, on the neoplastic cells of cutaneous anaplastic large cell lymphoma, with overexpression probably contributing to spontaneous regression

CD154 a protein, **CD40** ligand or CD40L, expressed on activated CD4+ lymphocytes, expression being essential for normal signalling to B cells, particularly for isotype switching; mutations in the CD154 gene are responsible for the X-linked immunodeficiency syndrome, the **hyperIgM syndrome**; expressed on monocytes, macrophages, eosinophils, basophils, NK cells, platelets, dendritic cells, epithelial cells, endothelial cells and fibroblasts; on platelet activation, CD154 moves to the surface membrane and has the potential to interact with CD40 on endothelial cells, leading to an inflammatory reaction, which is limited by binding of CD154 to co-expressed platelet CD40; CD154 stimulates myelopoiesis, particularly megakaryocytopoiesis by up-regulating flt3-ligand and thrombopoietin; CD154 expression on CD4+ lymphocytes is increased in HIV infection and may contribute to hyperimmunoglobulinaemia; CD154 in the supernatant may cause febrile reactions following platelet transfusion; monoclonal antibodies to CD154 have been used in the therapy of autoimmune thrombocytopenic purpura and to facilitate allogenic engraftment

CD154 is co-expressed with CD40 on some non-Hodgkin's cells so that an autocrine loop may occur; it is co-expressed with CD40 on cells of some cases of chronic lymphocytic leukaemia;

soluble CD154 is increased in chronic lymphocytic leukaemia and could promote cell survival; strongly expressed on hairy cells; transduction of the CD154 gene into autologous lymphoid cells has been used experimentally in immunotherapy of chronic lymphocytic leukaemia

CD155 a protein, polio virus receptor (PVR), a member of the immunoglobulin superfamily; expressed on B cells, monocytes and neural cells

CD156a a protein, previously designated CD156, also known as ADAM8, MS2 (mouse homologue); a zinc metalloprotease expressed on neutrophils and monocytes; upregulated by retinoic acid

CD156b a protein, **T**umour necrosis factor-**A**lpha (TNFα)-**C**onverting **E**nzyme, TACE, also known as ADAM 17; broadly expressed adhesion structures

CD157 a **glycosylphosphatidylinositol** (GPI)-anchored protein with structural similarities to **CD38**, **B**one marrow **St**romal cell antigen **1** (BST-1), a cyclic ADP-ribose hydrolase and ADP ribosyl cyclase; expressed on myeloid precursors, neutrophils, monocytes, mast cells, macrophages, follicular dendritic cells, endothelial cells, bone marrow stromal cells, gut epithelial cells, mesothelial cells, α and β cells of pancreas; over-expressed in bone marrow stromal cells and probably synovial cells in rheumatoid arthritis; interaction of CD157+ nurse-like cells with B cells may underlie the polyclonal B-cell activation in rheumatoid arthritis; soluble CD157 correlates with disease activity in rheumatoid arthritis

CD158a two proteins, p58.1 and p50.1, MHC class I-specific (HLA-C-specific) NK receptors; members of the KIR (**K**iller **I**nhibitory **R**eceptor) family and immunoglobulin gene super-family; expressed on a NK subset and rare T cells; p58.1 is inhibitory and p50.1 is stimulatory; following engagement of CD158a, inhibition of NK cell activity is seen

CD158b two proteins, p58.2 and p50.2, MHC class I-specific NK (HLA-C-specific) receptors; members of KIR family and immunoglobulin gene superfamily; expressed on a NK subset and rare T cells; T cells that express CD158b are CD3+, CD8+, TCRα/β+ and CD56+

CD159a   a protein, p70, NKG2A/KIR; a member of the KIR family and the immunoglobulin gene superfamily, expressed on NK cells

CD160   a protein, BY55, expressed on T-cell subset and NK cell subset; a co-stimulatory molecule

CD161   a lectin, NKRP-1, expressed on most NK cells, both mature and imma-ture, pre-NK cells, a subset of T cells and a subset of thymocytes

CD161 is expressed in aggressive and nasal type NK-cell leukaemia/lymphoma but not blastic NK-cell leukaemia/lymphoma

CD162   a cell surface glycoprotein, <u>P</u> <u>S</u>electin <u>G</u>lycoprotein <u>L</u>igand <u>1</u> (PSGL-1) or cutaneous leucocyte antigen, a mucin-like molecule; ligand for **CD42P** (P selectin), **CD62E** (E selectin) and **CD42L** (L selectin) and the bacterium which causes human granulocytic ehrlichiosis; expressed on haemopoietic progenitors and most myeloid cells, most T cells and some B cells; expressed more strongly on monocytes than on neutrophils; permits lymphocytes and neutrophils to roll on activated endothelium; binds haemopoi-etic precursors to P selectin; influences binding of neutrophils to activated platelets, polymorphic variants being implicated in susceptibility to cerebrovascular disease

CD162 is expressed more weakly on myeloblasts than mature neutrophils. Expression on monoblasts is similar to that on monocytes and is stronger than expression on myeloblasts

CD162R   a protein, PEN5, expressed on NK

CD163   a protein, M130; a member of the scavenger receptor superfamily, a scav-enger receptor for haemoglobin, binding to haemoglobin–haptoglobin complexes in plasma; expressed on macrophages and weakly on circulating monocytes (expression being up-regulated by activa-tion during infection and in myelopro-liferative disorders)

CD164   a   mucin-like   glycoprotein, MGC-24 (<u>M</u>ultiglycosylated <u>C</u>ore pro-tein of <u>24</u> kilodaltons), a transmembrane homodimer, expressed on haemopoietic progenitors, bone marrow stromal cells, endothelial cells and some epithelial cells; participates in the binding of CD34+ cells to bone marrow stroma and inhibits the recruitment of such cells into cell cycle; expressed on both CD34+ stem cells and on more primitive CD34– stem cells

CD165   an adhesion molecule, GP/37/ AD2, expressed on a subset of T lympho-cytes, immature thymocytes, monocytes and most platelets and expressed at a low level on most thymocytes and on thymic epithelium; may have a role in adhesion of thymocytes to thymic epithelium and the adhesion of T lymphocytes to epi-dermal keratinocytes; strongly expressed in many T-lineage acute lymphoblastic leukaemias

CD166   an adhesion molecule, <u>A</u>ctivated <u>L</u>eucocyte <u>C</u>ell <u>A</u>dhesion <u>M</u>olecule (ALCAM), also known as HCA, a mem-ber of the immunoglobulin gene super-family; expressed on thymic epithelial cells, activated T cells, monocytes, CD34+CD38+ haemopoietic progen-itors and a subset of stromal cells at sites of haemopoiesis; mediates homophilic and heterophilic adhesion by binding to its ligand, **CD6**; expressed on endothe-lium of yolk sac and dorsal aorta and has a crucial role in embryonic haemopoiesis and vasculoangiogenesis

CD167a   a receptor tyrosine kinase activ-ated by collagen, an adhesion structure, <u>D</u>iscoidin <u>D</u>omain <u>R</u>eceptor (DDR1); expressed on epithelial cells and myoblasts

CD168   an adhesion structure, RHAMM; expressed on thymocyte, T-cell subsets and monocytes; there are at least three splice variants; overexpressed in multiple myeloma, B-cell non-Hodgkin's lymphoma and chronic lymphocytic leukaemia

CD169   an adhesion structure, siaload-hesin; expressed on a macrophage subset; a ligand for MUC.1 (**CD227**) on breast epithelial cells

CD170   an adhesion structure, <u>S</u>ialic acid-binding <u>I</u>mmunoglobulin-like <u>Lec</u>tin <u>5</u> (siglec-5); expressed on a macrophage subset and neutrophils

CD171 an adhesion structure, L1-CAM; expressed on neurones, monocytes, a T-cell subset and B cells; mutations in the *L1-CAM* gene give rise to a spectrum of familial X-linked recessive neurological disorders collectively termed CRASH syndrome

CD172a an adhesion structure, SIRP alpha; expressed on monocytes, a T-cell subset and stem cells

CD173 a carbohydrate structure, blood group H, type 2; expressed on erythroid cells, a stem cell subset and platelets

CD174 a carbohydrate structure, Lewis y; expressed on a stem cell subset and epithelial cells

CD175 a carbohydrate structure, Tn; expressed on a stem cell subset

CD175s a carbohydrate structure, sialyl-Tn; expressed on erythroblasts

CD176 a carbohydrate structure, TF (Thomas-Friedrenreich antigen); expressed on a stem cell subset

CD177 a protein, NB1, expressed on a neutrophil subset; carries epitopes of the NB1 family of neutrophil alloantigens

CD178 Fas ligand, Tumour Necrosis Factor ligand Superfamily, member 6; (TNFSF6); expressed on activated T cells; mutations in the CD178 gene have been identified in patients with the **autoimmune lymphoproliferative syndrome** (*see also* **CD95**)

CD179a a protein, VpreB, expressed on very early B-cell precursors, pro-B and early pre-B cells where, together with **CD179b**, it complexes with **CD79a**, **CD79b** and μ immunoglobulin heavy chains to form the B-cell receptor; CD179a and CD179b are replaced, later in B-cell ontogeny, by immunoglobulin; expressed on about 0.1% of cells in normal bone marrow but on a larger proportion in regenerating marrow

CD179a is expressed in some cases of B-lineage acute lymphoblastic leukaemia

CD179b a protein, Lambda 5, expressed on B-cell precursors (*see* **CD179a**)

CD180 a protein, RP105/Bgp95, expressed on mantle and marginal zone B cells, monocytes and dendritic cells

CD183 chemokine receptor 3, CXCR3, a **chemokine receptor** expressed on activated T cells and activated NK cells; expressed by B-CLL cells

CD184 chemokine receptor 4, CXCR4, a **chemokine receptor** for chemokines of the CXC family, expressed on a T-cell subset, B cells, monocytes, dendritic cells and endothelial cells; it is a co-receptor for entry of certain T-cell tropic strains of HIV into CD4+ T cells

CD184 is expressed in B-lineage acute lymphoblastic leukaemia; high expression predicts extramedullary organ infiltration in childhood acute lymphoblastic leukaemia

CD195 CCR5, a **chemokine receptor** expressed on monocytes and a T-cell subset, which binds several β chemokines and, when expressed on macrophages, permits entry of macrophage-tropic strains of HIV; certain polymorphisms in the *CCR5* gene confer resistance to HIV infection; a polymorphism for the *CCR5* gene is associated with reduced likelihood of asthma, reduced severity of rheumatoid arthritis and improved survival of renal allografts

CDw197 CCR7, a **chemokine receptor** expressed on a T-cell subset

CD200 OX2, a cell surface glycoprotein, member of the immunoglobulin superfamily; expressed on thymocytes, B cells, activated T cells, neurons and endothelial cells; CD200 receptor is expressed on myeloid cells and CD200 may inhibit function of myeloid cells

CD201 Endothelial Protein C Receptor (EPCR), expressed on an endothelial cell subset; polymorphisms in the *EPCR* gene may be associated with late miscarriage and myocardial infarction

CD202b Tie2 (Tek), a receptor tyrosine kinase expressed on endothelial cells and stem cells; receptor for angiopoietin-1; polymorphisms in the *TIE2* gene are associated with familial multiple cutaneous and mucosal venous malformation syndromes

CD203c phosphodiesterase 3, NPP3/PDNP3, expressed on basophils and megakaryocytes

CD204   macrophage scavenger receptor, expressed on macrophages

CD205   a protein, DEC205, expressed on dendritic cells and thymic epithelium

CD206   macrophage mannose receptor, expressed on a dendritic cell subset, macrophages and monocytes

CD207   langerin, a lectin expressed on immature Langherhans cells

CD208   a protein, DC-LAMP, expressed on interdigitating dendritic cells

CD209   a protein, DK-SIGN, expressed on a dendritic cell subset

CDw210   1L10 receptor, expressed on T cells, B cells, NK cells, monocytes and macrophages
    CDw210 is expressed in chronic lymphocytic leukaemia

CD212   IL12 receptor, expressed on activated T cells and activated NK cells

CD213a1   IL13 receptor alpha 1, expressed on B cells, monocytes, fibroblasts and endothelial cells; upregulated in bronchial smooth muscle of asthmatics

CD213a2   IL13 receptor alpha 2, expressed on B cells and monocytes

CDw217   IL17 receptor, a broadly expressed molecule

CD220   insulin receptor α subunit, a broadly expressed molecule

CD221   IGF1 receptor, a broadly expressed molecule

CD222   mannose-6-phosphate/IGF2 receptor, a broadly expressed molecule

CD223   a protein, LAG-3, expressed on activated T cells and activated NK cells

CD224   gamma-glutamyl transferase, expressed on leucocytes and stem cells

CD225   a protein, Leu13, a broadly expressed molecule

CD226   a protein, **D**n**a**x **A**ccessory **M**olecule **1** (DNAM-1), also known as PTA1, expressed on T cells, NK cells, monocytes and platelets

CD227   MUC.1, a transmembrane glycoprotein, also known as epithelial membrane antigen, binds to **CD169**, expressed on a stem cell subset, immature erythroid cells, activated T cells, plasma cells, epithelial cells and glandular epithelium
    CD227 is expressed on adenocarcinoma cells, in most plasma cell neoplasms and by the cells of ALK-positive nodal (but not cutaneous) anaplastic large cell lymphoma

CD228   a protein, melanotransferrin, expressed on melanoma cells

CD229   a protein, Ly9, expressed on T cells and B cells

CD230   prion protein, broadly expressed; expressed in neurones and is thought to be involved in synaptic transmission; in prion diseases, such as bovine spongiform encephalopathy and Creutzfeldt–Jakob disease, the normal cellular prion protein alters its conformation on contact with infectious prion protein from another host

CD231   a protein, TALLA-1/A15, found in normal brain and skeletal muscle
    CD231 is expressed in T-cell leukaemia and on neuroblastoma cells

CD232   a protein, VESP receptor, a broadly expressed molecule

CD233   a protein, **band 3**, expressed on erythroid cells

CD234   Fy (**Duffy**)-glycoprotein (DARC), expressed on erythroid cells

CD235a   a glycoprotein, **glycophorin A**, expressed on erythroid cells

CD235b   a glycoprotein, **glycophorin B**, expressed on erythroid cells

CD235ab   glycophorin A/B cross-reactive monoclonal antibodies detecting antigens on erythroid cells

CD236   glycoproteins, **glycophorin C/D**, expressed on a stem cell subset and erythroid cells

CD236R   a glycoprotein, **glycophorin C**, expressed on a stem cell subset and erythroid cells

CD238   a protein, **Kell**, expressed on a stem cell subset and erythroid cells

CD239   a protein, **B**asal **C**ell **A**dhesion **M**olecule (B-CAM), expressed on keratinocyes and erythroid cells; carries the **Lutheran** (Lu) blood group antigens

CD240CE   a red cell antigen of the **Rh** system, Rh30CE

CD240D   a red cell antigen of the **Rh** system, Rh30D

CD240DCE   Rh30D/CE, cross-reactive monoclonal antibodies detecting **Rh** antigens on erythroid cells

CD241 RhAg, expressed on erythroid cells

CD242 Intercellular Adhesion Molecule-4 (ICAM-4), expressed on erythroid cells; the LW blood group glycoprotein

CD243 a protein, Multidrug Resistance 1 (MDR-1), expressed on stem cells and progenitor cells; its gene is amplified leading to overexpression in several drug resistant leukaemia cell lines

CD244 a protein, 2B4, expressed on NK cells and a T-cell subset, a receptor for the product of the *SAP* gene

CD245 a protein, p220/240, expressed on a T-cell subset

CD246 anaplastic lymphoma kinase, expressed by T cells

CD247 T-cell receptor zeta chain, expressed on T cells and NK cells

CDC2 see *CDK1*

CDCREL a gene, Cell Division Cycle Related; also known as *hCDCre* and peanut-like 1; gene map locus 22q11.2, encodes a member of the septin family of **GTPase** proteins which are thought to play a role in cytokinesis; the gene overlaps with that encoding platelet glycoprotein Ib, which is encoded on the same DNA strand in the same orientation; *CDCREL* contributes to the *MLL-hCDCre* fusion gene in acute myeloid leukaemia associated with t(11;22)(q23;q11.2)

CDK cyclin-dependent kinase

CDK1 a gene, Cyclin-Dependent Kinase 1, also known as Cell Cycle Controller *CDC2* (from the yeast homologue, cdc2— cell division cycle); gene map locus 10q21.1; universally expressed, encodes a catalytic subunit of a protein kinase complex, the M-phase promoting factor, that controls the transition from G1 to S phase and from G2 to the M phase of the **cell cycle**; activated by taxol which leads to G2/M phase arrest and apoptosis *in vitro*

CDK2 a gene, Cyclin-Dependent Kinase 2, also known as p33(CDK2); gene map locus 12q13; expressed late in G1 or in early S phase of the **cell cycle**, slightly before *CDC2*; small-molecule inhibitors of CDK2 have been investigated for prevention of chemotherapy-induced alopecia

CDK3 a gene, Cyclin-Dependent Kinase 3, gene map locus 17q22-qter, encodes a kinase activated by **cyclin E** which regulates G1-S transition during the **cell cycle**

CDK4 a gene, Cyclin-Dependent Kinase 4, gene map locus 12q14, encodes a protein kinase activated by the D-type cyclins and is involved in the control of cell proliferation during the G1 phase of the **cell cycle**; inhibited by p16(INK4A) (*see CDKN2A*); polymorphisms in the p16(INK4A) binding domain of CDK4 are associated with a predisposition to melanoma

CDK4B inhibitor Cyclin-Dependent Kinase 4 inhibitor B, *see CDKN2B*

CDK6 a gene, Cyclin-Dependent Kinase 6, also known as 'PLSTIRE' (after the practice of naming CDC2-related kinases on the basis of the amino acid sequence of the region corresponding to the conserved PSTAIRE motif of cdc2); gene map locus 7q21; encodes a protein activated by D-type cyclins, promoting transition from G1 to S phase of the **cell cycle**; dysregulated:
• by proximity to *IGH* in t(7;14)(q21;q32) associated with less than 5% of cases of splenic lymphoma with villous lymphocytes/splenic marginal zone lymphoma
• by proximity to κ in t(2;7)(p12;q21) associated with a lower percentage of cases

CDK7 a gene, Cyclin-Dependent Kinase 7, also known as kinase subunit of CAK, *CAK1*, gene map locus 2p15-cen, encodes a serine/threonine kinase; together with cyclin H, forms CDK-activating kinase (CAK), which phosphorylates several other CDKs and associates with the general transcription factor TFIIH

CDK8 a gene, Cyclin-Dependent Kinase 8, also known as *K35*, gene map locus 13q12; encodes a serine-threonine kinase which, along with cyclin C, forms part of the RNA polymerase II holoenzyme complex; associates with the **TAX** protein of human T-cell lymphotropic virus type I (HTLV-I)

CDK9 a gene, Cyclin-Dependent Kinase 9, also known as *PITALRE* (after the practice of naming cdc2-related kinases

Table 5   Cyclin-dependent kinase inhibitors – proteins and genes.

Family	CDKI Protein	Gene Preferred designation and location	Alternative designations
Cip/Kip family	p21^{Cip1/Waf1}	CDKN1A at 6p21.2	WAF1, CIP, CDKN1
	p27^{Kip1}	CDKN1B at 12p13	KIP1
	p57^{Kip2}	CDKN1C at 11p15.5	KIP2
INK4 family	p16^{INK4A}	CDKN2A at 9p21	p16(INK4A), CDK4 inhibitor, CDKN2
	p15^{INK4B}	CDKN2B at 9p21	p15(INK4B), CDK4B inhibitor
	p18^{INK4C}	CDKN2C at 1p32	p18(INK4C)
	p19^{INK4D}	CDKN2D at 19p13	P19(INK4D)

on the basis of the amino acid sequence of the region corresponding to the conserved PSTAIRE motif of cdc2), gene map locus 9q34.1; encodes a serine-threonine kinase which associates with **cyclin T1** to form transcription elongation factor, P-TEFb, an essential cofactor for the human immunodeficiency virus (HIV-1) transactivator, Tat; a target for flavopiridol and related anticancer drugs

CDKI   cyclin-dependent kinase inhibitor

CDKN1   *see CDKN1A*

CDKN1A   a gene, $\underline{C}$yclin-$\underline{D}$ependent $\underline{Ki}$nase $\underline{I}$nhibitor $\underline{1A}$, also known as $\underline{W}$ildtype p53-$\underline{A}$ctivated $\underline{F}$ragment $\underline{1}$—*WAF1*, $\underline{C}$dk-$\underline{I}$nteracting $\underline{P}$rotein 1—*CIP*, *CDKN1* and p21 (*see* Table 5); gene map locus 6p21.2; encodes a potent, tight-binding inhibitor of CDKs, p21^{Cip1/Waf1}; mediates a **p53**-induced G2 arrest in the **cell cycle** in response to DNA damage; expression in small cell lung cancer predicts a favourable outcome

CDKN1B   a gene, $\underline{C}$yclin-$\underline{D}$ependent $\underline{Ki}$nase $\underline{I}$nhibitor $\underline{1B}$, also known as *KIP1* and p27; gene map locus 12p13; encodes a CDK inhibitor, p27^{Kip1}, which regulates the G1/S transition of the **cell cycle** (*see* Table 5); expressed at high levels in quiescent cells, levels decline on mitogen induction; a major transcriptional target of AFX and other *forkhead* proteins; low levels of p27 protein have been linked with poor prognosis in gastric lymphoma

CDKN1C   a gene, $\underline{C}$yclin-$\underline{D}$ependent $\underline{Ki}$nase $\underline{I}$nhibitor $\underline{1C}$, also known as *KIP2*

and p57 (*see* Table 5); gene map locus 11p15.5, encodes p57^{Kip2}, an inhibitor of several cyclin G/CDK complexes; down-regulation of the gene is necessary for cells to enter **cell cycle**; the locus is genomically imprinted—the paternally inherited allele is transcriptionally repressed and methylated; mutations in this gene lead to Beckwith–Wiedemann syndrome, a familial disorder characterized by neonatal hypoglycaemia and subsequent mental retardation, macroglossia and other organomegaly, endocrine disorders and a propensity to rhabdomyosarcoma and hepatoblastoma

CDKN2   *see CDKN2A*

CDKN2A   a gene, $\underline{C}$yclin-$\underline{D}$ependent $\underline{Ki}$nase $\underline{I}$nhibitor $\underline{2A}$, also known as p14(ARF), p16(INK4A), CDK4 inhibitor, *CDKN2* and $\underline{M}$ultiple $\underline{T}$umour $\underline{S}$uppressor $\underline{1}$—*MTS1* (*see* Table 5); gene map locus 9p21, a candidate tumour suppressor gene; this locus gives rise to 2 transcripts from different promoters encoding p16^{INK4a} and p14^{ARF} (*see* **ARF**), each with a unique 5′ exon; the p16 protein binds to **CDK4**, inhibits its interaction with **cyclin D** and promotes passage through the G1 phase of the **cell cycle**; *CDKN2A* often undergoes homozygous deletion, together with deletion of *CDKN2B*, in B-lineage (15%) and, even more frequently, T-lineage (80%) acute lymphoblastic leukaemia; homozygous deletion is also common in lymphoid blast crisis of chronic granulocytic leukaemia and is associated with transformation of a low grade to a high grade lymphoma; hemizygous and homozygous deletions are common in mantle cell lymphoma; germline mutations at this locus (e.g. p16^Leiden) are seen in familial atypical multiple mole–melanoma syndrome, and in kindreds with familial melanoma and pancreatic cancer or neural tumours; together with *CDKN2B*. This gene is repressed by hypermethylation in a variety of haematological and solid tumours, the biological significance of this being unclear as hypermethylation is seen in some normal somatic tissues

CDKN2B a gene, Cyclin-Dependent Kinase inhibitor 2B, also known as p15(INK4B) and Multiple Tumour Suppressor 2—*MTS2* (*see* Table 5); gene map locus 9p21, a candidate tumour suppressor gene; encodes p15^INK4B, a protein that inhibits cyclin-CDK4 and cyclin CDK6 complexes and thus negatively regulates cell proliferation; often undergoes homozygous deletion, together with deletion of *CDKN2A*, in B-lineage and, even more frequently, T-lineage acute lymphoblastic leukaemia; homozygous deletion of both genes is also common in lymphoid blast crisis of chronic granulocytic leukaemia; occasionally deleted in multiple myeloma; together with *CDKN2A* this gene is repressed by hypermethylation in a variety of haematological and solid tumours, the biological significance of this being unclear as hypermethylation is seen in some normal somatic tissues

CDKN2C a gene, Cyclin-Dependent Kinase inhibitor 2C, also known p18(*INK4C*) (*see* Table 5); gene map locus 1p32; encodes p18^INK4C, a cyclin-dependent kinase inhibitor most abundant in skeletal muscle but present in other tissues; inhibits CDK6; homozygous deletion of this gene occurs in multiple myeloma but generally alterations of this gene in cancer are rare

CDKN2D a gene, Cyclin-Dependent Kinase inhibitor 2D, also known p19(*INK4D*) (*see* Table 5); gene map locus 19p13; encodes p19^INK4D, an inhibitor of **CDK4** and **CDK6**; alterations of this gene in cancer are rare

cDNA complementary DNA

CDX2 a gene, Caudal-type homeobox transcription factor 2, also known as *CDX3* and insulin-regulating transcription factor; gene map locus 13q12.3, encodes a homeobox transcription factor similar to the *Drosophila* gene, *caudal*; normally expressed in human jejunal, ileal and colonic mucosa, but not in gastric mucosa; expression in the stomach has been linked to intestinal metaplasia in atrophic gastritis; contributed to an *ETV6-CDX2* fusion gene in acute myeloid leukaemia associated with t(12;13)(p13;q12); also mutated in some cases of colorectal cancer

C/EBPε a gene at 14q11.2, CCAAT/Enhancer-Binding Protein gene ε, encoding **CCAAT/enhancer-binding protein**; homozygosity for mutations of the gene lead to **neutrophil specific granule protein deficiency**; up-regulated by the CBFα2–ETO fusion protein in AML with t(8;21)(q22;q22)

cell the basic unit of every living organism, whether a unicellular micro-organism or a complex multicellular organism such as man

cell cycle the progress of the cell though four phases of growth (G1), synthesis of DNA (S), further growth (G2) and mitosis (M); cells that are not in cycle are described as being in G0 (Fig. 15)

cell-mediated immunity immunity mediated by **T lymphocytes** and **natural killer cells**

cellular haemoglobin concentration mean (CHCM) an estimation of the concentration of haemoglobin in individual erythrocytes derived from determination of the optical characteristics of individual cells in an automated blood cell counter

centiMorgan (cM) the unit of genetic distance, the distance separating two **loci** that have 1% chance of recombination

central nervous system (CNS) the brain and the spinal cord

central retinal vein occlusion occlusion of the central vein of the retina, may result from **hyperviscosity** in multiple myeloma or other plasma cell dyscrasia, or from **hyperhomocysteinuria, factor V**

Figure 15   The cell cycle.
The phases of the cell cycle: G1 and G2 are phases of cell growth, G1 being to the 'Gap' before DNA synthesis and G2 being the 'Gap' before mitosis, S represents synthesis of DNA and M represents mitosis; cells in G0 are non-cycling.

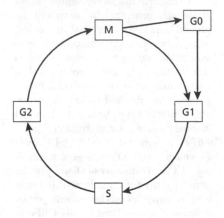

Leiden, the G20210A mutation in the *F2* (prothrombin) gene, **protein C deficiency, protein S deficiency** or **antithrombin deficiency** or the presence of a **lupus anticoagulant**

centroblast   a large, nucleolated follicle centre B lymphocyte (*see* Fig. 13, p. 30)

centroblastic/centrocytic lymphoma an alternative designation (in the **Kiel classification** and **the REAL classification**) of follicular lymphoma of the **WHO classification**; lymphoma cells resemble normal centrocytes and centroblasts

centroblastic lymphoma   a large cell lymphoma of B lineage with cells resembling normal centroblasts; a subtype of diffuse large B-cell lymphoma in the **WHO classification**

centrocyte   a small follicle centre B lymphocyte (*see* Fig. 13, p. 30)

centrocytic lymphoma   a somewhat ambiguous term including lymphomas with cells analogous to normal follicle centre cells but also sometimes used to refer to **mantle cell lymphoma** (designated 'diffuse centrocytic lymphoma' in the **Kiel classification**)

centromere   the constricted region of a nuclear **chromosome**, to which the spindle fibres attach during division; the junction of the long and short arms of a chromosome (*see* Fig. 9, p. 22)

centromeric   pertaining to the **centromere**

centromeric probe   a complementary oligonucleotide sequence capable of binding to the centromere of a specific chromosome

CEP1   a gene, **C**entrosomal **P**rotein **1**, also designated *FAN* and **C**entrosome-associated **P**rotein **110**—*CEP110*; gene map locus 9q33; encodes centrosome-associated protein 110; contributes to the *CEP100-FDGFR1* gene in the myeloproliferative disorder associated with t(8;9)(p12;q33) (*see* **8p11 syndrome**)

CEP110   *see CEP1*

cerebrospinal fluid (CSF)   the clear fluid surrounding the brain and spinal cord

CGD   **chronic granulomatous disease**

CGH   **comparative genomic hybridization**

CHAD   **chronic cold haemagglutinin disease**

Chagas' disease   a parasitic disease prevalent in South America, consequent on infection by *Trypanosoma cruzi*

Charcot–Leyden crystals   crystals in the shape of two elongated pyramids, in tissue section and bone marrow smears appearing like elongated diamonds, formed by crystallization of the granule contents of **eosinophils,** seen in tissues in reactive eosinophilia and eosinophilic leukaemia

CHCM   **cellular haemoglobin concentration mean**

Chédiak–Higashi syndrome   a serious, **autosomal recessive** condition characterized by giant lysosomes in various cells leading to large abnormally staining granules in granulocytes, monocytes and lymphocytes; other features include partial albinism, platelet dysfunction, recurrent infections and infection-triggered **haemophagocytosis**; it results from mutation in the *CHS1* gene (also known as *LYST*—**Lys**osomal **T**rafficking regulator gene)

cheilosis   scaling and fissuring of the lips (*see* **angular cheilosis**)

chemokine   a group of at least 46 small secreted polypeptides (8-14 kD) assigned to one of four chemokine families on the basis of the arrangement of the first two

Figure 16   Chromatin structure and physiology.
The DNA in the nucleus is packaged into a nucleoprotein structure called chromatin. The basic unit of chromatin is the nucleosome, which consists of 146bp of DNA wrapped around a core made of two copies of each of four histone proteins H2A, H2B, H3 and H4. The chromatin in untranscribed regions of the genome is densely packed (heterochromatin); that in transcriptionally active regions is more accessible (euchromatin). Every cell type has a pattern of chromatin packing that is unique to its spectrum of gene expression, and which is maintained after cell division. Chromatin must be decompacted in order for the transcriptional machinery to access genes and for transcription to occur. This reversible process is achieved by coregulator proteins, which either reposition nucleosomes to allow transcription factors access to promoter regions (nucleosome remodelling complexes, **NRCs**), or covalently modify histone proteins. Covalent modification includes acetylation and deacetylation, catalysed by histone acetylases (**HATs**) and histone deacetylases (**HDACs**) respectively; and arginine and lysine methylation, catalysed by histone arginine methyltransferases (**H-AMTs**) and histone lysine methyltransferases (**H-LMTs**). Histone acetylation and arginine methylation are associated with activation of transcription; deacetylation is associated with repression of transcription; lysine methylation can be associated with either activation or repression. It is not known whether methylation is reversible. The MOZ protein is an example of a histone acetylase; TEL and the TEL-AML1 fusion proteins can recruit histone deacetylases.

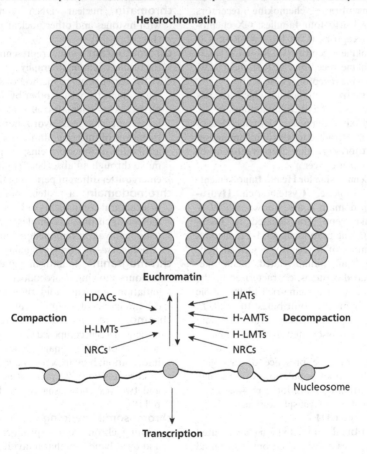

aminoterminal cysteine residues: CXC or α chemokines (CXCL1–CXCL16) which have two cysteines separated by another amino acid; CC or β chemokines (CCL1–CCL28) which have two adjoining cysteines; C (XCL1) and CX3C, which has cysteines separated by three amino acids (CX3CL1); the various chemokines bind chemokine receptors, thus mediating intravascular adhesion of leukocytes and migration of leucocytes into and within the intravascular space; they also influence angiogenesis

chemokine receptor   a group of seven transmembrane chemokine receptors grouped into four families: CX chemokine receptors (CXCR1–CXCR6); CC chemokine receptors (CCR1–CCR11), C chemokine receptor (XCR1) and CX3C chemokine receptor (CX3CR1)

chemotaxin   a molecule which attracts leucocytes to the site of inflammation

chemotaxis   the process by which leucocytes are attracted to sites of inflammation

chemotherapy   the drug treatment of infection or cancer

CHI   **Commission for Health Improvement**

CHIC2   a gene, **C**ysteine-rich **H**ydrophob**ic** domain **2**, also known as *BTL*—**B**rx-like gene **T**ranslocated in **L**eukaemia, gene map locus 4q11-12; encodes a member of a recently described family of small, palmitoylated, membrane-associated proteins, characterized by the presence of a cysteine-rich hydrophobic (CHIC) motif; contributes to a *BTL/CHIC2-ETV6* fusion gene in acute myeloid leukaemia associated with t(4;12)(q11-12;p13)

chimaerism   the presence of two genetically distinct populations of cells; may result from constitutional mosaicism or follow **stem cell transplantation**

CHIMP   *see* **CHI**

chlorambucil   an **alkylating agent** used in the treatment of chronic lymphoid leukaemias and low grade lymphomas

chloroacetate esterase   *see* **naphthol AS-D chloroacetate esterase**

chloroma   *see* **granulocytic sarcoma**

CHOP   a chemotherapeutic regimen commonly used in the treatment of high grade lymphoma comprising **C**yclophosphamide, **H**ydroxydaunorubicin (doxorubicin), vincristine ('**O**ncovin') and **P**rednisolone

Christmas disease   a haemorrhagic disorder resulting from **factor IX** deficiency, named after the first diagnosed patient (*see* **haemophilia B**)

chromatid   one of the two side by side replicas produced by chromosome replication in either **mitosis** or **meiosis** (*see* Fig. 9, p. 22); during the processes of mitosis and meiosis the two chromatids separate from each other and move to daughter cells

chromatin   nuclear DNA complexed with histones and other nuclear proteins (Fig. 16, p. 73)

chromatogram   visual representation of the results of **chromatography**

chromatography   a method of separating proteins from each other by means of physical characteristics, such as molecular weight, charge or hydrophobicity, or by means of differing affinity for lectins, antibodies or other proteins; the proteins move through an absorbent column and emerge after different periods of time

chromodomain   a protein motif found in structural components of large macromolecular chromatin complexes and proteins involved in remodelling chromatin structure (*see also* **bromodomain**)

chromogranin   an antigen expressed by tumours showing neuroendocrine differentiation, e.g. carcinoid tumour, small cell carcinoma of the lung, neuroblastoma

chromosome   a linear structure in the nucleus of a cell, composed of a long paired strands of DNA that carries genetic information; human beings have 23 pairs of chromosomes, 22 pairs of **autosomes** and two **sex chromosomes** (*see* Fig. 31, p. 110)

chromosome banding   a process of staining chromosomes, producing light and dark bands, so that individual chromosomes can be recognized (*see* **Q banding**, **G-banding** and Fig. 31, p. 110)

chromosome painting   a technique for identifying part or all of individual chromosomes by the use of a combination of probes that bind with a high level of specificity to all or part of a single pair of chromosomes

chronic developing over a period of time and progressing slowly

chronic cold haemagglutinin disease (CHAD) a chronic disease characterized by cold-induced peripheral vascular obstruction and haemolytic anaemia, consequent on production of a **cold agglutinin** by a clone of neoplastic B lymphocytes

chronic eosinophilic leukaemia a chronic leukaemia with predominantly eosinophilic differentiation

chronic granulocytic leukaemia a specific type of chronic myeloid leukaemia characterized by the presence of t(9;22) which leads to formation of the Philadelphia chromosome (22q–) (*see* Fig. 31, p. 110); often known as '**chronic myeloid leukaemia**'

chronic granulomatous disease an inherited defect in neutrophil function resulting from mutation in one of the four genes encoding phagocyte adenine dinucleotide phosphate (NADPH) oxidase subunits; complete absence or malfunction of NADPH oxidase leads to the lack of a respiratory burst and consequent defective killing of bacteria by neutrophils; genes implicated are *CYBB* (**sex-linked recessive** inheritance) and *CYBA*, *NCF1* and *NCF2* (**autosomal recessive** inheritance)

chronic leukaemia a type of leukaemia in which there is differentiation of leukaemic cells to mature cells and which causes death in months or years rather than in weeks

chronic lymphocytic leukaemia (CLL) a chronic lymphoid leukaemia of B lineage with characteristic cytological, histological, immunophenotypic and cytogenetic features

chronic lymphoid leukaemias a generic term for chronic leukaemias of B, T or NK lineage

chronic myelogenous leukaemia a synonym for **chronic granulocytic leukaemia** or **chronic myeloid leukaemia**

chronic myeloid leukaemia (CML) (i) an alternative designation of chronic granulocytic leukaemia (ii) a generic term for all chronic leukaemias of myeloid lineage

chronic myelomonocytic leukaemia (CMML) a chronic leukaemia with monocytic and usually also granulocytic differentiation, in the **FAB** classification one of the **myelodysplastic syndromes** and in the **WHO classification** one of the **myeloproliferative–myelodysplastic disorders**

chronic neutrophilic leukaemia a chronic leukaemia with predominantly neutrophilic differentiation

chronic obstructive airways disease (COAD) chronic bronchitis and emphysema, may lead to chronic **hypoxia** and **secondary polycythaemia**

chronic obstructive pulmonary disease (COPD) a synonym for **chronic obstructive airways disease**

CHS1 the gene, gene map locus 1q42.1-q42.2, also known as *LYST*, encoding a lysosomal trafficking regulator, mutations of which can lead to Chédiak–Higashi syndrome

Churg–Strauss syndrome a variant of polyarteritis nodosa characterized by eosinophilia and pulmonary infiltration

CIP1 *see CDKN1A*

cirrhosis chronic liver disease characterized by nodularity and scarring

cis on the same chromosome

cis-acting a DNA sequence that affects the expression of a gene on the same chromosome but not on the **homologous** chromosome

cisplatin an anti-cancer drug, used particularly in treating germ cell tumours

citrate a salt of citric acid, used as a calcium-binding anticoagulant for blood specimens for coagulation tests

cladribine a nucleoside analogue used in treating **hairy cell leukaemia**

class switching a process occurring in germinal centres in which B lymphocytes switch from expressing IgM/IgD to expressing IgG, IgA or IgE

clear cell carcinoma a carcinoma in which stained cells appear to have empty cytoplasm, often originating in the kidney

clinical governance a process through which NHS organizations are accountable for improving the quality of service, safeguarding high standards and creating an environment in which excellence in clinical care will flourish (UK)

clonal   pertaining to a **clone**

clonal selection   the process by which germinal centre B cells that have been exposed to antigen are rescued from apoptosis and thus selected for survival and proliferation if they produce antibody with a high affinity for the relevant antigen

clone   a population of cells derived from a single cell

cloning   production of a clone from a single cell; popularly indicates production of a new individual from a single cell

CLTC   a gene, **Cl**athrin, heavy polypeptide, gene map locus 17q23; one of two closely related genes encoding clathrin heavy chain, which is thought to contribute to a *CLTC-ALK* fusion gene, probably associated with t(2;17)(p23;q23), in a minority of patients with anaplastic large cell lymphoma

CLTCL   a gene, **Cl**athrin, heavy polypeptide-like 1 also known as clathrin, heavy polypeptide D, *CLTD* and *CLH22*; gene map locus 22q11.2; encodes a ubiquitously expressed protein very similar to *CLTC*, alternative transcripts have been identified in several tissues, but the significance of this is unclear; was thought to have contributed to a *CLTCL-ALK* fusion gene in anaplastic large cell lymphoma with a presumptive t(2;22)(p23;q11); in fact, this is now thought to have been a *CLTC-ALK* fusion gene, probably associated with t(2;17)(p23;q23); this usually ubiquitously expressed gene is not expressed in the majority of meningiomas

cM   a centiMorgan

CMV   **cytomegalovirus**

COAD   **chronic obstructive airways disease**

coagulation   blood clotting

coagulation cascade   a concept of how coagulation factors interact to cause blood clotting; each coagulation factor is conceived as initiating activation of another coagulation factor lower down the 'coagulation cascade' with amplification of the process at each step; the concept of the coagulation cascade is based on how

the coagulation factors appear to interact *in vitro* (Fig. 17)

coagulation factor   one of the plasma proteins required for clotting of blood, either *in vitro* or *in vivo*

coagulation network   a concept of how coagulation factors interact to cause blood clotting *in vivo* (Fig. 18, p. 78)

cobalamin   the common chemical structure of different forms of vitamin B_{12}, e.g. **hydroxocobalamin**, **cyanocobalamin**

coccidioidomycosis   a disease resulting from infection by the fungus *Coccidioides immitis*

codon   a triplet of nucleotides, in DNA or RNA, which codes for a specific amino acid or serves as a **termination signal**; there are 61 codons encoding 20 amino acids and 3 codons which act as termination or stop codons

coeliac disease   a disease resulting from hypersensitivity to the wheat protein, gluten, leading to chronic malabsorption and **splenic atropy**; may cause deficiency of **vitamin B_{12}**, **folic acid** or **iron** or haemorrhage as a result of **vitamin K** deficiency

cohesive   a growth pattern in which cells form a compact masses

cohort   a subgroup of individuals selected for study, born or recruited at the same time and followed up longitudinally

coiled coil   a protein motif characterized by an apolar residue occurring every seventh base; functions as a protein subunit oligomerization site

coincidence   occurring at the same time, e.g. when two cells pass through a counting chamber of a flow cytometer simultaneously

coincidence correction   correction of a cell count for **coincidence**

cold agglutinin   an agglutinating antibody with maximum activity at low temperatures

cold agglutinin disease (CHAD)   cold-induced haemolytic anaemia and vascular obstruction caused by the presence of a **cold agglutinin**

collagen   a fibrillar protein, synthesized by fibroblasts, which is apparent as eosinophilic fibres on a haematoxylin and eosin-stained tissue section

Figure 17   The coagulation cascade.

The coagulation cascade is the sequential *in vitro* activation of coagulation factors following interaction with a foreign surface. Factors XII, XI, IX, X and II are intrinsic pathways factors which are converted to serine proteases and act on subsequent factors in the cascade; factors VIII and V are cofactors; the extrinsic pathway is activated by the interaction of factor VII and tissue factor. The activated partial thromboplastin time tests the intrinsic pathway; coagulation is initiated by contact with particulate matter such as kaolin and a 'partial thromboplastin' (such as cephalin) acts as a substitute for platelet phospholipid (Phl). The prothrombin time tests the extrinsic pathway, coagulation being initiated by addition of a 'complete thromboplastin', which acts as a substitute for tissue factor. The thrombin time, in which thrombin is added to plasma, tests the final step of the common pathway, the conversion of fibrinogen to fibrin.

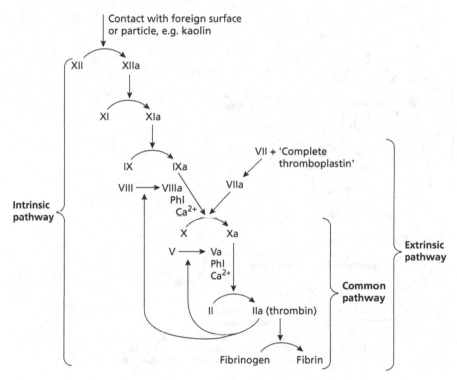

colloid   a suspension of fine insoluble particles; colloids for transfusion include human albumin or plasma protein fraction and various synthetic plasma substitutes

colony   a group of cells derived from a single cell when **progenitor cells** are cultured *in vitro*

colony-forming unit (CFU)   a **progenitor cell** which can give rise to a colony of cells on *in vitro* culture, e.g. CFU-E, CFU-G (*see* Fig. 41, p. 122), or when injected into an experimental animal

colony-forming unit-erythroid (CFU-E)   an erythroid **progenitor cell** that can give rise to a colony of erythroid cells when cultured *in vitro* (*see* Fig. 41, p. 122)

colony-forming unit-granulocyte (CFU-G)   a **progenitor cell** that can give rise to a colony of cells of granulocyte lineage when cultured *in vitro* (*see* Fig. 41, p. 122)

colony-forming unit-granulocyte/ macrophage (CFU-GM)   a **progenitor cell** that can give rise to a mixed colony of cells of both granulocyte and monocyte lineages when cultured *in vitro* (*see* Fig. 41, p. 122)

colony-forming unit-Mega (CFU-Mega)   a megakaryocyte progenitor that can give

Figure 18   The coagulation network.
A concept of how coagulation factors interact *in vivo*. The interaction of factor VII
and tissue factor leads to activation of both the extrinsic and intrinsic pathways,
which are more closely related than appears from *in vitro* tests of coagulation;
thrombin (factor IIa) is involved in three positive feedback loops that act on factors
of the intrinsic pathway; the net result is activation of factor XIII and conversion of
fibrinogen to fibrin monomer plus fibrinopeptides A and B; fibrin monomers
spontaneously associate to form fibrin polymer which is then stabilized by factor
XIIIa-mediated cross-linking between monomers.

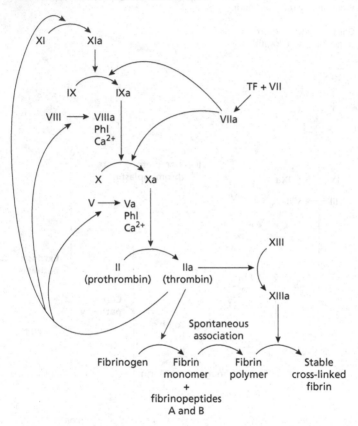

rise to a colony of cells of megakaryocyte
lineage when cultured *in vitro* (*see* Fig. 41,
p. 122)

colony-stimulating factor 1 (CSF1)
see **macrophage colony stimulating
factor**

combined esterase   a combined stain
for **chloroacetate esterase** and **non-specific
esterase**

**Commission for Health Improvement
(CHI or CHIMP)**   a public body (UK),
established with the aim of monitoring

and improving the quality of patient care
in England and Wales

**common acute lymphoblastic leuk-
aemia**   acute lymphoblastic lenkaemia
with expression of the common ALL
antigen, **CD10** (and, according to the
EGIL classification, without expression
of cytoplasmic μ chain)

**common lymphoid–myeloid progeni-
tor**   a stem cell capable of giving rise to
all lymphoid and myeloid cells, see also
pluripotent stem cell

common lymphoid progenitor a stem cell capable of giving rise to all lymphoid cells

common myeloid progenitor a stem cell capable of giving rise to all myeloid cells, see also **multipotent myeloid stem cell**

common pathway that part of the **coagulation cascade** that is common to the **intrinsic pathway** and the **extrinsic pathway**

common variable immunodeficiency genetically heterogeneous, late onset immunoglobulin deficiency; some patients have mutations in the X-linked agammaglobulinaemia gene (*XLA*), the X-linked (*X-HIM*) or autosomal hyperimmunoglobulin M (*HIM*) syndrome genes or the *SH2D1A* gene

compact bone solid bone with only small interstices, as in the cortex of a bone

comparative genomic hybridization (CGH) an *in situ* hybridization technique used in the characterization of unbalanced chromosomal abnormalities in tumour cells; a mixture of normal and test DNA, labelled with two different fluorochromes, is hybridized to normal human metaphase chromosomes, so that under- or over-representation of sequences of DNA can be detected as areas where one or other colour dominates; particularly useful for the analysis of archival and poor quality samples, and in tumours with complex karyotypes

compatible able to exist together, e.g. blood that an be transfused without giving rise to a transfusion reaction

competitive PCR a semi-quantitative PCR technique in which there is co-amplification of an internal control, the competitor, present in graded concentrations together with target gene

complement one or more components of the complement pathway (*see* **complement system**)

complement activation the sequential activation of complement components through the classical, alternate or mannose-binding lectin complement pathways (*see* Figs 19 and 20, pp. 80 and 81)

complementarity-determining region that part of an *IGH*, *IGK*, *IGL* or *TCR* locus that encodes the antigen-binding area of the **immunoglobulin** molecule or **T-cell receptor**

complementary DNA (cDNA) single-stranded DNA synthesized from a mRNA template by means of **reverse transcriptase**

complement fixation the process by which complement components are bound to the Fc part of antibody molecules, the antibody molecules being already either complexed to antigen or aggregated; complement can be fixed by IgM, IgG1, IgG3 and, to a lesser extent, IgG2 antibodies

complement system a group of plasma and cell surface proteins that participate in both innate and adaptive immune responses and act as a bridge between the two; the complement system also amplifies the B-cell response to antigens and helps remove immune complexes from plasma and both immune complexes and apoptotic cells from tissues; when antibodies aggregate or form an immune complex with antigens, there is sequential binding and activation of complement components, leading ultimately to damage or destruction of cells—the classical pathway of complement activation; the alternative and lectin pathways of complement activation are part of the body's innate immune responses, being activated by microbial cells walls and microbial carbohydrates respectively (Figs 19 and 20, pp. 80 and 81)

complete blood count (CBC) of a synonym for **full blood count (FBC)**, the latter being the internationally agreed terminology

complete remission (CR) the disappearance of all clinical and pathological signs of a disease, although minimal residual disease may still be detectable by immunophenotypic or molecular genetic techniques

compound heterozygote a person with two abnormal but different alleles of a given gene, e.g. compound heterozygosity for β^S and β^C, sickle cell/haemoglobin C disease

Figure 19   The classical complement pathway.

In the classical complement pathway the binding of immunoglobulin (IgG$_1$, IgG$_2$, IgG$_3$ or IgM) to antigen leads to binding of the Fc end of immunoglobulin molecules, if in close proximity, to the C1q,C1r,C1s complex with resultant activation of C1s. C1s, in turn, cleaves C4 and C2 with one product of each reaction combining to produce a C4b2a, a C3 convertase. C3 convertase cleaves C3 to C3a and C3b and then combines with C3b to form C4b2a3b, a C5 convertase. C5 convertase cleaves C5 to C5a and C5b. The latter initiates formation of the membrane attack complex by binding to C6, C7 and C8 with the complex then binding C9 and inserting it into the membrane of the cell bearing the antigen with resultant cell lysis. Cleavage products of various complement components have effects on neutrophils, macrophages, mast cells and smooth muscle cells. C3a and C5a are anaphylatoxins, which cause contraction of smooth muscle cells, degranulation of mast cells and increased vascular permeability. C5a is also chemotactic for neutrophils and macrophages. C3b not only contributes to the formation of C5 convertase but also binds to C3b receptor on neutrophils and macrophages, activating these cells.

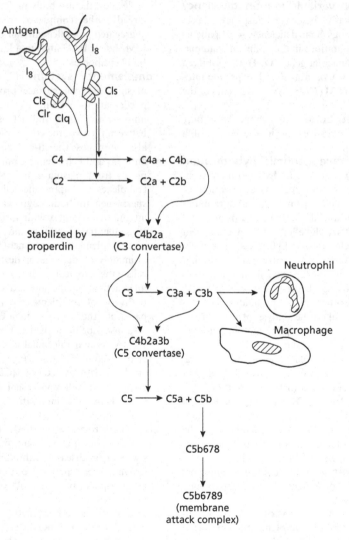

Figure 20 The alternative and mannose-binding lectin complement pathways.
The alternative complement pathway is initiated by the binding of trace amounts of C3b to the cell walls of
Gram-negative bacteria or fungi. C3b binds to factor B and factor D then cleaves bound factor B so that C3bBb
is formed. It is stabilized by properdin and acts as a C3 convertase. From this stage the pathway is the same as
the classical pathway (*see* Figure 19). The C3b which is generated can bind to bacterial cell walls thus creating a
positive feedback loop.

The mannose-binding lectin pathway can be activated by some parasites, fungi, viruses and bacteria with
cell walls containing mannose, which bind to mannose-binding lectin (MBL), in the presence of mannose-
binding lectin associated proteases 1 and 2 (MASP1 and MASP2). MASP2 is activated and it cleaves C4 and
C2 to produce a C3 convertase. It is possible that MASP 1 in the complex also has C3 convertase activity. Once
C3 convertase is formed, the pathway is the same as the classical pathway.

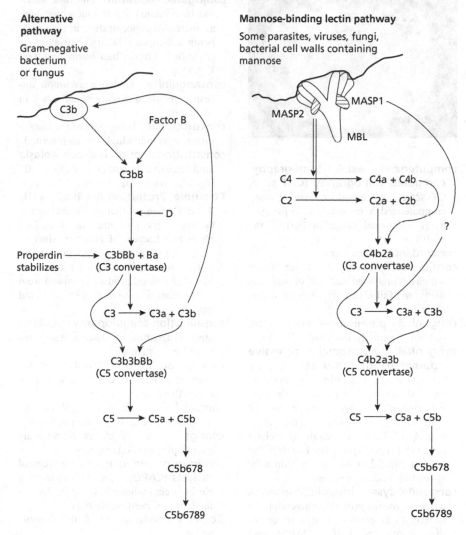

Figure 21   A CT scan of the abdomen.
A computerized axial tomogram (CT scan) of the abdomen showing massive enlargement of the kidneys, resulting from infiltration, in a child with acute lymphoblastic leukaemia.

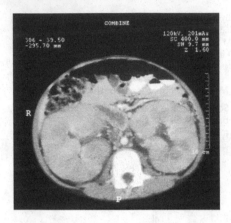

computerized axial tomography, computed tomography (CAT scan, CT scan) a method of imaging using computerized X-ray analysis to produce a cross-sectional image of part of the body (Fig. 21)

concordance agreement

confidence interval the range within which it is predicted that 95% of measurements will fall if repeated measurements are made

congenital present from birth; often, but not necessarily, inherited

congenital autosomal recessive agammaglobulinaemia severely reduced immunoglobulin synthesis and reduced humoral immunity, a genetically heterogeneous syndrome some cases of which result from a mutation of the µ chain gene at 14q32, the surrogate light chain gene (λ5/14) at 22q11.2, the Igα (CD79a) gene at 19q13.2 or the gene encoding the B-cell linker adaptor protein

congenital dyserythropoietic anaemia a heterogeneous group of congenital and inherited dyserythropoietic anaemias, divided into types I, II (**HEMPAS**) and III and various other less well-characterized subtypes

congenital non-spherocytic haemolytic anaemia a generic term used to designate a group of hereditary haemolytic anaemias with no distinguishing morphological features, mainly caused by defects in the **glycolytic pathway**

congenital X-linked agammaglobulinaemia an inherited immune deficiency syndrome resulting from a mutation in the *BTK* (Bruton tyrosine kinase) gene at Xq21.3

conjugated bilirubin bilirubin which has been conjugated to glucuronic acid, an increased concentration in the serum being indicative of biliary obstruction or cholestasis rather than haemolysis (*see* Fig. 11, p. 28)

consanguinity having a common ancestor and thus having some genes in common

constitutional being part of the constitution of an individual, implies inherited

constitutional pure red cell aplasia an alternative designation of Diamond–Blackfan syndrome

Consumer Protection Act 1987 a UK Act of Parliament that means that manufacturers—including manufacturers, suppliers and keepers of blood products—are liable for harm resulting from a defect in the product; it governs all aspects of blood and blood product provision from blood donation to the hospital blood bank

consumption coagulopathy an alternative designation of disseminated intravascular coagulation

contact activation activation of the **intrinsic pathway** of coagulation by contact with a foreign surface

contact factor a factor capable of initiating the intrinsic coagulation pathway

contigs groups of clones representing overlapping genomic regions

continuous ambulatory peritoneal dialysis (CAPD) a method of treating chronic renal failure by inserting dialysis fluid into the peritoneal cavity

Cooley's anaemia *see* β **thalassaemia major**

Coombs' test *see* **antiglobulin test**

COPD chronic obstructive pulmonary disease

cord blood transplantation transplantation of stem cells obtained from

Figure 22 Core binding factor.
The core binding factors (CBFs) comprise a group of heterodimeric transcription factors, some of which play a major role in the regulation of haemopoiesis: the genes encoding them are a common target for mutation in leukaemia. Each is composed of a non-DNA-binding CBFβ chain and a DNA-binding CBFα chain that contains a structural motif known as the *runt* domain. The *runt* domain permits DNA binding to a consensus YGYGGT (Y = C or T) sequence and is also involved in CBFα binding to CBFβ. The interaction of CBFα and CBFβ is thought to increase the DNA binding capacity of the *runt* domain. There are three CBFα-encoding genes in man, *RUNX1* encoding AML1/CBFα2, *RUNX2* encoding AML3/CBFα1 and *RUNX3* encoding AML2/CBFα3. CBFα2 is ubiquitously expressed but is expressed at very high levels in haemopoietic tissues, where it activates several genes and is critical for embryonic haemopoiesis. CBFα1 is expressed only in osteoblasts. The function of CBFα3 is unclear but it is known to activate several haemopoietic genes. Both CBFα2 and CBFα1 are known to interact with TLE family proteins (widely expressed transcriptional repressors) via a conserved motif located outside the *runt* domain. In addition, CBFα2 is known to activate CBP, a histone acetylase, suggesting inhibitory as well as activating functions for these proteins.

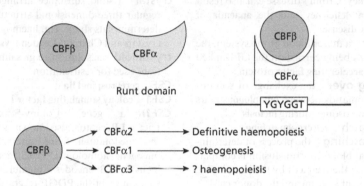

the umbilical cord after the placenta and cord have been separated from the neonate

core binding factor (CBF) a transcription factor complex which is a heterodimer, composed of CBFα (coded for by *AML1* —also known as *CBFA* and *RUNX1*) and CBFβ (encoded for by *CBFB*) (Fig. 22)

coronary artery disease atheroma affecting coronary arteries

coronary occlusion blockage of a coronary artery

coronary thrombosis blockage of a coronary artery by a blood clot, usually deposited on an atheromatous plaque

corpuscle a now little-used term for erythrocytes and leucocytes

correlation the relationship between two series of observations

correlation coefficient a mathematical expression of the closeness of the relationship between two series of figures; a

correlation coefficient of 1.0 indicates perfect correlation

cortex the outer part of an organ, e.g. the cortex of a lymph node, kidney, adrenal gland, bone; the cortex of bone is composed of compact bone, mainly with a lamellar structure

corticosteroids steroid hormones synthesized in the cortex of the adrenal gland, capable of causing **neutrophilia**, **lymphopenia** and **eosinopenia**

cosmid plasmid DNA containing Cos sites that enable it to be packaged into phage particles that can then enter bacteria; DNA sequences complementary to human DNA sequences serve as a probe

coumarin a class of oral anticoagulants, acting as **vitamin K** antagonists, of which warfarin is a commonly used example

CR complete remission

CR1 a gene at 1q32 encoding **CD35**, a complement regulatory protein, the C3b/

C4b receptor. that caries the Knops blood group antigens

C-reactive protein (CRP) an **acute phase reactant** produced by hepatocytes under the influence of **interleukin-6**

CRF an abbreviation for either chronic renal failure or corticotrophin-releasing factor

Crohn's disease an inflammatory disease of the distal small bowel; very extensive disease or, much more often, treatment by bowel resection may cause **vitamin B₁₂ deficiency**; Crohn's disease can also result in **iron deficiency** and the **anaemia of chronic disease**

Cromer a minor blood group system, the antigens being carried on the GPI-linked **decay accelerating factor** protein

crossing over the exchange of sections of chromatids between **homologous** pairs of chromosomes during **meiosis**

crossmatch *see* **crossmatching**

crossmatching the process of determining that blood for transfusion is compatible with the recipient by tests employing the patient's serum and the donor cells

cross-species fluorescence *in situ* hybridization (R$_x$FISH) fluorescence *in situ* hybridization analysis using probes for DNA of another species

CRP **C-reactive protein**

cryofibrinogen a precipitate that develops when plasma is chilled, composed mainly of fibrinogen and fibronectin, but also containing α_1 antitrypsin and α_2 macroglobulin and, in some individuals, polyclonal immunoglobulins

cryofibrinogenaemia the presence of cryofibrinogen in the plasma; in some individuals cryoglobulin is also present

cryoglobulin a protein which precipitates in the cold

cryoglobulinaemia the presence of a cryoglobulin in the circulating blood

cryoprecipitate a blood product that is prepared by freezing plasma rapidly to below –30°C then thawing it slowly overnight at 4°C; the resultant precipitate contains factor VIII, factor XIII and fibrinogen

cryosupernatant the depleted plasma that is removed when cryoprecipitate is prepared; in some circumstances it can be used for plasma exchange

cryptic hidden, as in 'cryptic translocation'

cryptic translocation a translocation that is detectable by molecular techniques but is not detectable by standard chromosome banding techniques, e.g. because of the similarities of the banding patterns of the two chromosomes implicated

cryptococcosis disease resulting from infection by the fungus *Cryptococcosis neoformans*

crystal a solid substance arranged in a regular three-dimensional structure that determines its shape, e.g. haemoglobin C crystals and Charcot–Leyden crystals

crystalloid a solution, e.g. saline solutions used for resuscitation

CSF cerebrospinal fluid

CSF1 colony stimulating factor 1

CSF1R a gene, Colony-Stimulating Factor 1 Receptor, also known as **CD115**, *fms* mcdonough feline sarcoma viral oncogene homologue, *FMS*; gene map locus 5q33.3; encodes a membrane tyrosine kinase of the PDGF receptor family that is the receptor for macrophage colony-stimulating factor; normally expressed by monocytes and macrophages; over-expressed in some types of acute myeloid leukaemia; allelic loss of *c-FMS* has been detected in both acute myeloid leukaemia and myelodysplastic syndromes though its prognostic significance is unclear

CT scan computerized tomography scan

CTIP2 a gene, COUP Transcription Factor Interacting Protein 2, *see* **BCL11B**

Cushing's syndrome a syndrome resulting from secretion of excess corticosteroids by the adrenal gland

cutaneous pertaining to the skin

cutaneous mastocytosis a disease resulting from infiltration of the skin by mast cells without apparent infiltration of other organs; the typical skin lesions are referred to as **urticaria pigmentosa**

cutaneous T-cell lymphoma a T-cell lymphoma of the skin; mainly **mycosis fungoides** or Sézary syndrome

cyanmethaemoglobin the form of haemoglobin produced by the addition of cyanide-containing reagents to blood, permitting accurate measurement of haemoglobin concentration

cyanocobalamin the form of **vitamin B$_{12}$** used for the **Schilling test**

cyanosis blueness of the skin and mucous membranes, can result from desaturation of haemoglobin (increased **deoxyhaemoglobin**) or the occurrence of **methaemoglobinaemia**

cyanotic heart disease congenital heart disease with mixing of venous (unsaturated) and arterial (saturated) blood; leads to **polycythaemia** as a consequence of tissue **hypoxia**

CYBA a gene, gene map locus 16q24, encoding cytochrome b$_{245}$ α polypeptide (p22^{phox}), mutation of which can lead to **chronic granulomatous disease**; the protein encoded is one of two subunits of flavocytochrome b$_{558}$ (the other subunit being gp91^{phox})

CYBB a gene, gene map locus Xp21.2, encoding cytochrome b$_{245}$ β polypeptide (gp91^{phox}), mutation of which can lead to **chronic granulomatous disease**; the protein encoded is one of two subunits of flavocytochrome b$_{558}$ (the other subunit being p22^{phox})

cyclical neutropenia periodically recurring neutropenia, usually with a cycle of 19–21 days

cyclin one of a class of proteins whose concentrations periodically rise and fall in step with the cell cycle; they interact with and activate cyclin-dependent kinases (CDKs) which regulate the transition between stages of the cell cycle; cyclin D1 plus CDK4 phosphorylates **pRB** and releases the transcription factor, E2F, and histone deacetylase, permitting the cell to progress from G1 to S (*see* Fig. 15, p. 72)

Cyclin D1 *see BCL1*; also known as *CCND1*

Cyclin D2 *see CCND2*

Cyclin D3 *see CCND3*

cyclin-dependent kinase (CDK) a group of negative regulators of cell cycling, e.g. CDK4, CDK6

cyclin-dependent kinase inhibitors (CDKI) two families of inhibitors of cyclin-dependent kinases, the Cip/Kip family inhibiting many CDKs and the INK4 family inhibiting specifically CDK4 and CDK6 (*see* Table 5, p. 70)

cyclophosphamide an **alkylating agent** used for immunosuppression and for treatment of lymphoma

cystinosis a metabolic disorder which leads to deposition of cystine crystals in tissues including the bone marrow

cytochemistry staining of cells by exposure to chemicals that react selectively with certain components of certain cells, thus aiding in the determining of cell lineage

cytogenetics the science of the study of chromosomes

cytokine a group of low molecular weight soluble proteins that act as messengers within the immune system and between the immune system and other systems, regulating haemopoiesis and mediating immune and inflammatory responses and wound healing; they include **interleukins, chemokines** and **interferons**

cytomegalovirus (CMV) a herpesvirus, which can cause an infectious mononucleosis-like illness and impaired bone marrow function, the latter mainly in immunosuppressed subjects

cytopenia reduction in the number of cells in the peripheral blood, e.g. **neutropenia, thrombocytopenia, pancytopenia**

cytoplasm that part of a cell which surrounds the nucleus, composed of the **cytosol** and various **organelles** and enclosed by a plasma membrane or cell surface membrane

cytoplasmic pertaining to the **cytoplasm**

cytosine a **pyrimidine** base of DNA and RNA, pairs with guanine

cytosine arabinoside an **antimetabolite** used in the treatment of **acute myeloid leukaemia**

cytoskeleton a protein network within the cytoplasm that gives a cell its shape, composed of **microfilaments, intermediate filaments** and **microtubules**

cytosol the gel-like mixture of water and proteins that, together with the **organelles** which it contains, makes up the cytoplasm of a cell

cytospin a method of preparing a single layer of cells for microscopic examination using a specialized centrifuge

Figure 23   Cytotoxic T-cell function.
The interactions between a cytotoxic T cell and its target. Activation of a cytotoxic T cell requires simultaneous signalling through the T-cell receptor and various other cell surface molecules. The antigen-presenting cell (APC), e.g. a virus infected autologous cell, processes an endogenous antigen to a peptide which is presented in a groove in the surface of an HLA class I molecule. It is recognized by the T-cell receptor–CD8 complex. CD54 (ICAM1) on the APC binds to CD11a/CD18 ($\alpha_2\beta_2$ integrin) on the T cell and CD58 binds to CD2. CD80 and CD86 on the APC are part of the innate immune system and are up-regulated when an APC recognizes a pathogen-associated molecule (e.g. lipopolysaccharide). They bind either to CD28, giving stimulatory signals, or to CD152 (CTLA4), giving inhibitory signals. CD40 binds to its ligand, CD154. Following binding and activation, the cytotoxic T cell inserts perforin into the membrane of the target cell, creating a pore through which granzymes enter, inducing apoptosis.

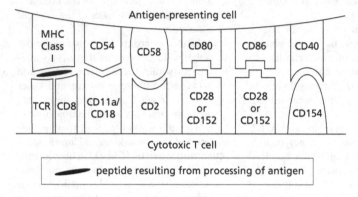

cytotoxic drug   a drug which is toxic to cancer cells (and also to normal cells); the term was initially synonymous with '**alkylating agent**' but is now used in a more general sense

cytotoxic T cell   a T cell that is able to recognize antigens, in an HLA class I context, and kill or damage cells bearing these antigens; cytotoxic T cells are important in defence against viral infections and in allograft rejection (Fig. 23)

D

δ chain (i) the δ globin chain which forms part of **haemoglobin A₂** (ii) the heavy chain of **immunoglobulin D**; two δ chains combine with two light chains (in a single molecule either κ or λ) to form a complete immunoglobulin molecule (ii) part of the γδ **T-cell receptor**, a surface membrane structure in T lymphocytes which permits antigen recognition

Da the abbreviation for **dalton**

dacrocyte a teardrop shaped poikilocyte

dactylitis a painful inflammation of the fingers and toes, may be a caused by bone **infarction** in **sickle cell disease**

DAF a gene at 1q32 which encodes the gly-cosylphosphatidyl inositol (GPI)-linked **decay accelerating factor**; this protein carries the Cromer blood group antigens

dalteparin a **low molecular weight heparin**

dalton (Da) the unit for measuring molecular weight, the weight of a hydro-gen atom

danaparoid a heparinoid with anti-factor Xa activity

dapsone an oxidant drug which often causes haemolysis

daunorubicin an anthracyclin used in the treatment of acute myeloid leukaemia

DBA-44 a monoclonal antibody which gives positive reactions with hairy cells, with cells of most cases of splenic lym-phoma with villous lymphocytes and with a subset of normal B cells

DCC a gene, **D**eleted in **C**olorectal **C**arcinoma also known as **C**olorectal **C**ancer-related chromosome sequence **18**, *CRC18*, and *CRCR1*, gene map locus 18q21.3; a candidate tumour suppressor gene; encodes a protein with sequence similarity to N-CAM (**CD56**); acts as a netrin-1 receptor, and is pro-apoptotic in the absence of this ligand; expression is absent in most metastatic colorectal car-cinomas, but is absent only in a minority of non-metastatic cancers; loss of expres-sion of *DCC* in colorectal carcinoma indi-cates a poor outcome; point mutations have been observed in colonic and oeso-phageal carcinoma; there is reduced ex-pression in about a third of cases of acute leukaemia and chronic granulocytic leuk-aemia, particularly in blast crisis

DDAVP 1-deamino-6-D-arginine vaso-pressin, **desmopressin acetate**

D-dimer a breakdown product of cross-linked **fibrin**; its presence in increased concentration in the plasma is indicative of local or disseminated intravascular coagulation

DDRT-PCR differential display PCR

DDX10 a gene, <u>DEAD</u>/H BO<u>X</u> <u>10</u>, gene map locus 11q22-q23; encodes a widely expressed RNA helicase which contains the evolutionarily conserved Asp-Glu-Ala-Asp (DEAD) box sequence; con-tributes to the *NUP98-DDX10* gene in inv(11)(p15q22) associated with *de novo* and therapy-related acute myeloid leuk-aemia and myelodysplastic syndromes

DEAD box a conserved motif (Asp-Glu-Ala-Asp—DEAD corresponds to the sin-gle letter amino acid code for this) found in ATP-dependent proteins involved in RNA splicing and transport

decompression sickness *see* **caisson disease**

deep vein thrombosis (DVT) forma-tion of a clot within the deep veins of the leg, thigh or pelvis

degenerate oligonucleotide poly-merase chain reaction (DOP-PCR)

a method of amplifying DNA using primers incorporating a short degenerate sequence, used for amplifying sequences non-specifically from sorted chromosomes, in order to develop **whole chromosome paints**

DEK a gene, gene map locus 6q23, encoding a ubiquitously expressed DNA-binding nuclear protein which is a component of the so-called 'exon–exon junction complex'; it contributes to the *DEK-CAN* fusion gene in t(6;9)(q23;q34) associated with acute myeloid leukaemia; the fusion protein localizes to the nucleus and functions as a transcription factor

del a cytogenetic abbreviation indicating a **deletion**

deletion (i) deletion of part of a chromosome, either part of the long arm or part of the short arm (del) (ii) deletion of a DNA sequence with the regions on either side being rejoined

dementia loss of higher cerebral functions, may result from **vitamin B$_{12}$ deficiency**

dendritic cell a specialized cell that presents antigen to B cells

dendritic cell leukaemia an acute leukaemia of cells analogous to normal dendritic cells

de novo arising, apparently spontaneously, without any preceding abnormality

densitometer a laboratory instrument that uses a photoelectric cell to measure differences in light transmission, can be used to measure the concentration of haemoglobin

deoxygenation the loss of oxygen from the blood or from haemoglobin

deoxyhaemoglobin haemoglobin which has given up oxygen to the tissues

deoxyribonucleic acid (DNA) the major constituent of the nucleus; a polynucleotide strand that is able to replicate and which codes for the majority of proteins synthesized by the cell; the DNA molecule is double-stranded, a double helix of two hydrogen-bonded complementary intertwined polynucleotides

der a cytogenetic abbreviation indicating a **derivative chromosome**

derivative chromosome (der) an abnormal chromosome derived from two

or more chromosomes, taking its name from the chromosome that contributes the **centromere**

dermatitis inflammation of the skin

dermatitis herpetiformis a chronic skin disease with blistering, associated with gluten hypersensitivity and the small bowel changes, and associated haematological features, of **coeliac disease**

dermis the deeper part of the skin

desirudin a recombinant form of **hirudin**

desmin an antigen expressed by normal muscle and **rhabdomyosarcoma** cells

desmopressin acetate (DDAVP) 1-deamino-6-D-arginine vasopressin, a vasopressin analogue that increases plasma concentration of **von Willebrand factor** and factor **VIII** and also increases **fibrinolysis**

DF2 an earlier name for the bacterium *Capnocytophaga canimorsus* which is transmitted by dog bites and can cause serious infection in hyposplenic subjects

DH the Department of Health (United Kingdom)

DHFR the gene encoding **dihydrofolate reductase**, amplification or mutation of which can render leukaemic cells resistant to **methotrexate**

diabetes mellitus an acquired inability to control the blood sugar concentration, as a result of inadequate secretion of insulin by the pancreas

Diamond–Blackfan syndrome constitutional **pure red cell aplasia**; some cases, both inherited and apparently sporadic, result from a mutation in the *RPS19* gene

diapedesis the passage of leucocytes through a vessel wall, occurring without damage to the vessel

dic a cytogenetic abbreviation indicating a **dicentric** chromosome

DIC **disseminated intravascular coagulation**

dicentric chromosome (dic) an abnormal chromosome with two **centromeres**

Diego a minor blood group system, antigens being encoded by the *AE1* (*SLC4A1*) gene at 17q21-q22 and expressed on membrane **band 3**

differential count quantification of the different types of leucocyte in the circulating blood, expressed either as percentages or as the absolute count of each cell type

differential display PCR (DDRT-PCR) a technique for the identification of differentially expressed genes using arbitrarily primed **RT-PCR**

differentiation (i) the process of commitment to one lineage rather than another (ii) maturation to cells typical of a certain lineage (iii) a stage in staining a blood film that permits the differentiation of various leucocytes from each other

diffuse evenly spread without any structure; in relation to lymphoma is used to indicate the absence of any follicular structure and also usually indicates that the marrow is heavily infiltrated by lymphoma cells (also referred to as a 'packed marrow' pattern); in relation to chromatin structure indicates an immature cell

dimer a molecule composed of two protein chains, which may be identical (**homodimer**) or dissimilar (**heterodimer**)

2,3-diphosphoglycerate (2,3-DPG) an intermediate in the **glycolytic pathway** that decreases the oxygen affinity of haemoglobin; **2,3-biphosphoglycerate** is now the preferred terminology (*see* Fig. 33, p. 113)

diploid having the normal complement of 46 chromosomes

direct antiglobulin test a test for the detection of immunoglobulin or complement components on the surface of erythrocytes, also referred to as a direct Coombs' test

discordant lymphoma histologically different lymphoma at two anatomical sites, which may be clonally identical

disease-free survival survival without recurrence of a disease *see also* **overall survival, event-free survival**)

disomic having the normal two copies of an **autosome**

disomy the presence of the normal two copies of an autosome

disseminated intravascular coagulation (DIC) widespread deposition of **fibrin** within blood vessels

DKC1 a gene, gene map locus Xq28, mutation of which is responsible for X-linked **dyskeratosis congenita**

DLI **donor lymphocyte infusion** (or donor leucocyte infusion)

dm a cytogenetic abbreviation indicating a **double minute chromosome**

DNA **deoxyribonucleic acid**

DNA ligase an enzyme that can repair breaks in a strand of **DNA**

DNA methylation the attaching of methyl groups to **DNA**, with resultant reduced expression of methylated genes

DNA polymerase an enzyme that catalyses the assembly of **DNA** by adding nucleotides to the growing 3′ end of the molecule

DO a gene on 12p encoding antigens of the Dombrock blood group system

Döhle body a weakly basophilic inclusion within the cytoplasm of a neutrophil composed of ribosomes

domain a discrete region of a protein with a specific structure

dominant inheritance a form of inheritance in which a single copy of a gene causes an evident effect or determines the phenotype, the other allele being **recessive**, *see* **autosomal dominant**

dominant negative effect the effect of a mutation in a gene which permits the gene to interfere with the function of a normal allelic gene

Donath–Landsteiner antibody an antibody, often with anti-**P** specificity, capable of binding to red cells in the cold and causing red cell lysis on rewarming; characteristic of **paroxysmal cold haemoglobinuria**

donor an individual who donates blood or tissue for use by another

donor lymphocyte infusion (DLI) the infusion of donor lymphocytes into a recipient of a haemopoietic stem cell transplant with the aim of recognizing and destroying residual leukaemic cells in the recipient

DOP-PCR **degenerate oligonucleotide polymerase chain reaction**

double blind a description of a **randomized controlled trial** comparing two or more forms of treatment in which neither the patient nor the doctor knows what treatment the patient is receiving until the trial is finished and a code is broken

double helix   the tertiary structure of DNA

double minute chromosome (dm) an abnormal chromosome with two **chromatids** and no **centromere**, i.e. an **acentric** fragment of a chromosome

down regulation a reduction in the number of receptors of a specific type on a cell surface as the result of reduced expression of the relevant gene

Down's syndrome a congenital syndrome of mental retardation with characteristic dysmorphic features as a consequence of trisomy 21 (or of triplication of a specific critical region of chromosome 21); in neonates may cause **polycythaemia** and **transient abnormal myelopoiesis**; in infants and older children is associated with an increased incidence of acute lymphoblastic leukaemia and acute myeloid leukaemia (particularly acute megakaryoblastic leukaemia)

doxorubicin an anthracycline antibiotic used in the treatment of lymphoma and various carcinomas and sarcomas

2,3-DPG   **2,3-diphosphoglycerate**

drumstick a nuclear appendage in females that contains the inactive X chromosome

dry tap jargon for an attempted bone marrow aspiration that yields nothing

dsDNA   **double-stranded DNA**

D^u   *see RHD*

Duffy a system of blood group antigens (**CD234**); Duffy antigens are receptors for *Plasmodium vivax* and for several classes of pro-inflammatory cytokines (*see also FY*)

Duncan's syndrome a **sex-linked recessive** condition in which there is abnormal susceptibility to **Epstein–Barr virus** infection, resulting from mutation of the *SAP* gene at Xq25, now generally known as the **X-linked lymphoproliferative syndrome**

duodenum the most proximal part of the small intestine that connects the stomach to the jejunum, the site of maximal iron absorption

dup a cytogenetic abbreviation indicating a **duplication**

duplication duplication of a gene or DNA sequence encompassing several genes or duplication of a segment of a chromosome, the latter detectable by conventional cytogenetic analysis and designated 'dup'

Dutcher body an intranuclear inclusion in a **plasma cell** caused by invagination of immunoglobulin-containing cytoplasm into the nucleus

DVT   **deep vein thrombosis**

dyscrasia a generic term used to refer to plasma cell and related neoplasms (**plasma cell dyscrasia**) or, more generally, to any disorder of the blood (blood dyscrasia)

dyserythropoiesis morphologically abnormal erythropoiesis

dysfibrinogenaemia presence of a dysfunctional **fibrinogen**, usually an inherited, **autosomal recessive** abnormality resulting from mutation in one of the three fibrinogen genes, *FGA*, *FGB* and *FGC* at 4q28

dysgranulopoiesis morphologically abnormal granulopoiesis

dyskeratosis congenita an inherited syndrome characterized by abnormal skin pigmentation, dystrophic nails, mucosal leukoplakia and **aplastic anaemia**; inheritance may be **X-linked recessive** (the great majority of cases), **autosomal recessive** or **autosomal dominant**; X-linked recessive cases can result from mutation in the *DKC1* gene and autosomal dominant cases from mutation in the *hTR* gene

dysmegakaryopoiesis dysplasia affecting **megakaryocytes** and **platelets**

dysmorphism abnormal development leading to abnormal physical characteristics

dysmyelopoiesis an alternative term for **myelodysplasia**

dysmyelopoietic syndromes an earlier designation of the **myelodysplastic syndromes**

dysplasia morphologically abnormal cells or tissues

E

ε the epsilon gene and epsilon globin chain, the latter being synthesized during early embryonic life and forming part of **haemoglobin Gower 1** and **haemoglobin Gower 2**

ε **(epsilon) aminocaproate** a cytochemical reaction which can be used to identify basophils

E2A a gene, <u>E</u>-box <u>2A</u>, correctly known as <u>T</u>ranscription <u>F</u>actor <u>3</u>, *TCF3*, also known as <u>I</u>mmunoglobulin <u>T</u>ranscription <u>F</u>actor <u>1</u>, *ITF1*, *E12* and *E47*; gene map locus 19p13.3, encodes two **bHLH** proteins, E12 and E47, by differential splicing; these proteins bind a motif in the immunoglobulin gene enhancer and are essential for B-cell development; *E2A* contributes to:
• the *E2A-PBX* fusion gene in B-lineage acute lymphoblastic leukaemia associated with t(1;19)(q23;p13)
• the *E2A-HLF* fusion gene in B-lineage acute lymphoblastic leukaemia associated with t(17;19)(q21-22;p13)
There are at least two types of *E2A-HLF* rearrangements at the molecular level, which result in different fusion proteins, both of which lead to arrested early B-cell development

E2F a gene, adenovirus <u>E2</u> promoter binding transcription <u>F</u>actor 1, gene map locus 20q11.2, encodes a widely expressed DNA-binding protein whose consensus binding sites are found in the promoters of many genes encoding proteins involved in cell proliferation and specifically in DNA synthesis; the archetypal member of a family of related proteins essential for the G1/S phase transition of the cell cycle; E2F proteins complex with unphosphorylated RB1; RB1–E2F com-

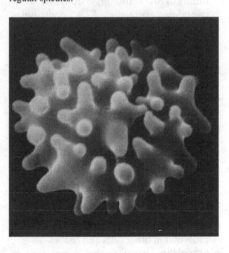

plexes actively repress transcription from promoters with E2F binding sites; deregulation of E2F1 activity is seen in a variety of neoplasms

EAP a gene, <u>E</u>pstein–<u>B</u>arr <u>A</u>ssociated <u>P</u>rotein, correctly known as <u>R</u>ibosomal <u>P</u>rotein <u>L22</u>, *RPL22*; gene map locus 3q26; encodes a ribosomal protein; *EAP* contributes to the *AML1-EAP* fusion gene in acute myeloid leukaemia, the myelodysplastic syndromes and blast crisis of chronic granulocytic leukaemia associated with t(3;21)(q26;q22)

EBV Epstein–Barr virus

ecchymosis a large subcutaneous haemorrhage, a form of **purpura**

echinocyte an erythrocyte the surface of which is covered by a large number of short regular spicules (Fig. 24)

eclampsia   pregnancy-associated hypertension complicated by convulsions, may cause **microangiopathic haemolytic anaemia**

ectasia   dilation, e.g. of a bone marrow **sinusoid**

EDTA   **ethylenediaminetetraacetic acid**

EEN   a gene, Extra Eleven Nineteen leukaemia fusion gene, correctly known as SH3 domain, Grb2-Like, 1, *SH3GL1*; gene map locus; 19p13, encodes a ubiquitously expressed adapter molecule involved in intracellular signalling; a member of a recently described subfamily of Src-homology-3 domain (SH3)-containing proteins; *EEN* contributes to the *MLL-EEN* fusion gene in acute myeloid leukaemia associated with t(11;19)(q23;p13)

EGIL   **European Group for the Immunological Characterization of Leukemias**

ehrlichiosis   disease caused by infection by *Ehrlichia* species

ELA2   gene, gene map locus 19p13.3, encoding **neutrophil elastase**, mutations of which may cause both **severe congenital neutropenia** (some autosomal cases and the majority of sporadic cases) and **cyclical neutropenia** (some autosomal dominant and some sporadic cases)

elastase   an enzyme present in neutrophils and in other cells and tissues

electrolyte   a solute that forms ions in solution and conducts electricity

electron   a negatively charged elementary particle associated with the nucleus of an atom

electronic issue   the issuing of ABO-compatible blood on the basis of a computer programme, identification of suitable units being by bar-code reading, applicable to patients with no atypical antibodies and with two concordant results for ABO and Rh groups, one of which is on a current sample

electron microscopy   the production of an image of a cell by using a beam of electrons, rather than light, to produce a photographic image (*see* **scanning electron microscopy, transmission electron microscopy**)

electrophoresis   separation of charged suspended particles such as proteins or nucleic acids by application to a membrane followed by exposure to a charge gradient, e.g. **serum protein electrophoresis** or **haemoglobin electrophoresis**; the separation of particles is determined mainly by their size and their charge

elephantiasis   non-pitting oedema, particularly of the legs, as a consequence of **filariasis**

ELISA   **enzyme-linked immunosorbent assay**

ELL   a gene, Eleven nineteen Lysine-rich Leukaemia gene, also known as *MEN*; gene map locus 19p13.1, encodes a ubiquitous transcription elongation factor which suppresses transient pauses by RNA polymerase II during transcription; *ELL* contributes to the *MLL-ELL* fusion gene in acute myeloid leukaemia associated with t(11;19)(q23;p13.1)

elliptocyte   an elliptical erythrocyte

elliptocytosis   presence of elliptical erythrocytes

elliptogenic   giving rise to elliptocytosis

eluate   a solution of a substance that is eluted

elution   (i) removal of an absorbed substance from a **chromatography** column (ii) removal of immunoglobulin from the surface membrane of an erythrocyte

EMA   **epithelial membrane antigen**

Embden–Meyerhof pathway   *see* **glycolytic pathway**

embolism   (i) the process of movement of a **thrombus** to another organ or site (ii) movement of a piece of tissue, such as bone marrow or atheromatous material, or extraneous material, such as air, through the bloodstream

embolus   (i) a blood clot that breaks free and is transported by the flowing blood to another organ or site (ii) any solid or cohesive material that moves through the bloodstream, usually causing obstruction of arteries

embryo   the earliest stage of development of the fertilized ovum, from implantation up to about 8 weeks

emesis   vomiting

emetic   causing vomiting

emperipolesis   active entry of haemopoietic cells into the surface-connected canalicular system of megakaryocytes

emphysema a chronic lung disease in which there is destruction of air sacs or alveoli leading to loss of oxygen-exchanging capacity; may lead to chronic **hypoxia** and therefore **secondary polycythaemia**

empirical based on experience without the scientific basis necessarily being understood

endemic constantly present in a community

endocrine secreting a **hormone** that has an effect on distant tissues or organs

endocytosis the process by which the surface membrane of a cell, usually with a specific particle bound to its receptor, is invaginated forming a vesicle containing the particle and some extracellular fluid; **phagocytosis** is a specialized form of endocytosis in which larger particles are engulfed

endogenous coming from within

endonuclease an enzyme that cleaves DNA or RNA within the strands rather than at the ends

endoplasmic reticulum a cytoplasmic organelle composed of a fluid-filled membrane system that is concerned with synthesis and transport of proteins and lipids; composed of the rough and the smooth endoplasmic reticulum

endosteal cells cells lining the inner surface of bone, **osteoblasts** and **osteoclasts**

endosteum the inner lining of bone

endothelial cells cells lining blood and lymphatic vessels

endotoxic shock an acute illness with hypotension mediated by **endotoxin**

endotoxin a toxin contained in the walls of certain bacteria

enhancer a DNA sequence that influences the **promoter** of a nearby gene to increase or decrease the initiation of **transcription**; an enhancer acts on a gene in *cis* and may be sited upstream, downstream or within a gene

ENL a gene, Eleven Nineteen Leukaemia gene also known as Mixed Lineage Leukaemia, Translocated to, 1, *MLLT1*; gene map locus 19p13.3, encodes a nuclear transactivating protein; *ENL* contributes to the *MLL-ENL* fusion gene in acute myeloid leukaemia and acute lymphoblastic leukaemia associated with t(11;19)(q23;p13.3)

enolase an enzyme in the erythrocyte **glycolytic pathway** (*see* Fig. 33, p. 113)

enoxaparin a low molecular weight **heparin**

enzyme a protein produced by living cells that catalyses chemical reactions

enzyme-linked immunosorbent assay (ELISA) a method of quantifying an **antigen** or an **antibody** by means of an enzyme-labelled immunoreactant and a solid-phase support

eosin an orange dye, named for Eos—the goddess of the dawn—used in **Romanowsky stains** of blood or bone marrow films and in **haematoxylin and eosin (H & E) stains** of histological sections

eosinopenia a reduction in the **eosinophil** count

eosinophil a granulocyte with acidophilic granules which stain orange with the acid stain, eosin

eosinophilia an increased **eosinophil** count

eosinophilic (i) showing increased uptake of **eosin** by a cell or tissue component (ii) pertaining to the **eosinophil** lineage

eosinophilic granuloma a form of **Langerhans cell histiocytosis** in which the lesions are infiltrated by eosinophils

eosinophilic leukaemia a leukaemia with prominent eosinophilic differentiation

eotaxin a chemokine (of the CC family), which is produced by eosinophils, some epithelial cells, lymphocytes and macrophages, and is a powerful chemoattractant for eosinophils

EPB41 a gene, gene map locus 1p33-34.2, encoding protein 4.1 of the red cell membrane (*see* Fig. 33, p. 113); mutation may result in **hereditary elliptocytosis**

EPB42 a gene, gene map locus 15q15, encoding **pallidin**, also known as protein 4.2 (*see* Fig. 33, p. 113), a component of the red cell membrane; mutations can result in **hereditary spherocytosis**

epidemic occurring in episodic outbreaks

epidermis the squamous cells forming the most superficial layer of the skin

epidermotropism having a tendency to infiltrate the **epidermis**

epinephrine adrenaline, the main hormone secreted by the adrenal medulla; a platelet **agonist**

epistaxis bleeding from the nose

epithelial cell the surface cell of skin or mucous membrane

epithelial membrane antigen (EMA) an antigen expressed by cells of epithelial origin and by cells of **anaplastic large cell lymphoma**

epithelioid cell an altered **macrophage** with abundant eosinophilic cytoplasm

epithelioid granuloma a cohesive collection of altered macrophages, referred to as **epithelioid cells**, with or without other cells; this term covers all granulomas with the exception of **lipid granulomas**

epithelium the surface covering of the body and of the gastrointestinal, respiratory and genitourinary tracts

epitope an antigenic determinant, part of an antigen which can be specifically recognized by a cell or antibody, e.g. by binding to a receptor on a B or T lymphocyte or by binding to a highly specific monoclonal antibody

EPO **erythropoietin**

EPOR the gene at 7q11-22, encoding the **erythropoietin receptor**, mutated in some types of familial **polycythaemia**

Epstein–Barr virus (EBV) a herpesvirus which causes **infectious mononucleosis** and is also one of the aetiological factors in a number of lymphomas including endemic **Burkitt's lymphoma**

Epstein's syndrome an inherited syndrome of renal failure, sensorineural deafness and thrombocytopenia resulting from a mutation in the non-muscle myosin heavy chain 9 gene (*NMMHC-A* or *MYH9*) at 22q11-13 (or 22q12.3-q13.2); a variant of **Alport's syndrome**

ERBB2 a gene, avian Erythroblastic Leukaemia viral oncogene homologue **2**, also known as **Her**statin (Her2), Neu and **T**yrosine **K**inase-type cell surface **R**eceptor, *TKR1*; gene map locus 17q21.1; encodes an orphan receptor tyrosine kinase of the EGF Receptor Family; amplification of this gene has been reported in a case of myelodysplastic syndrome transforming to acute myeloid leukaemia; expression has been reported in some cases of B-lineage acute lymphoblastic leukaemia; overexpression of *ERBB2* has been reported in prostate cancer and in 25–30% of breast cancer, where it confers Taxol resistance, increasing the aggressiveness of the tumour; however a recombinant monoclonal antibody against ERBB2 (trastuxumab) increases the clinical benefit of first-line chemotherapy in metastatic breast cancer that overexpresses the protein

ERFC **E-rosette forming cell**

ERG a gene, **E**arly **R**esponse **G**ene, also known as *v-ets*, avian erythroblastosis, avian **E**26 oncogene-**R**elated **G**ene, *ERG1* and *ERG2*; gene map locus 21q22.3; encodes an ETS family transcription factor which interacts in *in vitro* assays with SAP18, a transcriptional repressor in haemopoietic cells; *ERG* contributes to the *FUS-ERG* fusion gene in acute myeloid leukaemia associated with t(16;21)(p11;q22)

E-rosette forming cell (ERFC) a T cell, defined by its ability to form rosettes with sheep red blood cells; such cells express **CD2**

erythema redness of the skin or mucous membrane caused by vascular dilation

erythremic myelosis a neoplasm characterized by increased and abnormal erythropoiesis

erythroblast a nucleated red cell precursor

erythroblastic pertaining to **erythroblasts**

erythroblastic island a cluster of erythroblasts surrounding a central macrophage in the bone marrow

erythroblastosis fetalis an alternative designation of **haemolytic disease of the newborn**

erythrocyte a red cell, a non-nucleated peripheral blood cell containing haemoglobin and having oxygen transport as its major function

erythrocyte sedimentation rate (ESR) the rate at which erythrocytes sediment in

Figure 25   Erythropoiesis and granulopoiesis.
A diagrammatic representation of the various stages of erythropoiesis and granulopoiesis.

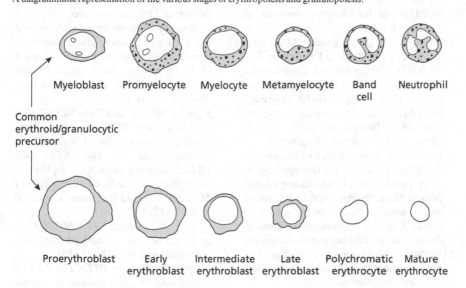

Myeloblast   Promyelocyte   Myelocyte   Metamyelocyte   Band cell   Neutrophil

Common erythroid/granulocytic precursor

Proerythroblast   Early erythroblast   Intermediate erythroblast   Late erythroblast   Polychromatic erythrocyte   Mature erythrocyte

anticoagulated blood; more precisely, the number of millimetres which red cells have sedimented after one hour

erythrocytosis an increased red cell count, haemoglobin and haematocrit; the term is synonymous with 'polycythaemia'

erythroderma an abnormality of the skin associated with redness, not due to simple vasodilation

erythroid pertaining to erythroblasts or erythropoiesis

erythroleukaemia acute myeloid leukaemia with prominent erythroid differentiation; as defined by the **FAB** group, erythroleukaemia or M6 AML is AML with more than 50% of bone marrow nucleated cells being erythroid (*see* Tables 3 and 4, pp. 7 and 8)

erythrophagocytosis phagocytosis of erythrocytes

erythropoiesis the process by which erythroid progenitors gives rise to mature erythrocytes or red cells (Fig. 25)

erythropoietin (EPO) a hormone, secreted mainly by the kidney, which promotes erythropoiesis, available in recombinant form for therapeutic use

erythropoietin receptor a receptor for **erythropoietin**, which is abundant on red cell precursors, encoded by the *EPOR* gene

ESR erythrocyte sedimentation rate

essential primary, having no recognized external cause

essential cryoglobulinaemia cryoglobulinaemia occurring as a manifestation of a **plasma cell neoplasm** which is otherwise occult

essential erythrocytosis polycythaemia for which no cause can be found; many cases represent an early stage of **polycythaemia rubra vera**

essential thrombocythaemia a myeloproliferative disorder with **thrombocytosis** without coexisting **polycythaemia**

ester a chemical compound formed by bonding of an alcohol and one or more organic acids; fats are esters

esterase an enzyme catalysing the hydrolysis of an **ester**

ET essential thrombocythaemia

ethnic origin deriving from a group with a common culture and sharing genetic characteristics

ethylenediaminetetraacetic acid (EDTA) a chelator of bivalent cations which is used, in the form of its sodium or potassium salt, as an anticoagulant for blood samples for a haemoglobin estimation and blood count

ETO a gene, **E**ight **T**wenty **O**ne, also known as **C**ore-**B**inding **F**actor (*see* Fig. 29, p.107), **A**lpha subunit **2**, **T**ranslocated to, **1** (*CBFA2T1*) and **M**yeloid **T**ranslocation **G**ene on **8**q22, *MTG8*; gene map locus 8q22; named for the chromosomes involved in the t(8;21)(q22;q22) translocation in which part of this gene is fused to part of the *AML1* gene to form *AML1-ETO*; homologous to the *Drosophila* gene *nervy*; encodes a non-DNA-binding nuclear protein normally expressed in gut, testes and central nervous system which is involved in the recruitment of histone deacetylases to the transcriptional complex

etoposide an anticancer drug, which is a **topoisomerase-II** interactive agent, used in treating lymphoma

ETS a family of transcription factor regulators related to the product of *v-ets* (**E**26-**T**ransformation **S**pecific), a viral oncogene encoded by the avian erythroblastosis virus; ETS proteins are characterized by a conserved winged helix-turn-helix DNA-binding domain (ETS domain) which binds DNA sequences centred over a core motif (EBS: ETS binding site); a subset of ETS proteins also carry an amino-terminal pointed (PNT) domain which permits interactions with distinct protein partners, thereby establishing unique biological functions within the family; ETS proteins are downstream effectors of RAS-MAPK signalling cascades—most ETS transcription factors are phosphorylated and activated by specific MAP kinases, however some, e.g. **ERG**, are inhibitory; they regulate varied physiological and pathophysiological processes such as haemopoiesis, apoptosis and tumorigenesis

ETV6 a gene, **Et**s **V**ariant gene **6**, homologous with *v-ets*, gene map locus 12p13, also known as *TEL*, encodes a transcription regulator; it belongs to the ETS family and has a pointed (PNT) domain and a 3′ ETS DNA binding domain; *ETV6* is ubiquitously expressed and exhibits context-dependent transcriptional activation and repression functions; it is essential for yolk sac angiogenesis and adult haemopoiesis; *ETV6* has been rearranged in at least 41 different translocations and many of the partner genes have been cloned; involvement of the PNT domain of *ETV6* in these fusion genes permits oligomerization of any resulting chimaeric proteins; *ETV6*:

• contributed to an *ETV6-ARNT* fusion gene in a case of M2 acute myeloid leukaemia associated with t(1;12)(q21;p13)

• contributed to the *ETV6-ARG (ABL2)* fusion gene in t(1;12)(q25;p13), occurring as a second event in a case of M3 acute myeloid leukaemia associated with t(15;17)

• contributed to the *ETV6-MDS1/EVI1* in a case of chronic myeloid leukaemia associated with t(3;12)(q26;p13)

• contributes to a *BTL/CHIC2-ETV6* fusion gene in acute myeloid leukaemia associated with t(4;12)(q11-12;p13)

• contributes to an *ETV6-ACS2* fusion gene in myelodysplastic syndrome and acute myeloid leukaemia associated with t(5;12)(q31;p13)

• contributes to the *ETV6-PDGFRB* fusion gene in chronic myelomonocytic leukaemia with eosinophilia associated with t(5;12)(q33;p13)

• contributed to an *ETV6-STL* fusion gene in a B-lineage acute lymphoblastic leukaemia cell line with t(6;12)(q23;p13)

• contributed to an *ETV6-AF7p15* fusion gene in a patient with acute myeloid leukaemia associated with t(7;12)(p15;p13)

• contributed to an *HLXB9-ETV6* fusion gene in infant acute myeloid leukaemia associated with t(7;12)(q36;p13)

• contributes to the *ETV6-JAK2* fusion gene is rare cases of acute lymphoblastic leukaemia or atypical chronic myeloid leukaemia associated with either t(9;12)(p24;p13) or with a complex chromosomal rearrangement with the same breakpoints

• contributed to an *ETV6-SYK* fusion gene in a patient with a myelodysplastic–myeloproliferative syndrome associated with t(9;12)(q22;p12)

• contributes to the *ETV6-ABL* fusion gene in rare cases of acute lymphoblas-

tic leukaemia, acute myeloid leukaemia and chronic myeloid leukaemia associated with t(9;12)(q34;p13) or a variant translocation
• contributes to an *ETV6-CDX2* fusion gene in acute myeloid leukaemia associated with t(12;13)(p13;q12)
• contributes to an *ETV6-TRKC* fusion gene in acute myeloid leukaemia and in familial fibrosarcoma associated with t(12;15)(p13;q25); the acute myeloid leukaemia and fibrosarcoma mutations differ at a molecular level
• contributes to the *ETV6-AML1* fusion gene in the 30% of cases of acute lymphoblastic leukaemia that are associated with a cryptic t(12;21)(p13;q22); there is generally loss of the normal *ETV6* allele suggesting that loss of *ETV6* function may contribute to oncogenesis
• contributes to the *MN1-ETV6* fusion gene in acute myeloid leukaemia associated with t(12;22)(p13;q11)
• contributed to *PAX5-ETV6* fusion gene in a case of acute lymphoblastic leukaemia

euchromatin diffuse or non-condensed transcriptionally active chromatin

eukaryocyte a cell with a nucleus

European Group for the Immunological Characterization of Leukemias (EGIL) a cooperative group that published guidelines on immunophenotyping

Evans' syndrome autoimmune haemolytic anaemia plus autoimmune thrombocytopenic purpura

event-free survival survival without disease relapse or the need to change to alternative treatment (*see also*, disease-free survival, overall survival)

EVI1 a gene, Ecotropic Viral Integration site 1, gene map locus 3q26; encodes a zinc finger nuclear protein which can repress transcription and recruits histone deacetylases; *EVI1*:
• is 5′ truncated and dysregulated by proximity to the enhancer elements of the ribophorin 1 gene and forms a *GR6-EVI1* fusion gene in acute myeloid leukaemia associated with inv(3)(q21q26) and t(3;3)(q21;q26)

• contributes to the fusion gene, *AML1-MDS1-EVI1*, in acute myeloid leukaemia associated with t(3;21)(q26;q23)
• contributes to the *ETV6-EVI1* fusion gene in acute myeloid leukaemia associated with t(3;12)(q26;p13)
• is involved in the translocations
t(2;3)(p13;q26)
t(2;3)(q23;p26)
t(3;17)(q26;q22)

exfoliative tending to lose layers of cells

exocrine pertaining to secretion of a substance which has an effect outside the tissues of the body, e.g. within the gastrointestinal tract or on the skin

exocytosis the process in which a secretory vesicle produced in the Golgi complex moves to the surface of the cell, fuses with the surface membrane and discharges its contents

exogenous coming from outside

exon a part of a gene which is represented in mature **messenger RNA**; most genes are composed of exons and non-transcribed **introns** (*see* Fig. 32, p. 111)

exonuclease an enzyme that breaks down DNA or RNA from the ends of the strands

extramedullary occurring outside the bone marrow

extramedullary haemopoiesis haemopoiesis occurring outside the bone marrow, usually in the liver and spleen

extramedullary myeloma extramedullary **plasmacytoma**, a plasma cell tumour occurring outside the bone marrow

extrinsic something which originates outside rather than being an essential part; the *extrinsic* pathway of coagulation involves activation of factor VII by tissue factor with subsequent activation of factors X and II and conversion of fibrinogen to fibrin; in contrast to the *intrinsic* pathway, the circulating blood does not contain all the factors necessary for the pathway (*see* Fig. 17, p. 77)

extrinsic pathway inhibitor *see* **tissue factor pathway inhibitor**

ex vivo a process which is detected in cells or tissues that have been removed from the body; the term should be contrasted with *in vivo* and *in vitro*

F

F2 the gene at 11p11-q12 that encodes **prothrombin** (factor II), a coagulation factor in both the intrinsic and extrinsic pathways, mutation of which can lead to **prothrombin deficiency** or **thrombophilia**

F5 the gene at 1q23 that encodes **factor V**, a coagulation factor in both the intrinsic and extrinsic pathways, mutation of which can lead to autosomal recessive **factor V deficiency** or to **factor V Leiden**, associated with **thrombophilia**

F7 the gene at 13q34 that encodes **factor VII**, a coagulation factor of the extrinsic pathway, mutation of which can lead to **factor VII deficiency**

F8C the gene at Xq28 that encodes **factor VIII**, a coagulation factor in the intrinsic pathway, mutation of which can lead to **haemophilia A**; about a third of mutations are new sporadic mutations

F9 the gene at Xq27.1-q27.2 that encodes **factor IX**, a coagulation factor in the intrinsic pathway, mutation of which can lead to **factor IX deficiency**

F10 the gene at 13q34 that encodes **factor X**, a coagulation factor in both the intrinsic and extrinsic pathways, mutation of which can lead to **factor X deficiency**

F11 the gene at 4q35 that encodes **factor XI**, a coagulation factor of the intrinsic pathway; mutations of this gene, which are prevalent among Ashkenazi Jews, can lead to **factor XI deficiency** in both **homozygotes** and **heterozygotes**

F12 the gene at 5q33-qter that encodes factor XII, the first factor of the intrinsic pathway of coagulation, mutation of which can lead to factor XII deficiency

F13A1 the gene at 6p25-p24 that encodes the A subunit of factor XIII

F13B the gene at 1q31-q32.1 that encodes the B subunit of factor XIII

Fab that part of an **immunoglobulin** molecule that is capable of binding to antigens (*see* Fig. 48, p. 139)

FAB pertaining to the **French–American–British** Cooperative Group and their classifications (*see* Table 3, p. 7)

Fabry's disease angiokeratosis corporis diffusum, an inherited disease in which phospholipids are stored in many parts of the body, particularly in blood vessels

FACS fluorescence-activated cell sorter or sorting

factitious false, not genuine, artefactual (of a laboratory test result), sometimes deliberately caused by an individual to simulate illness

factor I (roman numeral) fibrinogen, a plasma protein that is converted to **fibrin** by the action of **thrombin** thus leading to clot formation; the Aα, Bβ and γ chains are encoded respectively by the *FGA*, *FGB* and *FGG* genes; (not to be confused with **factor I** [upper case i] of the complement system)

factor II prothrombin, a **vitamin K**-dependent coagulation factor encoded by the *F2* gene; it is converted to **thrombin** by the action of activated factor X, in the presence of calcium, phospholipid and activated factor V (*see* Fig. 17, p. 77)

factor II: G20210A a variant form of factor II with a point mutation in the 3′ untranslated region, associated with increased plasma concentration of factor II and some increase in risk of thrombosis, present in 1–1.5% of some Caucasian populations

factor IIa activated factor II, **thrombin**

factor V a coagulation factor in the **common pathway** which also contributes to physiological anticoagulation; it is encoded by the *F5* gene; activated factor V, factor Va, is a cofactor in the conversion of **prothrombin** to **thrombin** by **factor Xa**; non-activated factor V is a cofactor with **protein S** in the inactivation of factor Va and factor VIIIa by activated **protein C** (*see* Figs 17 and 56, pp. 77 and 170)

factor Va activated factor V, a cofactor in the conversion of prothrombin to thrombin by factor Xa (*see* Fig. 17, p. 77)

factor V and factor VIII deficiency an inherited, **autosomal recessive**, deficiency of factors V and VIII resulting from a mutation in the *LMAN1* gene

factor V Leiden a variant form of factor V, also known as factor VR^{506}Q and factor VQ^{506}, resulting from a 1691G→A mutation in the *F5* gene; factor V Leiden has a prevalence of 3–15% in different Caucasian populations; the mutation leads to an alteration of protein structure at the point where factor V is cleaved by activated **protein C** and this renders factor V resistant to inactivation by activated protein C and also less effective as a cofactor for the inactivation of factor VIIIa by activated protein C (*see* Fig. 56, p. 170); there is mild **thrombophilia** and probably increased susceptibility to **thrombotic microangiopathy**

factor VII a **vitamin K**-dependent coagulation factor, the first factor in the **extrinsic pathway** of coagulation, which on vascular injury forms a 1:1 **stoichiometric** complex with **tissue factor** exposed on the endothelial cell; complexing of factor VII to tissue factor leads to its activation; activated factor VII initiates the extrinsic pathway of coagulation and also activates factor IX of the **intrinsic pathway** (*see* Fig. 18, p. 78)

factor VIIa activated factor VII, available as a recombinant coagulation factor

factor VIII anti-haemophiliac globulin, a coagulation factor in the **intrinsic pathway** encoded by the *F8C* gene, synthesized in the liver but requires **von Willebrand's factor** (synthesized in megakaryocytes and endothelial cells) for normal stability

in the plasma; it facilitates the activation of **factor X** by activated **factor IX** (*see* Figs 17 and 18, pp. 77 and 78)

factor VIIIa activated factor VIII

factor IX Christmas factor, a **vitamin K**-dependent factor in the **intrinsic pathway** encoded by the *F9* gene (*see* Figs 17 and 18, pp. 77 and 78)

factor IXa activated factor IX

factor X a **vitamin K**-dependent factor in the common coagulation pathway; factor X is activated both by factor VIIa and by factor IXa (in the presence of factor VIIIa in a calcium- and phospholipid-dependent reaction); in turn it activates prothrombin to thrombin, by a calcium- and phospholipid-dependent reaction in the presence of factor Va (*see* Figs 17 and 18, pp. 77 and 78)

factor Xa activated factor X

factor XI a factor in the **intrinsic pathway**, encoded by the *F11* gene; it is activated by **factor XIIa** *in vitro* and by thrombin *in vivo* and in turn it activates factor IX (*see* Figs 17 and 18, pp. 77 and 78)

factor XIa activated factor XI

factor XII Hageman factor, the first factor in the **intrinsic pathway**, encoded by the *F12* gene; after contact activation *in vitro*, it leads to activation of factor XI; deficiency causes marked abnormality of *in vitro* tests of the intrinsic pathway but *in vivo* is not associated with any haemorrhagic disorder (*see* Fig. 17, p. 77)

factor XIIa activated factor XII

factor XIII a factor composed of two A subunits and two B subunits, encoded by *F13A1* and *F13B* respectively that, when activated, causes stable cross-linking of **fibrin** (*see* Fig. 18, p. 78)

factor XIIIa activated factor XIII

factor B a protein in the alternative complement pathway (*see* Fig. 20, p. 81)

factor D a protein in the alternative complement pathway (*see* Fig. 20, p. 81)

factor H an glycoprotein encoded by a gene at 1q32 which inhibits complement activation; factor H competes with **factor B** for C3b and acts as a cofactor for **factor I** in the inactivation of C3b (*see* Fig. 20, p. 81); homozygous deficiency can be associated with familial or sporadic relapsing **haemolytic uraemic syndrome** and membranous glomerulonephritis

factor I (upper case i) an inhibitory protein in the complement system; homozygous deficiency can be associated with **haemolytic uraemic syndrome** and membranous glomerulonephritis

faggot cell a cell containing bundles of Auer rods, a feature of **hypergranular promyelocytic leukaemia** and its hypogranular/microgranular variant

falciparum malaria malaria caused by *Plasmodium falciparum*

false negative a negative result that should have been positive

false positive a positive result that should have been negative

familial occurring in families, by implication inherited

familial cold urticaria an **autosomal dominant** disorder resulting from a mutation in the *CIAS1* gene, resulting in a periodic cold-induced non-pruritic non-urticarial rash associated with neutrophilia

familial haemophagocytic lymphohistiocytosis (FHL) a familial syndrome, probably basically an immune deficiency syndrome, characterized by haemophagocytic syndromes occurring in childhood and often being fatal; two genetic mechanisms have been determined, linked to 10q21-22 in FHL1 and linked to 9q21.3-22 (*PERF1* gene) in FHL2.

familial Mediterranean fever an **autosomal recessive** disease, resulting from mutation in the *MEFV* gene, characterized by periodic fever and serositis

FAN see *CEP110*

FANCA a gene at 16q24.3, mutation of which explains 65–70% of cases of **Fanconi's anaemia**

FANCC a gene at 9q22.3, mutation of which explains 10–15% of cases of **Fanconi's anaemia**

FANCD2 a cloned gene that causes some cases of **Fanconi's anaemia**

FANCE a cloned gene that causes some cases of **Fanconi's anaemia**

FANCF a gene at 11p15, mutation of which explains <2% of cases of **Fanconi's anaemia**

FANCG a gene at 9p13, mutation of which explains about 10% of cases of **Fanconi's anaemia**

Fanconi's anaemia a recessively inherited, clinically and genetically heterogeneous chromosomal fragility syndrome, characterized by multiple congenital abnormalities, **aplastic anaemia** with onset usually in childhood and a predisposition to acute myeloid leukaemia and other tumours

FAS a gene, **T**umour **N**ecrosis **Fac**tor **R**eceptor **S**uper**f**amily, member **6**, *TNFRSF6*, **CD95**, gene map locus 10q24.1, encodes a transmembrane protein belonging to the TNF family that mediates apoptosis when trimerized by cross-linking to **Fas ligand**; *FAS* is mutated in about 10% of cases of multiple myeloma and in about 10% of cases of non-Hodgkin's lymphoma, particularly MALT-type non-Hodgkin's lymphoma and extranodal B-lineage diffuse large cell lymphoma

FBP17 a gene, **F**ormin **B**inding **P**rotein **17**, centromeric to 9q34; encodes a ubiquitously expressed protein which is believed to interact with SNX proteins, involved in EGF receptor trafficking; *FBP17* contributed to a *MLL-FBP17* fusion gene in an infant with M4 acute myeloid leukaemia

Fc the constant part of an immunoglobulin molecule that determines antibody class (G, A, M, E, D) and is responsible for fixation of **complement** and interaction with effector cells such as granulocytes, monocytes, mast cells and killer cells (*see* Fig. 48, p. 139)

Fc receptor a receptor for the Fc part of an **immunoglobulin** molecule (*see* **FcγR**, **FcεR**)

FcεR receptor for the Fc part of the **immunoglobulin E** molecule

FcγR receptor for the Fc part of the **immunoglobulin G** molecule: FcγRI, high affinity receptor on monocytes; FcγRII, lower affinity receptor on neutrophils, monocytes, eosinophils, platelets and B cells; FcγRIII, low affinity receptor on macrophages, neutrophils, eosinophils and NK cells

FCGRIIB a gene, low affinity Fc Gamma Receptor IIB, CD32, gene map locus 1q22; involved in the t(1;22)(q22;q11) rearrangement found in less than 1% of cases of follicular lymphoma and associated with transformation to high grade disease

FDPs fibrin degradation products

Fechtner's syndrome an inherited syndrome characterized by renal failure, sensorineural deafness, thrombocytopenia and neutrophil inclusions that resemble **Döhle bodies**; a variant of **Alport's syndrome** and **Epstein's syndrome** resulting from a mutation in the non-muscle myosin heavy chain 9 gene (*NMMHC-A* or *MYH9*) at 22q11-13 (or 22q12.3-q13.2)

Felty's syndrome hypersplenism causing pancytopenia in a patient with rheumatoid arthritis; there may be an underlying large granular lymphocyte leukaemia

ferric pertaining to trivalent iron (Fe^{3+})

ferritin a complex of iron and a protein, apoferritin; ferritin is present in the cytoplasm of erythroblasts; in macrophages it is converted into haemosiderin, the principal storage form of iron; small amounts are present in the plasma, and measurement of serum 'ferritin' (actually apoferritin) permits assessment of body iron stores

ferrous pertaining to bivalent iron (Fe^{2+}), the form of iron that is incorporated into protoporphyrin IX by ferrochelatase (*see* Fig. 34, p. 116)

ferrous sulphate an iron compound used to treat iron deficiency anaemia

fertilization the fusion of a spermatozoon with an ovum to form a zygote

fetal pertaining to the fetus

fetal haemoglobin haemoglobin F

fetus the unborn offspring after it has attained the particular form of the species, e.g. in man the unborn offspring beyond 8 weeks from fertilization

FFP fresh frozen plasma

FGA a gene at 4q28 encoding the Aα chain of fibrinogen, mutation of which can lead to dysfibrinogenaemia

FGB a gene at 4q28 encoding the Bβ chain of fibrinogen, mutation of which can lead to dysfibrinogenaemia

FGFR1 a gene, Fibroblast Growth Factor Receptor 1, gene map locus 8p11.2-p11.1, encodes a receptor tyrosine kinase; contributes to:
• a *ZNF198-FGFR1* fusion gene in a syndrome of chronic myelomonocytic leukaemia with eosinophilia/T-lineage lymphoblastic lymphoma, sometimes referred to as the **8p11 syndrome** or the stem cell leukaemia–lymphoma syndrome, associated with t(8;13)(p11;q11-12)
• the *FOP-FGFR1* fusion gene in a similar disorder associated with t(6;8)(q27;p11)
• the *CEP110-FGFR1* fusion gene in t(8;9)(p11-12;q33) associated with the same syndrome
• the *BCR-FGFR1* fusion gene in association with chronic myeloid leukaemia and t(8;22)(p11;q11)

FGFR1 was also found to be rearranged in a case of chronic myeloid leukaemia associated with systemic mastocytosis

FGFR3 a gene, Fibroblast Growth Factor Receptor 3, gene map locus 4p16.3; encodes a receptor tyrosine kinase which is dysregulated, by proximity to the *IGH* Cα enhancer on chromosome 14, in t(4;14)(p16.3;q32), a cryptic translocation associated with multiple myeloma

FGG a gene at 4q28 encoding the γ chain of fibrinogen, mutation of which can lead to dysfibrinogenaemia

FHIT a gene, Fragile Histidine Triad gene, also known as AP3A hydrolase, gene map locus 3p14.2; the FRA 3B fragile site; the gene is composed of 10 exons distributed over at least 500 kb, and encodes a widely expressed enzyme involved in the regulation of DNA replication; deletions and structural rearrangements in FRA 3B have been observed in many epithelial malignancies; loss of *FHIT* function is important in the development and/or progression of head and neck squamous cell cancers, and cervical, oesophageal and lung cancers; *FHIT* expression is reduced in a majority of cases of acute lymphoblastic leukaemia and in a significant proportion of cases of chronic myeloid leukaemia, the significance of this being unclear

Figure 26 The fibrinogen molecule.
A diagrammatic representation of the fibrinogen molecule showing the Aα, Bβ and γ chains, the sites of cleavage by thrombin to produce fibrinopeptides A and B (black) and the sites of cleavage by plasmin.

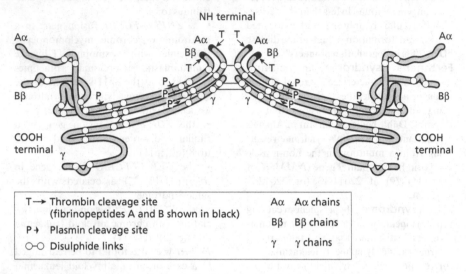

T→	Thrombin cleavage site (fibrinopeptides A and B shown in black)	Aα	Aα chains
P→	Plasmin cleavage site	Bβ	Bβ chains
O—O	Disulphide links	γ	γ chains

FHL familial haemophagocytic lymphohistiocytosis

fibre FISH a **FISH** technique using very elongated genomic DNA

fibrin a fibrillar protein, the formation of which is the basis of blood coagulation; fibrin is formed by polymerization and cross-linking of fibrin monomers, which are produced by the action of **thrombin** on **fibrinogen**

fibrin degradation products (FDPs) breakdown products of **fibrin** which are present in the plasma in increased concentration in the presence of extensive or **disseminated intravascular coagulation** or increased **fibrinolysis**; **D-dimer** is a specific fibrin degradation product

fibrinogen a soluble plasma protein (Fig. 26) that is converted, by the action of thrombin, into fibrin monomers, which polymerize and are cross-linked to form a stable, insoluble fibrin polymer, thus leading to blood clotting: also known as factor I

fibrinolysis the process by which **plasmin** breaks down **fibrin** (Fig. 27)

fibrinolytic pertaining to **fibrinolysis**

fibroblast the cell that is responsible for synthesis and deposition of collagen; small numbers of fibroblasts are present in the bone marrow

fibrosis the replacement of normal tissue, e.g. the bone marrow, by **fibroblasts** and **collagen**; the term 'fibrosis' may also be used to refer to **reticulin** deposition but a distinction should be drawn between reticulin deposition and collagen deposition

filariasis a disease resulting from infection by filarial parasites such as *Loa loa, Wuchereria bancrofti* and *Brugia malayi*

filgrastim recombinant **granulocyte colony-stimulating factor**

FIM a gene, **F**used **I**n **M**yeloproliferative disorders, *see ZNF198*

FISH fluorescence *in situ* hybridization

fixation (i) the process by which cells are killed and tissues and cells are preserved by exposure to chemicals such as ethanol, methanol, acetone or formalin (ii) the process by which **complement** components are bound to immunoglobulin that has already formed a complex with antigen

FKHR a gene, **F**or**k**head bo**x** **O1A**, *FOXO1A*, gene map locus 13q14.1;

Figure 27   The fibrinolytic pathways.

Major pathways are shown by a solid arrow and minor pathways by a dotted arrow. Two lines across an arrow indicate a negative effect, either inhibition or destruction. Dashed crossed lines indicate proteolysis with resultant reduction inactivity of the target protein. Thrombin activation and fibrin deposition lead to activation of fibrinolysis. Fibrin binds plasminogen and plasminogen is converted to plasmin by tissue plasminogen activator (tPA) released from activated endothelial cells. Plasmin breaks down fibrin and the fact that plasmin is formed from plasminogen bound to fibrin means that, normally, fibrinolysis is preferentially focused in the area of fibrin deposition. However if there is excess free plasmin, fibrinogen, factor Va and factor VIIIa can all be degraded. α2 antiplasmin (α$_2$AP) and α2 macroglobulin (α$_2$M) inhibit the action of plasmin, particularly circulating plasmin. Plasminogen activator inhibitors 1 and 2 (PAI1 and PAI2) inhibit the action of tPA, thus reducing fibrinolysis. Thrombin production also leads to activation of protein C which, to some extent, breaks down PAI1, thus enhancing fibrinolysis. However, thrombin also activates thrombin-activatable fibrinolysis inhibitor (TAFI), which inhibits the action of plasmin on fibrin. There is thus a delicately balanced system of positive and negative controls of fibrinolysis.

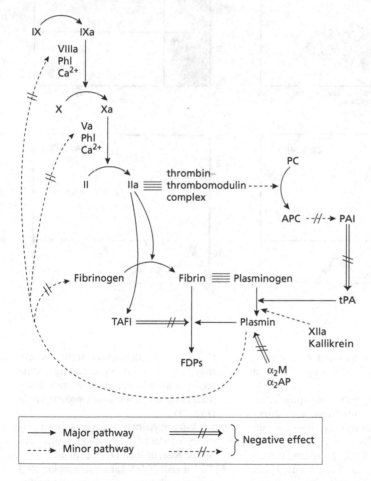

encodes a forkhead domain transcription factor that is negatively regulated by protein kinase B signalling (see *AKT*) and is essential for the completion of mitosis; contributes to the *PAX3-FKHR* and *PAX7-*

FKHR fusion genes, in t(2;13)(q35;q14) and t(1;13)(p36;q14) respectively, in alveolar rhabdomyosarcoma

FL a gene at 13q12-13 that encodes flk2/flt3 ligand

Figure 28 Flow cytometry immunophenotyping.
The results of immunophenotyping performed by flow cytometry on the peripheral blood cells of a patient with lymphocytosis. Forward and sideways light scatter have been used to gate on lymphocytes (top left), which have then been further analysed. The lymphocytosis resulted from an increase of CD8-positive lymphocytes (bottom left) with a reversal of the normal CD4:CD8 ratio. However, in addition, there is a population of lambda-positive B cells with a striking reversal of the normal kappa:lambda ratio. The patient had both a post-splenectomy lymphocytosis and circulating follicular lymphoma cells.

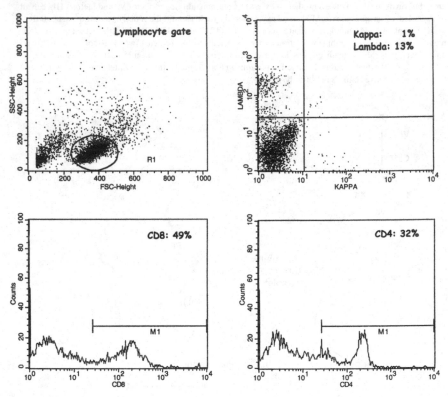

flag jargon for an automated instrument indication that a blood sample shows an abnormality

flagging jargon indicating production of 'flags' by an automated instrument, indicating abnormal or possibly unreliable test results

FLI1 a gene, Friend Leukaemia virus Integration 1, gene map locus 11q24, encodes an ETS transcription factor; contributes to a EWS-FLI1 fusion gene in Ewing's sarcoma associated with t(11;22)(q24;q12)

flow cytometry the process of evaluating characteristics of cells, in suspension, that are flowing through a detection device; may be based on fluorescence, light scatter, light absorbance or impedance measurements; used for **immunophenotyping** (Fig. 28)

flow karyotyping the use of flow cytometry to identify/separate chromosomes on the basis of their DNA content

FLT3 a gene, FMS-Like Tyrosine kinase 3 receptor, also known as stem cell tyrosine kinase, gene map locus 13q12, encodes a receptor tyrosine kinase of the PDGFR superfamily and is the receptor for flt3 ligand; expression in human blood and bone marrow cells is restricted to CD34+

cells; in frame internal tandem duplications affecting the JM domain of the flt3 protein are found in blast cell genomic DNA from approximately 20% of adult patients with acute myeloid leukaemia, across all FAB subtypes, usually in the absence of detectable cytogenetic abnormalities; *FLT3* mutations are associated with a worse prognosis; mutations are also present in some patients with myelodysplastic syndromes

fludarabine a **nucleoside analogue** used in treating **chronic lymphocytic leukaemia**

fluorescence activated cell sorter (FACS) an instrument that can sort cells into those that have bound or not bound a **fluorochrome**-labelled antibody

fluorescence *in situ* hybridization (FISH) identification of DNA or RNA sequences in cells in **metaphase** or **interphase** following hybridization with complementary RNA or DNA probes that have been labelled with a **fluorochrome**

fluorescence resonance energy transfer (FRET) the non-radiative transfer of energy from a fluorophore in an excited state to a nearby acceptor fluorophore; the farther apart the two molecules are, the weaker the transfer efficiency; so the technique is useful in assessing the interaction between two different (labelled) macromolecules

fluorochrome a **fluorescent chemical**

FMC7 a monoclonal antibody which gives positive reactions with cells of most non-Hodgkin's lymphomas but not with the cells of chronic lymphocytic leukaemia, acute lymphoblastic leukaemia or lymphoblastic lymphoma, thought to recognize a conformational epitope of **CD20**

FMS *see CSF1R*

FN1 a gene, Fibronectin, also known as Large, External, Transformation-Sensitive protein, *LETS*; gene map locus 2q31, encodes a high molecular weight cell surface glycoprotein that also represents about 1% of serum protein, and is required by most cells to bind to collagen; *FN1* contributed to a *NUP98-FN1* fusion gene, one of two fusion genes present in a case of M2 acute myeloid leukaemia;

fibronectin deficiency has been identified in association with Ehlers-Danlos syndrome (type X).

foamy macrophage a macrophage with heavily vacuolated cytoplasm, usually indicative of the presence of lipid

folate a generic term for **folic acid** and related compounds which are essential for normal DNA synthesis

folic acid pteroylglutamic acid, one of the B group of vitamins, essential for nucleic acid synthesis

folinic acid N^5-formyltetrahydrofolic acid, a form of folate that can circumvent the block in folate metabolism caused by dihydrofolate reductase inhibitors such as methotrexate

follicle centre cell a type of mature B lymphocyte found in the follicles of lymph nodes; includes **centrocytes** (small cells with condensed chromatin) and **centroblasts** (larger cells which may be nucleolated)

follicle centre cell lymphoma *see* **follicular lymphoma**

follicular dendritic cell an antigen-presenting cell in lymphoid follicles that presents antigen to germinal centre B lymphocytes

follicular lymphoma a lymphoma composed of cells analogous to those in the follicles of normal lymph nodes; such lymphomas usually have a follicular structure but sometimes the growth pattern is diffuse

fondaparinux a synthetic **factor Xa** inhibitor

FOP a gene, *FGFR1* **O**ncogene **P**artner; gene map locus 6q27, encodes a ubiquitously expressed leucine rich repeat (LRR) protein, that contributes to the *FOP-FGFR1* fusion gene in the lymphoproliferative–myeloproliferative disorder associated with t(6;8)(q27;p11) (*see also* **8p11 syndrome**)

foreign body giant cell a giant cell of monocyte/macrophage lineage with multiple nuclei spread through the cytoplasm

forkhead domain a phosphoprotein binding motif originally identified in a group of forkhead transcription factors e.g. FKHR, but also present in a wide variety of other proteins e.g. the nuclear proliferative antigen Ki-67 which is involved in centrosome separation during mitosis

formalin a solution of formaldehyde, used for fixing tissues

FOS a transcription factor of the leucine zipper family

FOS a gene, Finkel-Biskis-Jinkins (FBJ) murine Osteosarcoma viral oncogene homologue, gene map locus 14q24.3, encodes a major component of the activator protein-1 (AP-1) transcription factor complex; expressed at high levels in term placenta and trophoblastic cells; transforms cells through alterations in DNA methylation and in histone deacetylation; expression in chronic granulocytic leukaemia correlates with interferon-alpha responsiveness

fragment (of red cell) a schistocyte or erythrocyte fragment

frame-shift mutation a deletion or insertion of a number of base pairs that is not either 3 or a multiple of 3, into a DNA molecule, so that the **reading frame** is altered

French–American–British (FAB) Co-operative Group an international cooperative group of haematologists who proposed a number of widely accepted classifications of leukaemia and myelodysplastic syndromes

fresh frozen plasma (FFP) plasma from a single blood donation that has been frozen, shortly after separation from red cells, to a core temperature of below –30°C and which therefore retains normal levels of coagulation factors

FRET fluorescence resonance energy transfer

fusion the process of joining together to form a fusion gene, composed of parts of two genes, or a fusion protein, the product of such a gene (Fig. 29)

FUS a gene, Fusion, derived from 12-16 translocation, malignant liposarcoma; gene map locus 16p11.2, also known as Translocated in Liposarcoma (*TLS*);

encodes a glycine-rich protein which is a component of nuclear riboprotein complexes that plays a role in genomic stability; contributes to the *FUS-ERG* fusion gene in acute myeloid leukaemia associated with t(16;21)(p11;q22)

FUT1 a locus on chromosome 19 with two alleles relevant to ABH blood group antigens: the *H* allele encodes α-2-fucosyltransferase, which converts the h antigen to the H antigen; the *h* allele does not encode a transferase (*see* Fig. 3, p. 4)

FUT2 a locus at 19q13 with two alleles relevant to **secretor** status and **Lewis blood group** antigens (Fig. 30, p. 108) : the *Se* allele encodes α-2-L-fucosyltransferase, which converts a precursor type 1 disaccharide on a plasma glycosphingolipid molecule to the H type 1 antigen without which the Le^b antigen cannot be synthesized; the s*e* allele does not encode a transferase; individuals who are *SeSe* or *Sese* have ABH antigens in saliva and other body fluids whereas *sese* individuals do not; the former are referred to as 'secretors' and the latter as 'non-secretors'; homozygosity for *Se* also leads to an increased plasma concentration of **von Willebrand factor**

FUT3 a locus at 19p13.3 with two alleles relevant to **Lewis blood group** antigens (*see* Fig. 30, p. 108): the *Le* allele encodes α-3/4-L-fucosyltransferase, which converts a precursor type 1 disaccharide on a glycosphingolipid molecule to the Le^a antigen, H type 1 antigen to Le^b and A type 1 or B type 1 to ALe^b or BLe^b respectively; the *le* allele does not encode a transferase

FY a locus at 1q21-22 where allelic genes encode antigens of the Duffy blood group system; the genes at this locus are Fy^a, Fy^b, Fy^x and *Fy*; Fy^x leads to weak expression of the Fyb antigen; *Fy* has a **promoter** mutation and when this gene is homozygously present the phenotype is Fy(a-b-)

Figure 29   Fusion genes and fusion proteins.
Two fusion genes involving *CBFA2* and *CBFB*, encoding CBFα2 and CBFβ respectively illustrate the role of fusion genes and chimaeric proteins in oncogenesis.

(a) CBFα2 and CBFβ together form a heterodimeric haemopoietic transcription factor, Core Binding Factor (CBF). CBFβ does not itself bind to DNA but interacts via its CBFα binding domain (CBFα BD) with CBFα2. This interaction occurs in the runt domain of CBFα2 and increases the ability of another part of the runt domain to bind the consensus DNA sequence YGYGGT. Once bound to DNA, CBF can activate transcription of a large number of haemopoietic genes. In certain circumstances it can act as a repressor via the VWRPY motif at the carboxy terminus of CBFα2 which interacts with the transcriptional repressor, TLE. Normally, CBFα2 is sequestered in the nucleus due to its nuclear matrix-binding domain NMTS.

(b) The acquired chromosomal abnormality inv(16)(p13q32) seen in a specific subtype of AML, leads to the fusion of most of the *CBFB* gene to the region encoding the tail domain of the smooth muscle myosin heavy chain (*SMMHC* or *MYH11*) gene. Several variants of a CBFB-SMMHC fusion transcript have been detected in AMLs with inv(16). Most lead to a fusion protein containing a fully functional CBFα BD fused to the α-helical tail of SMMHC. The fusion protein is able to form multimers because of this tail, which can be visualized as nuclear and cytoplasmic speckles. It is believed that multimeric CBFβ-SMMHC sequesters CBFα2 subunits and so reduces DNA binding by CBF.

(c) The translocation t(8;21)(q22;q22) seen in another subtype of AML, leads to the fusion of the runt domain of the *CBFA2* gene to the majority of *ETO* which encodes a non-DNA binding nuclear protein involved in the recruitment of histone deacetylses. The ETO protein has 'nervy' domains that permit interactions with transcriptional repressors. The CBFα2-ETO fusion protein is able to interact with CBFβ and does so with greater affinity than wild-type CBFα2, but the ETO moiety leads to the repression of transcription. This leads to a differentiation arrest in myeloid cells.

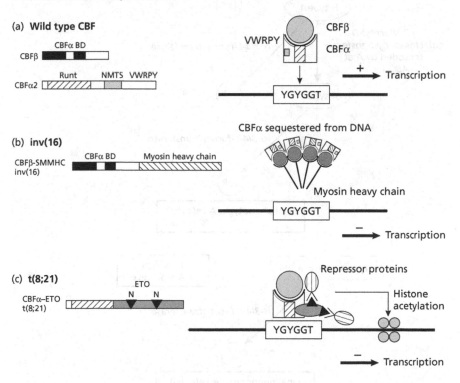

Figure 30   The Lewis blood group system.

The interaction between transferases encoded by three sets of allelic genes to produce Lewis blood group antigens: (a) In an individual who is A positive (genotype either *AA* or *AO*), Le positive (genotype *LeLe* or *Lele*) and who is a 'secretor' (genotype *SeSe* or *Sese*). The *Le* allele at the *FUT3* locus encodes a transferase that converts a precursor to Le^a antigen whereas the *Se* allele at the *FUT1* locus produces H type 1 which can be converted by the transferase encoded by *Le* into Le^b. In the presence of the transferase encoded by the *A* allele at the *ABO* locus A Le^b is also produced. The phenotype is A Le(a+b+).

(b) In an individual who is A positive (genotype either *AA* or *AO*) and Le positive (genotype *LeLe* or *Lele*) but who is a 'non-secretor' (genotype *sese*) Le^a is the only Lewis antigen produced. The phenotype is A Le(a+b−).

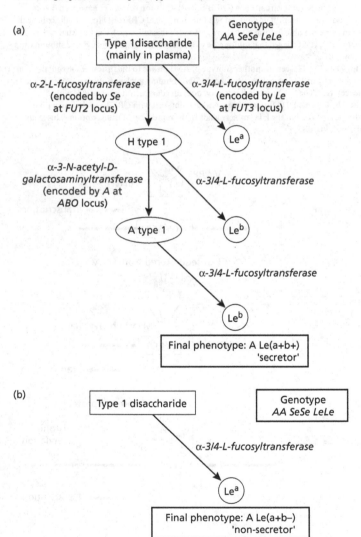

G

γ the Greek letter gamma

γ chain (i) the γ globin chain which forms part of haemoglobin F (ii) the heavy chain of an **immunoglobulin G** molecule; two γ chains combine with two light chains, in an individual molecule either κ or λ, to form an immunoglobulin molecule (iii) part of the γδ **T-cell receptor**, a surface membrane structure which permits antigen recognition

γ-glutamyl cysteine synthetase (an enzyme of the pentose shunt) hexose monophosphate shunt (*see* Fig. 59, p. 182)

γ heavy chain disease a **plasma cell dyscrasia** in which there is secretion of monoclonal γ chain

G an abbreviation for the purine, guanine

G0, G1 and G2 three phases of the **cell cycle** (*see* Fig. 15, p. 72)

G6PD **glucose-6-phosphate dehydrogenase**

G6PD the gene at Xq28 encoding **glucose-6-phosphate dehydrogenase**; mutation may lead to **glucose-6-phosphate dehydrogenase deficiency** with intermittent or, much less often, chronic, haemolysis

gallium scan an imaging technique using ^{67}Ga-single photon emission computerized tomography to detect metabolic activity in residual areas of active lymphoma

gamete a germ cell, a spermatozoon or an ovum

GAP GTP-ase activating protein

GAS1 a gene, Growth Arrest-Specific 1; gene map locus 9q21.3-q22.1; encodes a plasma membrane protein which is a homologue of the iron protein subunit of Complex I of the mitochondrial electron transport chain; expressed in non-transformed cells in response to stimuli driving cells into G0 phase; deleted in many myeloid neoplasms

GAS2 a gene, Growth Arrest-Specific 2; gene map locus 11p15.2-p14.3; encodes a ubiquitously expressed component of the microfilament system which increases susceptibility to **p53**-dependent apoptosis

GAS6 a gene, Growth Arrest-Specific 6, also known as **Axl** receptor tyrosine kinase Ligand, *AXLLG*; gene map locus 13q34; encodes a vitamin K-dependent protein homologous to **protein** S which is the ligand for the receptor tyrosine kinase **AXL**

GAS7 a gene, Growth Arrest-Specific 7; gene map locus 17p13, encodes a putative transcription factor expressed normally in the brain, that contributed to a *MLL-GAS7* fusion gene in a case of therapy-related M4 acute myeloid leukaemia with a cryptic t(11;17)(q23;p13) translocation

GAS41 a gene, Glioma-Associated Sequence 41, gene map locus 12q13-q15, encodes a putative transcription factor that has homology with *AF9* and *ENL*; *GAS41* amplified in high-grade glioma

GATA-1 a gene encoding a **transcription factor** that is important in erythropoiesis and critical in megakaryocyte differentiation

Gaucher cell the characteristic altered macrophage of **Gaucher's disease**

Gaucher's disease hereditary glucosyl ceramide lipidosis, a heterogeneous group of inherited diseases resulting from various mutations in the glucocerebrosidase gene; these mutations lead to accumulation of glucocerebroside in characteristic macrophages, designated **Gaucher cells**; may be diagnosed by bone marrow aspiration

Figure 31   G banding.
A karyogram of G-banded chromosomes of a patient with chronic granulocytic leukaemia. The banding pattern produced by the Giemsa stain, together with a consideration of the size of the chromosome and the position of the centromere, permits the identification of individual chromosomes, normal and abnormal. There is a t(9;22)(q34;q11); this is a balanced translocation between chromosomes 9 and 22 with breakpoints at 9q34 and 22q11 respectively.

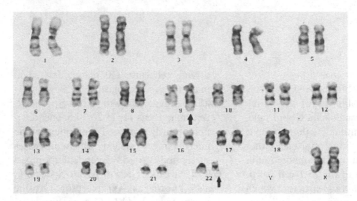

Gaussian a description of data that, when plotted as **a histogram**, have a bell-shaped distribution; also referred to as a 'normal distribution' (*see* Fig. 45, p. 128)

GBA the gene encoding glucocerebrosidase, mutated in **Gaucher's disease**

G-banding a technique for staining **metaphase** spreads of chromosomes with a Giemsa stain to produce a unique banding pattern that permits the identification of individual chromosomes (Fig. 31)

G-CFU granulocyte colony-forming unit

G-CSF granulocyte colony-stimulating factor

GCSFR a gene, Granulocyte Colony-Stimulating Factor Receptor, also known as Colony-Stimulating Factor 3 Receptor, *CSF3R*, **CD114**; gene map locus 1p35-p34.3; encodes the G-CSF receptor; point mutations in this gene have been reported in some patients with severe congenital neutropenia (Kostmann's syndrome), these patients being at greatest risk of developing myelodysplastic syndrome or acute myeloid leukaemia; mutation leading to synthesis of a truncated protein has also been implicated in acute myeloid leukaemia complicating Kostmann's syndrome

GDP guanosine diphosphate

GEF guanine nucleotide exchange factor

gelatinous transformation deposition of acid mucopolysaccharide in bone marrow, replacing haemopoietic tissue

gene the segment of DNA that is involved in producing a polypeptide chain; it includes regions preceding and following the coding region (5′ and 3′ untranslated regions) as well as intervening sequences (**introns**) between individual coding segments (**exons**) (Fig. 32); genes mediate inheritance; they are located on nuclear chromosome or, rarely, on a **mitochondrion**

gene expression the **transcription** of a gene into **tRNA, rRNA** or **mRNA**, in the latter case with subsequent **translation** to protein

gene profiling *see* **microarray analysis**

genetic pertaining to inheritance by genes

genetic code the relationship between a triplet of bases, called a codon, and the amino acid which it encodes

genome the complete DNA sequence of an individual or a species

genomic pertaining to a gene or genes

genotype the genetic makeup of an individual, cf. **phenotype**

Figure 32 Gene structure and function.
A gene is a segment of DNA that is involved in producing a protein. It is also known as a transcriptional unit and includes not only coding regions (exons), but also non-coding sequences which lie between exons (introns), and before and after the coding segments (5' and 3' untranslated regions). Transcription is the enzymatic process whereby RNA is synthesized from a DNA template. The promoter is the section of DNA where the transcriptional machinery binds before transcription can start. It is defined by certain highly conserved sequences, e.g. the TATA box which is found 25bp 'upstream' from (i.e. 5' to) the transcriptional start site, and the CAAT box, found 75bp upstream. Transcriptional termination signals lie in the 3'UTR and trigger the 3' cleavage of newly formed RNA (*see* Figure 65, p. 202). The first coding triplet in a gene is referred to as the start codon and is usually ATG (encoding methionine); the coding sequence always ends in a termination signal (a codon which does not encode an amino acid); this can be TAG, TGA or TAA. Translation is the synthesis of a protein from a messenger RNA (mRNA) template; this always proceeds from a start codon to a stop codon. Some genes have multiple promoters and may have introns spanning several Kb. There are many examples of overlapping genes and of transcription in either orientation occurring from different promoters in the same segment of DNA. The flanking sequences on either side or within the transcriptional unit may contain enhancers, which are sequences of DNA involved in the binding of positive or negative transcriptional regulatory proteins.

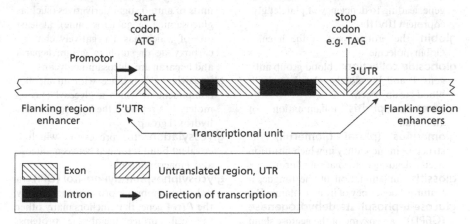

Gerbich antigen an erythrocyte membrane antigen, carried on **glycophorin C**; monoclonal antibodies to this antigen can be used for the identification of erythroid cells

germ cell a gamete, a spermatozoon or an ovum

germinal centre a specialized structure in a lymph node or other lymphoid tissue in which follicular dendritic cells present antigen to B lymphocytes

ghost cell an erythrocyte which contains negligible amounts of haemoglobin

giant cell arteritis inflammation of arteries with the inflammatory cells including giant cells, usually associated with a high **erythrocyte sedimentation rate**, which can therefore be used as a diagnostic aid

giant metamyelocyte a metamyelocyte which is two to three times normal size and often has a nucleus of abnormal shape, characteristic of **megaloblastic erythropoiesis**

Giemsa stain a Romanowsky type stain which can be used for staining blood and bone marrow cells and tissue sections and is also used for staining preparations of chromosomes (*see* **G-banding**); one component of a **May–Grünwald–Giemsa** stain

GIFT granulocyte immunofluorescence test

Gilbert's syndrome a common syndrome resulting from **homozygosity** for a polymorphism in the **promoter** region of the gene encoding bilirubin UDP glucuronosyl transferase-1, *UGT1*, leading to unconjugated hyperbilirubinaemia; it causes neonatal jaundice in infants with **G6PD deficiency** and aggravates jaundice in adults with haemolytic anaemias

gingivitis inflammation of the gums, can be a feature of acute leukaemia with monocytic differentiation

gland (i) specialized epithelial tissue capable of secretion (ii) a popular term for a **lymph node**

glandular fever *see* **infectious mononucleosis**

Glanzmann's thrombasthenia a severe, autosomal recessive, inherited defect of platelet function, resulting from mutation in either the *ITGA2B* or the *ITGB3* gene, leading to deficiency of platelet glycoprotein IIb/IIIa

globin the protein part of the haemoglobin molecule

globoside collection blood group antigens, P and P^k, closely related to the P blood group system

glomerulonephritis inflammation of glomeruli

glomerulus (plural glomeruli) the structure in the kidney in which filtration occurs, leading to formation of urine

glossitis inflammation of the tongue, a feature of deficiency of iron or vitamin B$_{12}$

glucose-6-phosphate dehydrogenase (G6PD) an enzyme of the **pentose shunt** which protects red cells from oxidant damage (*see* Fig. 59, p. 182)

glucose-6-phosphate dehydrogenase (G6PD) deficiency reduced glucose-6-phosphate dehydrogenase activity in red cells leading to susceptibility to oxidant-induced haemolysis

glucose phosphate isomerase an enzyme in the erythrocyte **glycolytic pathway** (Fig. 33)

glutathione synthetase an enzyme related to the **pentose shunt** (*see* Fig. 59, p. 182)

glycogen a complex carbohydrate

glycolipid a sugar-containing lipid in which a monosaccharide is linked to a lipid via glycosidic bond

glycolysis the process by which glucose is metabolized, providing energy for a cell

glycolytic pathway (Embden–Meyerhof pathway) the metabolic pathway in erythrocytes and other cells in which glucose is broken down to provide energy for the cell (Fig. 33)

glycophorin a group of red cell membrane proteins, glycophorins A, B, C and D (**CD235a, CD235b, CD236, CD236R**), antibodies to which can be used to identify cells of erythroid lineage (*see* Fig. 64, p. 199, and *see also GYPA, GYPB, GYPC*)

glycoprotein a post-translationally modified protein in which a carbohydrate is covalently linked to an amino acid residue

glycosaminoglycan a polysaccharide consisting of repeating disaccharide units of amino sugar derivatives (such as glucosamine or galactosamine), at least one of which has a negatively charged carboxylate or sulphate group; **heparin** and heparan are glycosaminoglycans

glycoside a substance with an alcohol component in which a glycosyl (sugar) moiety has replaced the hydrogen in the hydroxyl group

glycosylation the process in which a covalent bond is formed between glucose and a macromolecule

glycosylphosphatidylinositol (GPI) a red cell membrane protein, encoded by the *PIGA* gene, that anchors many other red cell surface membrane proteins, including **CD55, CD58** and **CD59**

GM-CFU granulocyte/macrophage colony-forming unit

GM-CSF granulocyte/macrophage colony-stimulating factor

GMPS a gene, Guanosine-5′-Monophosphate Synthetase, gene map locus 3q24, encodes the enzyme that catalyses the amination of xanthylate (XMP) to guanylate (GMP) in the purine synthesis pathway; contributed to an *MLL-GMPS* fusion gene in a patient with M4 acute myeloid leukaemia associated with t(3;11)(q25;q23); in the resulting chimaeric proteins the catalytic domain of GMPS was intact

GMS stain Grocott's methenamine silver stain

Golgi apparatus or Golgi complex stacks of flattened membranous sacs receiving newly synthesized proteins from

Figure 33 The glycolytic pathway.
The glycolytic pathway provides energy for body cells including erythrocytes. Enzymes are shown in italics and enzyme products in upright script. Pyruvate kinase deficiency is the most common inherited defect of the glycolytic pathway.

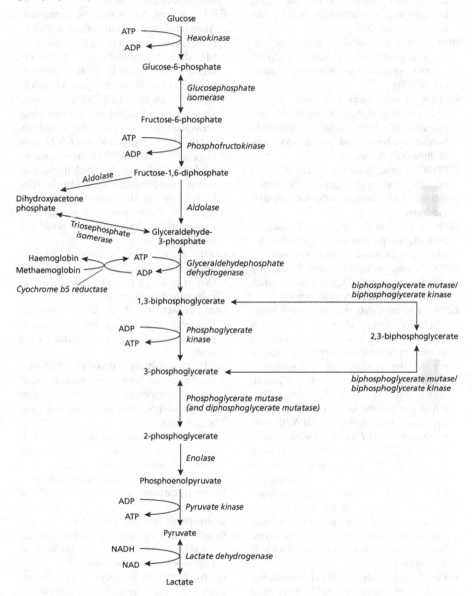

the **endoplasmic reticulum**, responsible for modification, packaging and distribution of proteins

Golgi zone the area of a cell, usually adjacent to the nucleus, where the **Golgi complex** is located; in cells with a well developed Golgi apparatus the Golgi zone appears as a pale area

Good Clinical Practice a standard for the design, conduct, performance, monitoring, auditing, recording and reporting of clinical trials that provides assurance that the data and reported results are credible and accurate and that the rights, integrity and confidentiality of trial subjects are protected

gout acute crystal arthropathy secondary to urate deposition; may be a feature of **myeloproliferative disorders**, causes **neutrophilia**

GP1BA a gene, gene map locus 17pter-p12, encoding platelet glycoprotein Ibα, mutation of which can lead to **Bernard–Soulier syndrome** and **platelet-type von Willebrand's disease**

GP1BB a gene, gene map locus 22q11.2, encoding platelet glycoprotein Ibβ, mutation of which can lead to **Bernard–Soulier syndrome**

GPV a gene on chromosome 3 encoding platelet glycoprotein V, mutation of which can lead to **Bernard–Soulier syndrome**

GPIX a gene on chromosome 3 encoding platelet glycoprotein IX, mutation of which can lead to **Bernard–Soulier syndrome**

GPH a gene, **G**ep**h**yrin, gene map locus 14q24, encodes gephyrin—a protein expressed in the brain which is involved in anchoring the inhibitory glycine receptor to the postsynaptic cytoskeleton; several alternative transcripts are known which differ at their 5′ termini, but which encode the same 3′ tubulin binding site; also known as *GPNH*; contributed to a *MLL-GPNH* fusion gene in t(11;14)(q23;q24) in a patient with M5b acute myeloid leukaemia and in a patient with 'undifferentiated' acute leukaemia following therapy with a **topoisomerase** II-interactive drug in which the fusion protein retained the gephyrin tubulin binding site; autoantibodies to gephyrin have been observed in a patient with stiff man syndrome

GR6 a gene located within the leukaemia breakpoint region of 3q21, gene map locus 3q21, expressed in early fetal development but not in adult peripheral blood cells; has no known homologies; *GR6* contributes to an *GR6-EVI1* fusion gene in acute myeloid leukaemia and myelo-

dysplastic syndrome associated with t(3;3)(q21;q26) and inv(3)(q21q26)

grade an expression of the degree of malignancy of a tumour

GRAF a gene, RhoA **G**TPase **R**egulation **A**ssociated with **F**ocal adhesion kinase pp125, gene map locus 5q31, encodes an SH3 domain-containing protein which is highly homologous to *BCR*; a member of the GTPase-activating protein (GAP) family; binds to pp125(FAK), a tyrosine kinase involved in the integrin signalling transduction pathway, also stimulates the GTPase activity of **RhoA**; *GRAF* contributed to a *MLL-GRAF* fusion gene in a child with juvenile myelomonocytic leukaemia associated with t(5;11)(q31;q23); both alleles of the gene were also disrupted in three cases of acute myeloid leukaemia–myelodysplastic syndrome associated with 5q–

graft a tissue that is transplanted into another individual or, less accurately, that is removed from an individual and subsequently returned

graft rejection the process by which a transplanted tissue, e.g. bone marrow, is recognized as foreign and rejected by the body

graft-versus-host disease (GVHD) the illness resulting from engraftment of immunocompetent lymphoid cells that recognize host tissues as foreign and attack them

graft-versus-leukaemia (GVL) the ability of engrafted tissue to exert a specific anti-leukaemic effect that is different from the generalized graft-versus-host effect

Gram-negative non-staining with a Gram stain

Gram-positive staining with a Gram stain

Gram stain a stain used for staining bacteria, which are then classified as Gram-positive or Gram-negative

granulocyte a leucocyte with a lobed nucleus and granular cytoplasm—a **neutrophil, eosinophil** or **basophil**

granulocyte-colony forming unit (G-CFU) a **progenitor cell** that can give rise to a colony of granulocytes when cultured *in vitro*

granulocyte-colony stimulating factor (G-CSF) a cytokine that promotes granulopoiesis, leading to an increased neutrophil count *in vivo* and supporting growth of granulocyte colonies *in vitro*, encoded by a gene at 17q11.2-21; recombinant G-CSF is available as a therapeutic product

granulocyte immunofluorescence test (GIFT) a test for anti-neutrophil antibodies

granulocyte/macrophage colony-forming unit (GM-CFU) a progenitor cell which can give rise to a mixed colony of granulocytes and macrophages on *in vitro* culture

granulocyte/macrophage colony-stimulating factor (GM-CSF) a haemopoietic growth factor, synthesized by B cells, T cells, NK cells and macrophages, which stimulates production of granulocytes and macrophages, leading to neutrophilia and monocytosis *in vivo* and sustaining growth of, mixed granulocyte/macrophage colonies *in vitro*, encoded by a gene at 5q31

granulocytic sarcoma chloroma, a soft tissue tumour composed of leukaemic myeloblasts with or without maturing cells

granuloma (i) a cohesive cluster of epithelioid macrophages with or without lymphocytes and other inflammatory cells (ii) a cohesive cluster of altered macrophages containing lipid vacuoles

granulomere the granular part of a platelet

granulopoiesis the process by which granulocytes are produced (*see* Fig. 25, p. 95)

grey platelet syndrome an inherited platelet defect in which platelets lack α granules and thus, when stained, appear pale blue or grey and agranular

Griscelli syndrome partial albinism with immunodeficiency—defective **natural killer cell** function, absent delayed hypersensitivity reactions and sometimes secondary **hypogammaglobulinaemia**

Grocott's methenamine silver (GMS) stain a stain used for the detection of fungi

growth factor a protein secreted by one cell that promotes growth of cells of another lineage

GSH2 a gene, gene map locus 4q11, encoding a brain-specific homeobox gene homologous to the *Drosophila* gene '*intermediate neuroblasts defective*' (*ind*); *GSH2* is upstream of the *CHIC2-ETV6/TEL* fusion gene and is dysregulated in acute myeloid leukaemia associated with t(4;12)(q11;p13)

GTP guanosine triphosphate

guanine a **purine** base of DNA or RNA, pairs with cytosine

guanine nucleotide exchange factors (GEFs) a family of molecules that bind to inactive **GTPases**, e.g. Rho, RAS and RAC, and induce conformational changes allowing **GDP** release and replacement by **GTP** (*see also RAS*)

GVHD graft-versus-host disease

GVL graft-versus-leukaemia

GYPA a gene at 4q28.2-q31.1, also known as *GPA* and *MN* locus, encoding glycophorin A; the M and N antigens are encoded by alleles of *GYPA*

GYPB a gene at 4q28.2-q31.1, also known as *GPB* and *Ss* locus, encoding **glycophorin B**; the S and s antigens are encoded by alleles of *GYPB*

GYPC a gene at 2q14-q24 encoding **glycophorin C** and **glycophorin D**, which carries the Gerbich blood group antigens

H

H4(10S170) a gene, gene map locus
10q21, encoding a leucine zipper protein
the function of which is unknown; contributes to:
• a fusion gene, *H4(10S17)-PDGFRB*,
in atypical chronic myeloid leukaemia
associated with t(5;10)(q33;q22);
• an *H4-BCL6* fusion gene in non-
Hodgkin's lymphoma;
The leucine zipper domain is present
in the chimaeric proteins generated in
each of these cases and permits their
oligomerization

H & E haematoxylin and eosin stain

HAART highly active antiretroviral
therapy

haem a porphyrin structure that contains iron and that forms part of the
haemoglobin molecule; it is synthesized
partly within **mitochondria** and partly in
the **cytosol** (Fig. 34)

haematemesis the vomiting of blood

haematocrit (Hct) the proportion of a
column of centrifuged blood which is
occupied by erythrocytes or an equivalent estimation produced by an automated blood counter

haematogone a primitive lymphoid cell
which morphologically resembles a lymphoblast but is a normal reactive cell

haematology the study of blood and its
diseases

haematopoiesis a synonym for **haemopoiesis**, this term being generally used in
the USA

haematopoietic pertaining to **haematopoiesis**, a synonym for **haemopoietic**,
this term being generally used in the USA

haematoxylin a basic dye used in cytology
and to stain parasites; used in combination with eosin to stain tissue sections

Figure 34 Haem synthesis.
The process by which haem is synthesized. Enzymes
are shown in italics and enzyme products in upright
script.

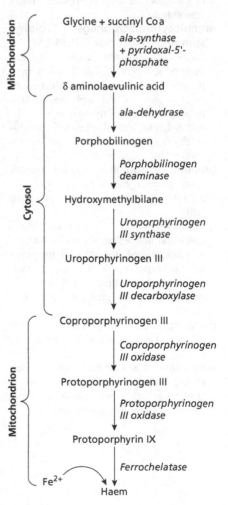

haematoxylin and eosin (H & E) the standard stain used for staining tissue sections, a mixture of basic **haematoxylin** and acidic **eosin**

haematuria the presence of red cells in the urine

haemiglobin cyanide an alternative designation of cyanmethaemoglobin, the form of haemoglobin which results from interaction with cyanide in the cyanmethaemoglobin method for estimation of haemoglobin concentration

haemochromatosis *see* **hereditary haemochromatosis**

haemocytometer a counting chamber for counting blood cells

haemodialysis a method of treating acute or chronic renal failure by passing the patient's blood through a dialysis machine; blood and dialysis fluid are separated by a semipermeable membrane so that exchange of solutes can occur

haemoflagellates flagellated blood parasites such as trypanosomes and leishmania

haemoglobin a complex molecule composed of four globin chains, each of which partially encloses a haem molecule (Fig. 35), which has as its major function the transport of oxygen from the lungs to the tissues

haemoglobin A the major haemoglobin component present in most adults, having two α chains and two β chains

haemoglobin A$_2$ a minor haemoglobin component present in adults and, as an even lower proportion of total haemoglobin, in neonates and infants; it has two α chains and two δ chains

haemoglobin Bart's an abnormal haemoglobin with four γ chains and no α chains, present as the major haemoglobin component in **haemoglobin Bart's hydrops fetalis** and as a minor component in neonates with **haemoglobin H disease** or **alpha thalassaemia trait**

haemoglobin Bart's hydrops fetalis a fatal condition of a fetus or neonate, resulting from **homozygosity** or **compound heterozygosity** for α⁰ **thalassaemia** (Fig. 36); as there are no alpha genes there can be no production of haemoglobin A, A$_2$ or F

Figure 35 **The haemoglobin molecule.** A sketch of the haemoglobin molecule showing that it is composed of two α globin chains and two β globin chains, each enclosing a haem moiety.

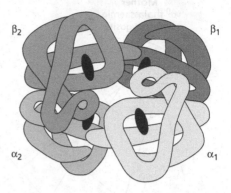

haemoglobin C a variant haemoglobin with an amino acid substitution in the beta chain, mainly found in those of African ancestry

haemoglobin Constant Spring a variant haemoglobin with a structurally abnormal alpha chain which is synthesized at a reduced rate, leading to **α thalassaemia**

haemoglobin D the designation of a group of haemoglobin variants, some α chain variants and some β chain variants, that have the same mobility as **haemoglobin S** on **haemoglobin electrophoresis** at alkaline pH

haemoglobin dissociation curve a plot of percentage saturation of haemoglobin against partial pressure of oxygen (Fig. 37)

Haemoglobin Distribution Width (HDW) a measurement made by some automated blood counters that indicates the amount of variation in haemoglobin concentration between erythrocytes; an increased HDW correlates with anisochromasia on a blood film

haemoglobin E a variant haemoglobin with an amino acid substitution in the beta chain, mainly found in South-east Asia and parts of the Indian subcontinent

haemoglobin electrophoresis a method of separating normal and variant

Figure 36   haemoglobin Bart's hydrops fetalis.
A diagrammatic representation of the possible outcomes in a family at risk of
producing a fetus with haemoglobin Bart's hydrops fetalis.

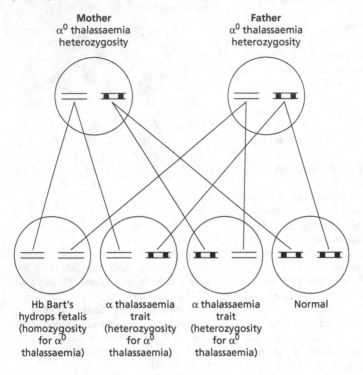

Mother
α^0 thalassaemia
heterozygosity

Father
α^0 thalassaemia
heterozygosity

Hb Bart's
hydrops fetalis
(homozygosity
for α^0
thalassaemia)

α thalassaemia
trait
(heterozygosity
for α^0
thalassaemia)

α thalassaemia
trait
(heterozygosity
for α^0
thalassaemia)

Normal

Figure 37   A haemoglobin dissociation curve.
A haemoglobin dissociation curve showing the
sigmoid form of the normal dissociation curve and
the factors which shift the curve to the left or right.

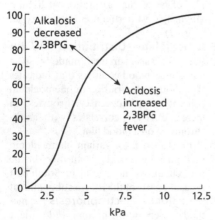

Alkalosis
decreased
2,3BPG

Acidosis
increased
2,3BPG
fever

kPa

haemoglobins from each by applying a
haemolysate to a membrane or gel across
which there is an electrical gradient; the
pH and the nature of the membrane or gel
determines the rate at which different
haemoglobins migrate in the electrical
field (Fig. 38)

haemoglobin F   fetal haemoglobin, the
major haemoglobin of the fetus and
neonate (Fig. 39), which is present as a
very minor component in most adults
and in higher amounts in a minority;
adult levels have usually been reached by
about one year of age

haemoglobin G   the designation of a
group of haemoglobin variants, some of
which are alpha chain variants and some
of which are beta chain variants, that
have the same mobility as **haemoglobin S**
on **haemoglobin electrophoresis** at alkaline pH; whether a variant haemoglobin

Figure 38 Haemoglobin electrophoresis.
The results of haemoglobin electrophoresis on a cellulose acetate membrane at alkaline pH. Haemoglobins S, D and G move together, as do haemoglobins C, E and A_2: (a) haemoglobins S and C; (b) haemoglobin S; (c) haemoglobins A and C; (d) haemoglobin S; (e) haemoglobins A and C; (f) haemoglobins S and C; (g) haemoglobins A and C; (AFSC) control sample containing haemoglobins A, F, S and C.

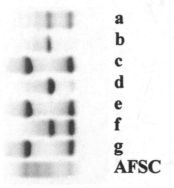

is designated **haemoglobin D** or haemoglobin G is completely arbitrary

haemoglobin Gower an embryonic haemoglobin; haemoglobin Gower 1 is $\zeta_2\varepsilon_2$ and haemoglobin Gower 2 is $\alpha_2\varepsilon_2$

haemoglobin H a variant haemoglobin with four β chains and no α chains, present in **haemoglobin H disease** and, in small quantities, in **α thalassaemia trait**

haemoglobin H disease a thalassaemic condition caused by marked underproduction of α chains, often but not always resulting from compound heterozygosity for **α^+ thalassaemia** and **α^0 thalassaemia** with consequent lack of three of the four alpha genes (Fig. 40)

haemoglobin H inclusions small round evenly dispersed erythrocyte inclusions composed of **haemoglobin H**; they can be stained with vital dyes

haemoglobin Lepore a variant haemoglobin resulting from the fusion of part of a δ globin gene with part of

Figure 39 Changes if haemoglobin F percentage during development.
The proportions of haemoglobin F and other normal haemoglobins present in the embryo, fetus, neonate and infant.

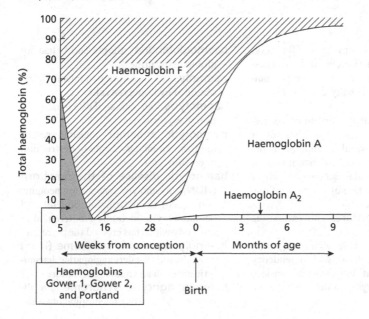

Figure 40   Haemoglobin H disease.
A diagrammatic representation of the possible outcomes in a family at risk of
producing a child with haemoglobin H disease.

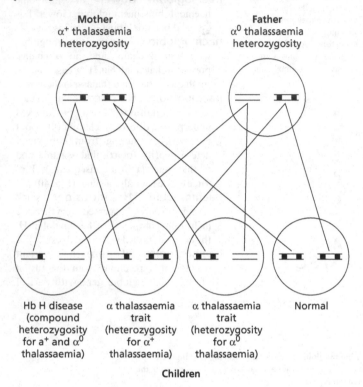

Mother
α⁺ thalassaemia
heterozygosity

Father
α⁰ thalassaemia
heterozygosity

Hb H disease
(compound
heterozygosity
for a⁺ and α⁰
thalassaemia)

α thalassaemia
trait
(heterozygosity
for α⁺
thalassaemia)

α thalassaemia
trait
(heterozygosity
for α⁰
thalassaemia)

Normal

Children

a β globin gene, giving a δβ fusion gene and fusion protein; it is synthesized at a slower rate than the β chain and thus is functionally equivalent to a β thalassaemia

haemoglobinopathy   an inherited disorder resulting from synthesis of a structurally abnormal haemoglobin; the term can also be used to encompass, in addition, the thalassaemias in which there is a reduced rate of synthesis of one of the globin chains

haemoglobin Portland   an embryonic haemoglobin, ζ₂γ₂

haemoglobin S   sickle cell haemoglobin, a variant haemoglobin with a tendency to polymerize at low oxygen tension, causing erythrocytes to deform into the shape of a sickle

haemoglobinuria   the presence of haemoglobin in the urine

haemolysate   a solution of haemoglobin obtained by lysing red cells

haemolysis   an increased rate of destruction of erythrocytes

haemolytic anaemia   anaemia resulting from an increased rate of destruction of erythrocytes

haemolytic disease of the newborn (HDN)   haemolytic anaemia in a neonate, consequent on destruction of fetal and neonatal erythrocytes by a maternal alloantibody which has crossed the placenta

haemolytic uraemic syndrome (HUS) a syndrome of **microangiopathic haemolytic anaemia** and acute renal failure

haemophagocytic syndrome   an illness resulting from haemophagocytosis, characterized by **pancytopenia** and sometimes **hepatomegaly, splenomegaly** and fever, *see also* **familial haemophagocytic lymphohistiocytosis**

haemophagocytosis phagocytosis of haemopoietic cells and their progeny

haemophilia an inherited haemorrhagic disorder resulting from deficiency of **factor VIII** (haemophilia A, resulting from a mutation in the *F8C* gene) or **factor IX** (haemophilia B, resulting from a mutation in the *F9* gene)

haemophilia A an **X-linked recessive** inherited bleeding disorder (*see* Fig. 68, p. 207) resulting from a mutation, most often an inversion that splits the gene, involving the *F8C* gene

haemophilia B an **X-linked recessive** inherited bleeding disorder, previously known as Christmas disease, resulting from a mutation, most often a point mutation, in the *F9* gene

haemophilia B Leiden a variant of **haemophilia B**, resulting from one of a number of point mutations in the promoter region of the *F9* gene, in which **factor IX** concentration rises at puberty with improvement of the bleeding tendency; the likely explanation is that the mutations affect a binding region for androgen-sensitive transcription factors

haemopoiesis the process of production of blood cells (Fig. 41)

haemopoietic pertaining to **haemopoiesis**

haemopoietic cell a precursor cell giving rise ultimately to granulocytes, monocytes, erythrocytes and platelets

haemopoietic growth factor a protein, often a glycoprotein, that promotes growth and differentiation of **haemopoietic cells**, e.g. erythropoietin, thrombopoietin

haemorrhage bleeding; may be a normal phenomenon, e.g. following injury, or the result of an inherited or acquired haemorrhagic disorder

haemorrhagic disease of the newborn a haemorrhagic disorder of neonates consequent on **vitamin K** deficiency

haemosiderin the major storage form of iron, present in **macrophages**

haemostasis the process by which haemorrhage is arrested

hairy cell an abnormal B-lymphocyte present in **hairy cell leukaemia**, analogous to a late B cell

hairy cell leukaemia a chronic B-lineage leukaemia with neoplastic cells which are morphologically and immunophenotypically distinctive

hairy cell leukaemia variant a chronic B-lineage leukaemia with neoplastic cells which resemble the cells of hairy cell leukaemia morphologically but with there being differences in immunophenotype and haematological and clinical features

Ham test *see* **acid lysis test**

HAM HTLV-I-associated myelopathy

hand mirror cell a blast cell shaped like a mirror, may be of lymphoid or myeloid lineage

Hand–Schüller–Christian disease part of the clinical spectrum of **Langerhans cell histiocytosis**

haploid a description of cells with a complement of 23 chromosomes, one copy of each autosome and either an X or a Y chromosome; normal sperm and ova are haploid but in **somatic** cells haploidy is highly abnormal

haploidy the state of having a **haploid** complement of chromosomes

haplo-insufficiency an abnormal phenotype or predisposition to disease as a result of loss of one allele of a gene or loss of a longer DNA sequence from one of a pair of chromosomes

haplotype genotype of a group of alleles from two or more closely linked loci, e.g. the β^S gene occurs in association with several different haplotypes

hapten a small antigen that becomes immunogenic when complexed with a larger protein

HC2 a monoclonal antibody which gives positive reactions with hairy cells and occasionally with cells of other chronic lymphoproliferative disorders

hCDCre *see CDCREL*

Hct haematocrit

HDN haemolytic disease of the newborn

HDW Haemoglobin Distribution Width

heavy chain the longer of the two polypeptide chains of a dimer, usually refers to the heavy chain of an immunoglobulin

Figure 41   Haemopoiesis.

A diagrammatic representation of haemopoiesis showing the stem cell/progenitor cell hierarchy and the growth factors that are thought to act at each stage of development.

Abbreviations for cell names: PSC, pluripotent stem cell (also known as HSC, haemopoietic stem cell); CLP, common lymphoid progenitor; T, T cell; B, B cell; NK, natural killer cell; LDC, lymphoid dendritic cell; CMP, common myeloid progenitor (also known as multipotent myeloid stem cell); CFU-GM, colony-forming unit–granulocyte-macrophage; CFU-G, colony-forming unit–granulocyte; CFU-M, colony-forming unit–macrophage; MDC, myeloid dendritic cell; CFU-Eo, colony-forming unit–eosinophil; CFU-Baso, colony-forming unit–basophil; CFU-Mast, colony-forming unit–mast cell; BFU-E, burst-forming unit–erythroid; CFU-E, colony-forming unit–erythroid; BFU-Mega, burst-forming unit–megakaryocyte; CFU-Mega, colony-forming unit–megakaryocyte; HSC, haematopoietic stem cell.

Abbreviations for growth factors: SCF, stem cell factor; FLT3L, FLT3 ligand; IL, interleukin; GM-CSF, granulocyte-macrophage colony-stimulating factor; G-CSF, granulocyte colony-stimulating factor; M-CSF, macrophage colony-stimulating factor; EPO, erythropoietin; TPO, thrombopoietin.

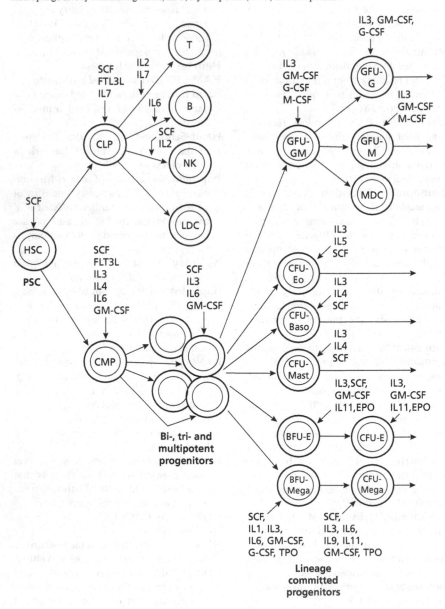

Figure 42   Helper T cell.
A diagrammatic representation of the interaction between a helper T cell and a B cell. The B cell binds an exogenous antigen, by means of its membrane immunoglobulin–CD79a complex, and processes it to a peptide which it presents, in a groove of an HLA type II molecule, to a helper T cell. The peptide, in its HLA type II context, is recognized by the CD3–T cell receptor (TCR)–CD4 complex. Other specialized antigen-presenting cells (e.g. macrophages and dendritic cells) can similarly present processed antigen to helper T cells. Binding of the helper T cell to the B cell also involves binding of CD2 on the T cell to CD58 on the B cell. CD54 is up-regulated on activated B cells and binds to CD11a/CD18 on T cells. In addition, there is binding of CD28 on the T cell to CD80 or CD86 on the B cell, giving stimulatory signals, or binding of CD152 to CD80 or CD86 on the B cell, giving inhibitory signals. CD154 (CD40 ligand) on the T cell binds to CD40 on the B cell, giving signals for somatic hypermutation and immunoglobulin class switching. Signalling is bidirectional. The B cell signals to the helper T cell to become activated and proliferate while the T cell signals to the B cell to mature into a plasma cell and switch from secreting IgM to secreting other classes of immunoglobulin. The progeny of the helper T cell that has been activated by an antigen-presenting B cell can migrate to other tissues where they initiate a cytotoxic or inflammatory response if they encounter target cells expressing the appropriate antigen.

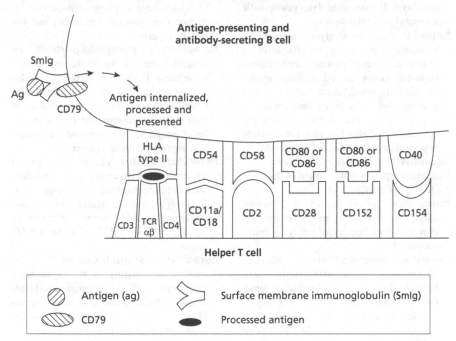

molecule; each immunoglobulin molecule has two light chains (κ or λ) and two heavy chains (γ, α, μ, ε or δ)

heavy chain disease   a lymphoproliferative disorder or **plasma cell dyscrasia** in which there is synthesis of **heavy chain** (γ, α or μ) rather than synthesis of complete immunoglobulin molecules

Heinz body   an erythrocyte inclusion composed of denatured haemoglobin, detected by exposure to vital dyes such as methyl violet

helix–loop–helix   *see* bHLH

HELLP syndrome   a syndrome occurring in pregnancy comprising Haemolysis, Elevated Liver enzymes and Low Platelets

helper T cell   a T lymphocyte that promotes antigen secretion by B lymphocytes (*see* type 1 and type 2 helper T cell) (Fig. 42)

hemighost   an erythrocyte in which all the haemoglobin appears retracted into one half of the cell leaving the remainder of the cell as an empty membrane; hemighosts are characteristic of oxidant damage and the presence of an unstable haemoglobin

hemizygosity having a single copy of a gene on a single X chromosome, e.g. hemizygosity for G6PD deficiency

hemizygote an individual having one copy of a gene on a single X chromosome, e.g. a male with a singe copy of a mutant *G6PD* gene

HEMPAS Hereditary Erythroid Multinuclearity with Positive Acidified Serum test—type II **congenital dyserythropoietic anaemia** (*see* **acid lysis test**)

heparin a sulphated **glycosaminoglycan**, a naturally occurring anticoagulant in human and animal tissues, which inhibits **thrombin**, **factor Xa** and activated intrinsic pathway coagulation factors *in vivo* and *in vitro*; as a therapeutic product, it has usually been extracted from pig intestines (*see* also **low molecular weight heparin** and **unfractionated heparin**)

hepatitis inflammation of the liver

hepatomegaly enlargement of the liver

HER2 *see ERBB2*

hereditary passed down from a parent, usually by means of genes located on chromosomes but occasionally by mitochondrial genes

hereditary elliptocytosis an inherited abnormality of the erythrocyte membrane leading to elliptical red cells, sometimes to haemolysis and occasionally to a haemolytic anaemia, resulting from mutations in the *SPTA1*, *SPTB*, *AE1* or *EPB41* genes

hereditary glucosyl ceramide lipidosis *see* **Gaucher's disease**

hereditary haemochromatosis a hereditary condition leading to iron overload; in adults, the condition usually results from mutation in the *HFE* gene but in a minority it results from mutation in the *TFR2* gene; the juvenile form results from mutation of a gene on chromosome 1q

hereditary hyperferritinaemia–cataract syndrome a constitutional abnormality with **autosomal dominant** inheritance, characterized by cataracts and elevated serum **ferritin** without any elevation of serum iron concentration or any tissue iron overload; the cataracts may be congenital or may develop during childhood or adult life; the underlying defect is in synthesis of L type ferritin, which is increased and poorly regulated as a result of a mutation affecting the **iron-responsive element** of L ferritin **mRNA**; serum ferritin is L type rather than a mixture of L and H.

hereditary persistence of fetal haemoglobin an inherited condition in which fetal haemoglobin persists at higher than normal levels beyond the neonatal period

hereditary pyropoikilocytosis an inherited abnormality of the erythrocyte membrane leading to striking poikilocytosis and severe haemolytic anaemia, usually consequent on inheritance of two different elliptogenic mutations or an elliptogenic mutation and a common low expression allele, α spectrin^{LELY}

hereditary spherocytosis an inherited abnormality of the erythrocyte membrane leading to spherical red cells, compensated haemolysis and sometimes haemolytic anaemia, resulting from mutations in *ANK1*, *SPTA1*, *SPTB*, *EA1* or *EPB42* genes

hereditary stomatocytosis an inherited abnormality of the erythrocyte membrane leading to formation of bowl-shaped cells, referred to as **stomatocytes** (Fig. 43), and either compensated haemolysis or haemolytic anaemia

hereditary xerocytosis an inherited abnormality of the erythrocyte membrane leading to increased cation flux and either compensated haemolysis or haemolytic anaemia

Hermansky–Pudlak syndrome a heterogeneous inherited syndrome with **autosomal recessive** inheritance characterized by oculocutaneous albinism and defective platelet function, the latter resulting from a storage pool defect; some cases result from mutation of the *HPS1* gene on chromosome 10; there is increased lipofuscin in bone marrow macrophages

Figure 43 Stomatocytes.
Three stomatocytes, showing that in three dimensions a stomatocyte is bowl shaped.

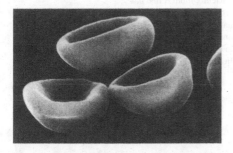

herpesviruses a group of viruses including chicken pox/varicella, the Epstein–Barr virus and cytomegalovirus

herpes zoster shingles, recrudescence of varicella-zoster virus infection, causing a vesicular rash in the distribution of a peripheral nerve

heterochromatin condensed, genetically inactive chromatin

heterodimer a **dimer** composed of two dissimilar polypeptide chains

heterogeneous irregularly distributed

heterophile antibody an antibody recognizing antigens on cells of another species

heteroplasmy the presence in a cell of mutated and non-mutated mitochondrial DNA

heterozygote an individual who has a single copy of a specified autosomal or (in a female) X chromosome gene

heterozygous having a single copy of a specified autosomal or (in a female) X chromosome gene

hexokinase an enzyme in the erythrocyte **glycolytic pathway** (*see* Fig. 33, p. 113)

HFE a gene on chromosome 6, mutation of which can cause **hereditary haemochromatosis** in **homozygotes** and **compound heterozygotes**; previously known as *HLA-H*; it encodes a protein that interacts with the transferrin receptor (product of the *TFRC* gene), negatively affecting cellular iron uptake from transferrin; the HFE protein binds to β_2-microglobulin, binding being essential for transport of the HFE product to the cell surface where it combines with transferrin receptor, reducing its affinity for iron; the C282Y mutation, present in most patients with haemochromatosis, prevents the binding of the HFE product to β_2-microglobulin

high grade a term used to describe aggressive, highly malignant lymphomas

high hyperdiploid having between 51–60 chromosomes

highly active antiretroviral therapy (HAART) triple-drug antiretroviral therapy for HIV infection employing a combination of drugs from three classes: (i) nucleoside-analogue reverse-transcriptase inhibitors, non-nucleoside-analogue reverse-transcriptase inhibitors and protease inhibitors

high performance liquid chromatography (HPLC) a method of separating proteins, such as haemoglobin variants, from each other on the basis of characteristics such as size, hydrophobicity and ionic strength; a solution of proteins is passed through a specially designed column with different proteins emerging after a characteristic period of time, referred to as the retention time (Fig. 44)

HIP a gene, **H**untingtin **I**nteracting **P**rotein 1, gene map locus 7q11.2; encodes a protein which interacts with Huntingtin and F-actin, and is involved in dopamine receptor endocytosis at clathrin coated pits; Huntingtin is the product of the gene that is mutated in Huntington's disease; *HIP* contributes to the *HIP1-PDGFRB* fusion gene in chronic myelomonocytic leukaemia associated with t(5;7)(q33;q11.2); in the resulting fusion protein the extracellular domains of PDGFRβ are replaced with almost the entire HIP1 molecule, leading to constitutive receptor oligomerization and activation.

hirudin an antithrombotic substance produced in the salivary glands of the medicinal leech, *Hirudo medicinalis*; recombinant forms are **desirudin** and **lepirudin**

histamine an inflammatory mediator secreted by **mast cells** and **basophils**

histidine-rich glycoprotein a plasma protein, synthesized by platelets, that binds to plasminogen, thus reducing the amount of circulating plasminogen avail-

Figure 44   High performance liquid chromatography.
Separation of normal haemoglobins from each other by high performance liquid
chromatography (HPLC): (a) normal adult showing, from left to right, haemoglobin
F (shaded), glycosylated haemoglobin (long black arrow), haemoglobin A that has
undergone post-translational modification (short black arrow), haemoglobin
A (hollow arrow) and haemoglobin A_2 (shaded); (b) premature baby showing, from
left to right, haemoglobin F which has undergone post-translational modification
(short arrows), haemoglobin F (shaded), and haemoglobin A (hollow arrow); note
that in this premature baby there is negligible haemoglobin A_2.

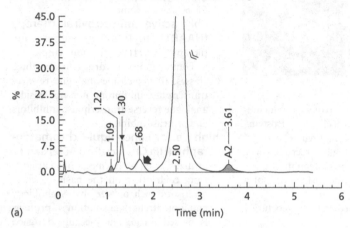

(a)

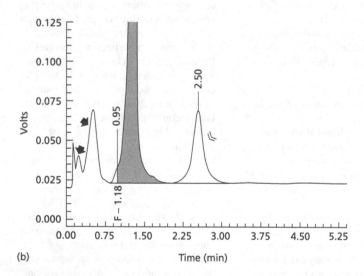

(b)

able for conversion to plasmin; it therefore has an antifibrinolytic effect and
deficiency, which is very rare, is associated with an increased likelihood of
thrombosis

histiocyte   an alternative designation of
a **macrophage**; neoplasms of histiocytic

and related lineages are designated in **the
WHO classification** as shown in Table 6

histiocytic lymphoma   an outmoded
designation of large cell lymphoma of
B- or T-lymphocyte lineage rather than
of histiocyte lineage; to avoid confusion,
a tumour resembling a lymphoma but

Table 6 The WHO classification of histiocytic and dendritic cell neoplasms.

Histiocytic sarcoma
Langerhans cell histiocytosis
Langerhans cell sarcoma
Interdigitating dendritic cell sarcoma/tumour
Follicular dendritic cell sarcoma/tumour
Dendritic cell sarcoma, not otherwise classified

composed of histiocytes should be referred to as a 'histiocytic sarcoma' (*see* Table 6)

histiocytic medullary reticulosis a disease characterized by infiltration of tissues including the bone marrow by strikingly haemophagocytic histiocytes; once thought to be a histiocyte malignancy, it is now known that at least the majority of cases are reactive

histiocytosis increased macrophages in bone marrow or other tissues

histiocytosis X a former designation of **Langerhans cell histiocytosis**, a neoplasm of **Langerhans cells** (*see* Table 6)

histogram a graphical representation of the distribution of measurements using rectangular bars to represent the relative frequency of a certain measured value (Fig. 45)

histology the study of the structure of tissues by examination of stained tissue sections

histones proteins bound to **DNA** in chromosomes

histoplasmosis a disease caused by infection by the fungus, *Histoplasma capsulatum*

HIV the **human immunodeficiency virus**

HLA a complex of genes at 6p21.3 encoding the α chain of class I HLA antigens and the α and β chains of class II HLA molecules

HLA human leucocyte antigen

HLA type I deficiency an immune deficiency syndrome (*see* **bare lymphocyte syndrome**) in which a mutation in either the *TAP1* or *TAP2* genes at 6p21.3 means that there is defective delivery of peptides to developing type I HLA molecules, which are therefore unstable and are not efficiently transported to the cell surface

HLA type II deficiency an immune deficiency syndrome (*see* **bare lymphocyte syndrome**) resulting from a mutation in

genes that regulate the transcription of type II HLA genes: either the transactivator gene, *CIITA* at 16p13, or transcription factor genes—*RFXAP* on 13q, *RFX5* at 1q21 or *RFXANK*; numbers of CD4+ T cells are greatly reduced

HLF a gene, **H**epatic **L**eukaemic **F**actor, gene map locus 17q21-22, encodes a leucine zipper transcription factor which is normally expressed in liver, kidney and neurones within the central nervous system; *HLF* contributes to the *E2A-HLF* fusion gene in B-lineage acute lymphoblastic leukaemia associated with t(17;19)(q21-22;p13); two different rearrangements between *E2A* and *HLF* are known; in each case, the chimeric protein comprises the amino-terminal transactivation domain of **E2A** (TCF3) and the carboxyl-terminal leucine zipper dimerization domain of HLF; both fusion proteins induce expression of the zinc finger transcriptional repressor slug, which in turn down-regulates the expression of pro-apoptotic proteins

HLXB9 homeobox gene HB9, gene map locus 7q36, encodes a homeobox transcription factor which is expressed in CD34+ but not in CD34− bone marrow cells and is down-regulated during lineage commitment; *HLXB9* contributes to an *HLXB9-ETV6* fusion gene in infants with acute myeloid leukaemia associated with t(7;12)(q36;p13); germline mutations in this gene are associated with the currarino triad (sacral agenesis, ureteric and perianal dysgenesis)

hMRE11 a gene, gene map locus 11q21; encodes a DNA repair enzyme expressed in all proliferating cells; *hMRE11* is mutated in ataxia-telangiectasia-like disorder

Figure 45   Histograms.

Two histograms showing the distribution of serum vitamin B_{12} concentrations in
80 healthy volunteers: (a) plotted on an arithmetic scale, showing that the distribution
is not Gaussian; (b) re-plotted on a logarithmic scale, showing that the distribution of
the data is now Gaussian, i.e. the data have a log normal distribution.

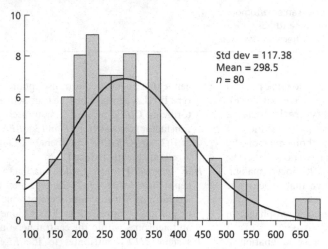

Std dev = 117.38
Mean = 298.5
n = 80

(a) ACB12

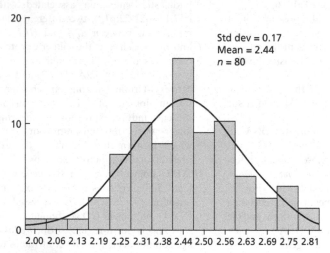

Std dev = 0.17
Mean = 2.44
n = 80

(b) LOGACB12

Hodgkin's cell   a mononuclear giant cell with a large nucleolus that is part of the neoplastic population in Hodgkin's disease

Hodgkin's disease or Hodgkin lymphoma   a lymphoma characterized by certain histological features, specifically by the presence of **Reed–Sternberg cells** and mononuclear **Hodgkin's cells** in an appropriate background of lymphocytes, eosinophils and fibroblasts with variable collagen fibrosis; the neoplastic cells are almost always B lymphocytes (but in 1–2% of patients are T lymphocytes); designated in the **WHO classification** as shown in Table 7, the disease characteristically

Table 7 The WHO classification of Hodgkin Lymphoma (Hodgkin's disease).

Nodular lymphocyte-predominant Hodgkin lymphoma
Classical Hodgkin lymphoma
Lymphocyte-rich classical Hodgkin lymphoma
Nodular sclerosis classical Hodgkin lymphoma
Mixed cellularity classical Hodgkin lymphoma
Lymphocyte-depleted classical Hodgkin lymphoma

presents with enlargement of lymph nodes (*see* Figs 61 and 70, pp. 188 and 210)

hof a German term indicating the hollow in a nucleus in which the Golgi apparatus is located

homeobox a DNA binding domain characteristic of a family of transcription factors that included PBX1 and HOX11; *see also HOX* genes

homeodomain *see HOX* genes

homocysteine an amino acid, increased plasma levels of which, whether inherited or acquired in origin, are associated with an increased thrombotic risk

homodimer a **dimer** with two identical chains

homogeneous evenly distributed

homogeneously staining region (hsr) a segment of a chromosome that stains homogeneously, indicating amplification of DNA sequences

homologous structurally similar, in some circumstances suggesting a common origin in the remote past (e.g. homologous genes in different species)

homologous chromosomes a matching pair of chromosomes, one derived from each parent of the individual

homology having structural similarity

homotypic having the same nature, e.g. homotypic adhesion is adhesion of cells to other cells of the same type

homozygous having identical **alleles** at a given locus

hookworm a parasitic intestinal round worm which may cause **eosinophilia** and **iron deficiency anaemia**

hormone a long distance chemical mediator

horned cell a **keratocyte**, an erythrocyte with two or four symmetrical spicules (*see* Fig. 50, p. 147)

host the recipient of a transplant (or an individual harbouring a parasite)

Howell–Jolly body a nuclear inclusion in an erythrocyte

Howship's lacuna a hollow on the surface of a bony spicule occupied by an **osteoclast**

HOX **genes** genes encoding a superfamily of evolutionarily conserved transcription factors which share a 60 amino-acid DNA-binding domain, the homeodomain; they fall into two classes—I and II; class I genes are organized into 4 clusters (A,B,C,D) located on chromosomes 7, 17, 12 and 2 respectively; class II genes are dispersed throughout the genome and may have divergent homeodomain sequences; clusters B and C play a role in erythropoiesis, whilst members of cluster A are predominantly expressed in cells of granulocytic lineage; virtually all *HOX* genes of the A, B and C clusters are expressed in pluripotent haemopoietic stem cells—a feature lost with the onset of lineage commitment; several non-cluster *HOX* genes are also important in normal haemopoiesis

HOX11 a gene, **H**omeobo**x** **11**, also known as **T**-**C**ell **L**eukaemia **3**, *TCL3*, and *TLX1*; gene map locus 10q24, which encodes a non-cluster homeobox transcription factor which is thought to play a role in splanchnic development; *HOX11* is dysregulated:

- by proximity to the *TCRAD* (αδ) locus in T-lineage acute lymphoblastic leukaemia associated with t(10;14)(q24;q11)
- by proximity to the *TCRB* gene at 7q35 in T-lineage acute lymphoblastic leukaemia associated with t(7;10)(q35;q24)

HOX11L2 a gene, **H**omeobo**x** **11**-**L**ike **2**, also known as **T**-cell **L**eukaemia homeobo**x**

3 (*TLX3*), and **R**espiratory **N**eurone homeobox (*RNX*); gene map locus 5q35.1; encodes a non-cluster homeobox transcription factor which is thought to play a role in the development of the medulla oblongata; is transcriptionally activated, probably by proximity to the transcription regulatory elements of *BCL11B*, in a quite common t(5;14)(q35;q32) cryptic translocation in T-acute lymphoblastic leukaemia

HOXA9   a gene, **Ho**meobox **A9**; gene map locus 7p15-p14.2, encodes a class I homeobox transcription factor that is thought to be important in myeloid differentiation; *HOXA9* contributes to the *NUP98-HOXA9* fusion gene in M2 acute myeloid leukaemia associated with t(7;11)(p15;p15) (*see also NUP98*); the fusion protein functions as a transcription factor; in acute myeloid leukaemia *HOXA9* expression correlates strongly with a worse prognosis

HOXA11   a gene, **Ho**meobox **A11**, gene map locus 7p15-p14.2, encodes a class I homeobox transcription factor that is important in myeloid differentiation; contributed to a *NUP98-HOXA11* fusion gene in a patient with Ph-negative chronic myeloid leukaemia transforming rapidly to M2 acute myeloid leukaemia; germline mutations in the homeodomain of *HOXA11* are seen in radioulnar synostosis in association with amegakaryocytic thrombocytopenia.

HOXD13   a gene, **Ho**meobox **D13**, also known as *HOX4I*, gene map locus 2q31-q32, encodes a class I homeobox transcription factor that is not normally expressed in haemopoietic tissues; it contributes to a *NUP98-HOXD13* fusion gene, one of two fusion genes present in therapy-related and *de novo* acute myeloid leukaemia associated with t(2;11)(q31;p15); germline mutations in this gene are associated with synpolydactyly with foot anomalies

Hoyerall–Hreidarsson syndrome   a syndrome of **aplastic anaemia**, immunodeficiency, microcephaly and cerebellar hypoplasia resulting from a mutation in the *DKC1* gene; a severe variant of X-linked **dyskeratosis congenita**

HPA   **human platelet antigen**

HPLC   **high performance liquid chromatography** (previously 'high pressure liquid chromatography')

HPRT   an X chromosome gene encoding **hypoxanthine-guanine phosphoribosyltransferase**, mutation of which can convey resistance to 6-thioguanine therapy; it is sometimes used for clonality studies

HSP89A   a gene, **H**eat **S**hock **P**rotein **89 A**lpha, gene map locus unknown, encodes heat shock protein 89α; the gene contributed to an *HSP89A-BCL6* fusion gene in a high grade gastric B-cell lymphoma

hsr   a cytogenetic abbreviation indicating a **homogeneously staining region**

HTLV-I   **human T-cell lymphotropic virus I**

HTLV-I-associated myelopathy (HAM)   a myelopathy caused by HTLV-I, the retrovirus which also causes **adult T-cell leukaemia/lymphoma**

hTR   the gene encoding telomerase RNA, mutation of which can lead to autosomal dominant **dyskeratosis congenita**

human herpesvirus 8 (HHV8)   a herpesvirus that has an aetiological role in **primary effusion lymphoma** and **Cattleman's disease**

human immunodeficiency virus (HIV)   the retrovirus that causes the **acquired immune deficiency syndrome** (AIDS)

human leucocyte antigen (HLA)   a group of highly polymorphic cell surface antigens, encoded by genes at 6p21.3, involved in self and non-self recognition, tolerance, rejection of **allografts** and **graft-versus-host disease**, divided into HLA class I, class II and class III antigens

human leucocyte antigens, class I (HLA class I)   molecules that are mainly involved in the presentation of endogenous antigen-derived peptides to CD8+ cytotoxic T cells and NK cells; expressed on most somatic cells but to a varying degree; expressed on all leucocytes and on platelets but negative or weakly expressed on erythrocytes; composed of a heavy chain that is encoded by genes at 6p21.3 and a common light chain, β2 **microglobulin**, which is encoded by a gene on chromosome 15; there are

Table 8 Human neutrophil antigens – recommended terminology and the proteins on which they are expressed.

System	Antigen	Protein on which antigen is located
HNA-1	HNA-1a (previously NA1)	FcγRIII (CD16)
	HNA-1b (previously NA2)	
	HNA-1c (previously SH)	
HNA-2	HNA-2a (previously NB1)	Gp58–64, a GPI-linked glycoprotein
HNA-3	HNA-3a (previously5b)	Gp70–95
HNA-4	HNA-4a (previously MART)	CD11b
HNA-5	HNA-5a (previously CND)	CD11a

Table 9 Human platelet antigens – recommended terminology and the platelet glycoproteins on which they are expressed.

System	Antigens	Glycoprotein on which antigens are carried
HPA-1	HPA-1a (previously Pl^{A1}, Zw^a)	IIIa
	HPA-1b (previously Pl^{A2}, Zw^b)	
HPA-2	HPA-2a (previously Ko^b)	Ibα
	HPA-2b (previously Ko^a, Sib^a)	
HPA-3	HPA-3a (previously Bak^a, Lek^a)	IIb
	HPA-3b (previously Bak^b)	
HPA-4	HPA-4a (previously Yuk^b, Pen^a)	IIIa
	HPA-4b (previously Yuk^a, Pen^b)	
HPA-5	HPA-5a (previously Br^b, Zav^b)	Ia
	HPA-5b (previously Br^a, Zav^a, Hc^a)	
HPA-6w	HPA-6bw (previously Ca^a, Tu^a)	IIIa
HPA-7w	HPA-7bw (previously Mo)	IIIa
HPA-8w	HPA-8bw (previously Sr^a)	IIIa
HPA-9w	HPA-9bw (previously Max^a)	IIb
HPA-10w	HPA-10bw (previously La^a)	IIIa
HPA-11w	HPA-11bw (previously Gro^a)	IIIa
HPA-12w	HPA-12bw (previously Iy^a)	Ibβ
HPA-13w	HPA-13bw (previously Sit^a)	GP1a

three classical HLA class I groups of antigens (HLA-A, HLA-B and HLA-C) and three non-classical (HLA-D, HLA-E and HLA-F)

human leucocyte antigens, class II (HLA class II) molecules that are mainly involved in the presentation of exogenous antigen-derived peptides to CD4+ helper T cells; expressed on B cells, activated T cells, monocytes, macrophages, dendritic cells, activated neutrophils and thymic epithelium; class II antigens are heterodimers encoded by genes at 6p21.3, falling into HLA-DM, HLA-DO, HLA-DP, HLA-DQ and HLA-DR groups

human neutrophil antigen (HNA) neutrophil-specific **alloantigens** encoded by genes at 5 loci (Table 8)

human platelet antigen (HPA) platelet-specific alloantigens encoded by genes found at at least 13 loci; the **ISBT** has agreed a standardized nomenclature (Table 9)

human T-cell lymphotropic virus I (HTLV-I) a retrovirus that causes **adult**

T-cell leukaemia/lymphoma and **HTLV-I-associated myelopathy**

humoral immunity antibody-mediated immunity

HUT11 a locus at 18q12-q21 where various alleles encode antigens of the Kidd blood group antigen system which also function as the human erythroid urea transporter; genes at this locus are the codominant *Jka* and *Jkb* and various *Jk null* alleles that result from mutation of the wild type *Jka* or *Jkb*; a Jk(a-b-) phenotype (rare except in Finns and Polynesians) can result from homozygosity or compound heterozygosity for *Jk null* alleles or from inheritance of the dominant unlinked *In* inhibitor gene, *In(JK)*

hyalomere the agranular periphery of a platelet

hybridization the annealing of complementary sequences of DNA or RNA, e.g. Southern and Northern blotting

hybridoma a clone of cells capable of producing a monoclonal antibody, produced by fusion of an antibody-producing cell with a mouse myeloma cell

hydrops fetalis severe oedema and serous effusions in a fetus or neonate; may be caused by severe anaemia, as in **haemoglobin Bart's hydrops fetalis**, severe **haemolytic disease of the newborn** and intrauterine **parvovirus B19** infection

hydroxocobalamin the form of **vitamin B₁₂** used for therapy

hydroxyurea an **antimetabolite** used to treat chronic myeloid leukaemias and myeloproliferative disorders

hyperbetalipoproteinaemia increased concentration of plasma beta lipoproteins

hyperbilirubinaemia increased plasma bilirubin concentration

hypercalcaemia increased plasma calcium concentration

hypercholesterolaemia increased serum cholesterol concentration

hyperchromatic showing increased uptake of stain, thus appearing dense

hyperchromia (i) increased staining of red cells reflecting an increased haemoglobin concentration within individual red cells (ii) increased staining of nuclei, consequent on altered chromatin structure

hyperchylomicronaemia increased plasma concentration of chylomicrons

hyperdiploid having more than 46 chromosomes

hyperendemic constantly present in a community and having a high prevalence

hypereosinophilic syndrome a syndrome of cardiac and other tissue damage resulting from an increased eosinophil count with tissue damage consequent on the release of eosinophil granule contents (*see* **idiopathic hypereosinophilic syndrome**)

hyperferritinaemia with congenital cataracts *see* **hereditary hyperferritinaemia-cataract syndrome**

hypergammaglobulinaemia increased concentration of serum immunoglobulins

hypergranular promyelocytic leukaemia acute myeloid leukaemia with arrest of maturation at the promyelocyte stage with the promyelocytes being hypergranular

hyperhomocysteinaemia an inherited metabolic defect resulting from deficiency of cystathionine β-synthase, associated with an increased risk of thrombosis

hyperimmunoglobulin D syndrome an **autosomal recessive** condition, resulting from mutation in the mevalonate kinase gene, characterized by periodic fever with leucocytosis and an acute phase response

hyperimmunoglobulin E syndrome a congenital immunodeficiency syndrome characterized by abscesses, osteopenia, eosinophilia and unusual facial features; it maps to chromosome 4

hyperimmunoglobulin M syndrome either (i) an X-linked immune deficiency syndrome in which a mutation in the gene at Xq26.3-27.1 encoding **CD154** results in failure of **helper T-cells** to express CD154: helper T cells therefore cannot bind to **CD40** on antigen-presenting B cells (*see* Fig. 42, p. 123), leading to a failure of class switching and susceptibility to cancer and autoimmune disease or (ii) an autosomal recessive syndrome, some cases resulting from mutation in the activation-induced cytidine deaminase gene at 12p13, an mRNA-editing enzyme, with resultant IgG and IgA deficiency with normal or elevated IgM

hyperkalaemia increased plasma potassium concentration

hyperlipaemia increased concentration of blood lipids

hypermutation *see* **somatic hypermutation**

hypernatraemia increased plasma sodium concentration

hyperparathyroidism increased activity of the parathyroid glands

hyperplasia increase of the number of cells of a certain lineage or tissue

hyperreactive malarial splenomegaly splenomegaly and increased polyclonal IgM as a consequence of chronic malaria, previously referred to as tropical splenomegaly

hypersplenism **splenomegaly** leading to **pancytopenia** as a consequence of pooling of cells in the spleen and a decreased erythrocyte lifespan

hypertension increase of blood pressure

hyperthyroidism overactivity of the thyroid gland

hypertonic having an osmolarity greater than normal; more concentrated than normal

hypertrophy overdevelopment of an organ or tissue; increased size rather than increased number of cells

hyperuricaemia increased serum uric acid concentration

hyperviscosity a pathological increase in the viscosity of the blood or plasma, may be a feature of multiple myeloma or **Waldenström's macroglobulinaemia**

hyperviscosity syndrome a clinical syndrome resulting from hyperviscosity; clinical features may include mental changes and reduced level of consciousness, visual changes resulting from effects on the retina, congestive cardiac failure and bleeding; may result from **multiple myeloma** or **Waldenström's macroglobuli-**

naemia or, less often, from a marked increased in polyclonal immunoglobulins

hyphaema bleeding into the anterior chamber of the eye

hypochromia reduced staining of erythrocytes

hypodiploid having fewer than 46 but more than 23 chromosomes

hypogranular neutrophil neutrophil with reduced secondary granules

hypogranular variant of promyelocytic leukaemia a variant form of hypergranular promyelocytic leukaemia in which the leukaemic promyelocytes appear hypogranular rather than hypergranular; the leukaemic cells have characteristic bilobed nuclei

hyponatraemia reduced plasma sodium concentration

hypoparathyroidism reduced activity of the parathyroid glands

hypoplasia underdevelopment or regression of an organ, tissue or cell lineage

hypoplastic acute myeloid leukaemia acute myeloid leukaemia that is unusual in that the bone marrow is hypocellular rather than hypercellular

hypoplastic anaemia an anaemia, usually pancytopenia, as a consequence of bone marrow hypoplasia; usually part of the spectrum of **aplastic anaemia**

hypopyon accumulation of leucocytes in the anterior chamber of the eye, a rare complication of leukaemia

hyposplenism reduced or absent splenic function

hypothyroidism reduced activity of the thyroid gland

hypotonic having an osmolarity less than normal; more dilute than normal

hypoventilation reduced breathing

hypoxanthine-guanine phosphoribosyltransferase a purine salvage enzyme encoded by *HPRT*

hypoxia inadequate supply of oxygen to cells

I

i an antigen composed of repeats of linear poly-N-acetyllactosaminoglycan, expressed on fetal red cells, in adults largely converted to the I antigen, branched poly-N-acetyllactosaminoglycan, by the action of β-1,6-N acetylglucosaminyl transferase

i (or iso) an **isochromosome**

i phenotype the null phenotype of the I blood group, resulting from deletion or mutation of the *IgnT* gene, in Asians associated with congenital cataract

I an antigen composed of repeats of branched poly-N-acetyllactosaminoglycan, on adult red cells, produced by the action of β-1,6-N acetylglucosaminyl transferase on i antigen

I-branching β-1,6-N acetylglucosaminyl transferase an enzyme encoded by the *I* or *IgnT* gene at 9q21, which converts the i antigen to the I antigen

I cell disease a congenital metabolic disorder, associated with vacuolated lymphocytes

ICSH International Council (previously Committee) for Standardization in Haematology

idiopathic literally 'of unknown cause' but the term often continues in use long after the cause of a disorder is known

idiopathic hypereosinophilic syndrome a syndrome defined as a hypereosinophilia of unknown cause, persisting for at least six months and with associated tissue damage

idiopathic myelofibrosis bone marrow fibrosis consequent on a chronic myeloproliferative disorder (but conventionally excluding cases following polycythaemia, rubra vera, essential thrombocythaemia and chronic granulocytic leukaemia, which are more likely to be designated, for example, 'post-polycythaemia myelofibrosis')

idiopathic thrombocytopenic purpura (ITP) a previous designation of **autoimmune thrombocytopenic purpura**

idiotype the specific surface antigens which permit a clone of lymphocytes or plasma cells to be recognized, dependent on the specific immunoglobulin which is expressed on the surface membrane

Ig immunoglobulin, e.g. IgG, IgA, IgM, IgE or IgD

IGH the Immunoglobulin Heavy chain locus, at 14q32 encoding the heavy chains of immunoglobulin; there are multiple V (variable), D (diversity), J (joining) and C (constant) gene segments; rearrangement of gene segments at the *IGH* locus occurs, producing a gene encoding a specific heavy chain (Fig. 46); the *IGH* enhancer can contribute to oncogenesis by dysregulating many other genes such as *BCL2*, *BCL3*, *BCL6*, *BCL7A*, *BCL8*, *BCL9*, *BCL10*, *BCL11A*, *CDK6*, *C4ST1*, *Cyclin D1*, *Cyclin D2*, *FCγRIIB*, *FGFR3*, *IL3*, *IRF4*, *MMSET*, *MAF*, *MUM2*, *MUM3*, *MYC*, *NF-κB2*, *PAFAH2*, *PAX5* and *RCK*.

IGK the locus at 2p12 encoding the κ light chain of immunoglobulin

IGL the locus at 22q11 encoding the λ light chain of immunoglobulin

IKAROS a gene, also known as Zinc Finger protein, subfamily 1A, member 1, *ZNFN1A1*, gene map locus 7p13-p11.2, encodes the archetypal member of a family of lymphoid-restricted zinc finger transcription factors that are considered master regulators of lymphocyte differentiation; there are at least 8 alternatively spliced transcripts encoding isoforms with

Figure 46 The *IGH* locus and the generation of antigen receptor diversity.

Antigen receptors for B cells (immunoglobulins, Igs) and T cells (T cell receptors, TCRs) are heterodimers in which each polypeptide is composed of an amino terminal variable (V) region joined to a constant (C) region. Ig and TCR genes are similar in organization and permit the generation of proteins with V domains that are unique to the cells that make them. The V domains of IgH chains (and TCR β or δ chains) are encoded by a combination of V_H, D and J segments; the partner polypeptide (Ig light chains or TCR α or γ) is assembled from V and J segments only. There are a few hundred such segments at the *IGH* locus (and a similar number at each Ig light chain locus) and of these, about 30% are pseudogenes; yet it is estimated that the total diversity for human immunoglobulins is 10^{14}. Two strategies allow for the generation of such huge diversity from so few genes:

(i) T and B cells use a site-specific DNA recombination mechanism called V(D)J recombination to assemble a V region gene from germ line DNA by cutting and joining together randomly chosen combinations of one of each of the segments. The intervening DNA is excised and lost from the genome of the mature lymphocyte. This process is catalysed by RAG proteins (encoded by <u>R</u>ecombination <u>A</u>ctivating <u>G</u>enes) which recognize recombination signal sequences (RSSs) flanking each segment. The RSSs ensure the correct order of V(D)J recombination is followed and prevent V–V or D–D joining. The recombination process is imprecise and leads to small deletions and random insertions (*) at the V–D and D–J junctions of functional *IGH* loci, adding additional diversity.

(ii) Mature B cells exhibit the phenomenon of somatic hypermutation, whereby random single base changes are directed to gene segments encoding antigen binding pockets in rearranged VDJ genes (▲). This may either increase or decrease the specificity of the expressed Ig for its antigen. The mechanism of this process is obscure.

(iii) In the case of *IGH* genes, the same V region can be joined to several different C regions in the descendants of an original B cell (isotype or class switching), so permitting the same antigen specificity to be utilized in different biological contexts. The mechanism of this is unclear.

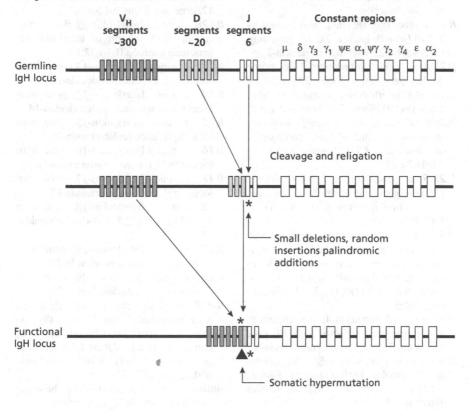

common N-terminal and C-terminal domains (Ik1 through Ik8); an in-frame deletion of 10 amino acids upstream of the transcription activation domain and adjacent to the C-terminal zinc fingers of Ik-2, Ik-4, Ik-7, and Ik-8 has been reported in childhood acute lymphoblastic leukaemia; *IKAROS* fuses to *BCL6* as a result of the t(3;7)(q27;p12) translocation in diffuse large B-cell lymphoma; *IKAROS* mutations and decreased activity are associated with disease progression in chronic granulocytic leukaemia

IL interleukin

IL1A, IL1B two genes, gene map locus 2q14, encoding Interleukin-1α (acidic) and Interleukin-1β (neutral); a TATA box mutation in the *IL1B* promoter is associated with an increased risk of hypochlorhydria and gastric cancer after *H. pylori* infection

IL2 a gene, Interleukin-2, also known as T-Cell Growth Factor, *TCGF*, gene map locus 4q26-q27, encodes **interleukin-2**

IL2RA a gene, Interleukin-2 Receptor Alpha, gene map locus 22q11.2-q13, encodes **interleukin-2 receptor** α, also known as **CD25** and Tac (Activated T cell)

IL2RB a gene, Interleukin-2 Receptor Beta, encodes interleukin-2 receptor β, also known as **CD122**, gene map locus 22q11.2-q13

IL2RG a gene, Interleukin-2 Receptor Gamma, gene map locus Xq13, encodes interleukin-2 receptor γ, also known as **CD132**

IL3 a gene, Interleukin-3, gene map locus 5q31, encodes **interleukin-3**; *IL3* is dysregulated by proximity to the *IGH* locus in acute lymphoblastic leukaemia associated with t(5;14)(q31;q32) leading to eosinophilia

IL4 a gene, Interleukin-4, also known as B-cell Stimulatory Factor 1, *BSF1*; gene map locus 5q31.1; encodes **interleukin-4**

IL5 a gene, Interleukin-5; also known as Eosinophil Differentiation Factor, *EDF*; gene map locus 5q31.1; encodes **interleukin-5**

IL6 a gene, Interleukin-6, also known as interferon beta 2, Hepatocyte Stimulatory Factor, *HSF* and B-cell Stimulatory

Factor 2, *BSF2*; gene map locus 7p21; encodes **interleukin-6**

IL7 a gene, Interleukin-7, gene map locus 8q12-q13, encodes **interleukin-7**

IL8 a gene, Interleukin-8, also known as chemokine ligand 8, *CXCL8* and Neutrophil-Activating Peptide 1, *NAP1*; gene map locus 4q12-q13; encodes **interleukin-8**

IL9 a gene, Interleukin-9, also known as T-cell/mast cell growth factor P40, gene map locus 5q31.1, encodes **interleukin-9**

IL10 a gene, Interleukin-10, also known as Cytokine Synthesis Inhibitory Factor, *CSIF*, gene map locus 1q31-q32, encodes **interleukin-10**

IL11 a gene, Interleukin-11, gene map locus 19q13.3-13.4, encodes **interleukin-11**

IL12A a gene, Interleukin-12 Alpha chain, encodes p35 subunit of **interleukin-12**, gene map locus 3p12-q13.2

IL12B a gene, Interleukin-12 Beta chain, encodes p40 subunit of **interleukin-12**, gene map locus 5q31.1-q33.1

IL13 a gene, Interleukin-13, gene map locus 5q31, encodes **interleukin-13**

IL14 a gene, Interleukin-14, gene map locus unknown, encodes **interleukin-14**

IL15 a gene, Interleukin-15, gene map locus 4q31, encodes **interleukin-15**

IL16 a gene, Interleukin-16, gene map locus 15q26.1, encodes **interleukin-16**

IL17 a gene, Interleukin-17, gene map locus 2q31, encodes **interleukin-17**

IL18 a gene, Interleukin-18, gene map locus 11q22.2-q22.3, encodes **interleukin-18**

IL19 a gene, Interleukin-19, gene map locus 1q32, encodes **interleukin-19**

IL20 a gene, Interleukin-20, gene map locus 1q32, encodes **interleukin-20**

IL21R a gene, Interleukin-21 Receptor, gene map locus 16p11, normally expressed by peripheral blood NK cells; contributes to a *IL21R-BCL6* fusion gene in B-lineage non-Hodgkin's lymphoma with t(3;16)(q27;p11)

ileum the distal small intestine, the site of maximum **vitamin B$_{12}$** absorption

iliac pertaining to the ilium

ilium one of the bones of the pelvis; the posterior superior iliac spine, which is

Table 10 WHO classification of B-cell neoplasms*.

Precursor B-cell neoplasms
  Precursor B lymphoblastic leukaemia/lymphoma
Mature B-cell neoplasms
  B-cell chronic lymphocytic leukaemia/small lymphocytic lymphoma (*morphological variant – μ heavy chain disease*)
  B-cell prolymphocytic leukaemia
  Lymphoplasmacytic lymphoma/Waldenström macroglobulinaemia (*morphological variant – γ heavy chain disease*)
  Mantle cell lymphoma
  Splenic marginal zone lymphoma (including splenic lymphoma with villous lymphocyte)
  Hairy cell leukaemia (*morphological variant – hairy cell variant leukaemia*)
  Plasma cell myeloma
  Monoclonal gammopathy of undetermined significance (MGUS)
  Solitary plasmacytoma of bone
  Extraosseous plasmacytoma
  Primary amyloidosis
  Heavy chain disease
  Extranodal marginal zone B-cell lymphoma of mucosa-associated lymphoid tissues (MALT-lymphoma)
  Nodal marginal zone B-cell lymphoma
  Follicular lymphoma
  Mantle cell lymphoma (*morphological* variants – blastoid variants and variants resembling small cell lymphoma and marginal zone B-cell lymphoma).
  Diffuse large B-cell lymphoma (*morphological* variants – centroblastic, immunoblastic, T-cell/histiocyte-rich, anaplastic, *grade III lymphomatoid papulosis**)
  Mediastinal (thymic) large B-cell lymphoma
  Intravascular large B-cell lymphoma
  Primary effusion lymphoma
  Burkitt lymphoma/leukaemia:

* In addition, two entities of 'uncertain malignant potential' are recognized: lymphomatoid granulomatosis and post-transplant lymphoproliferative disorder, polymorphic.

part of the ilium, is often used for bone marrow aspiration and trephine biopsy

imatinib mesylate a specific inhibitor of BCR-ABL tyrosine kinase and of platelet-derived growth factor β, used in the treatment of chronic granulocytic leukaemia and other chronic myeloid leukaemias involving *PDGFRB*; imatinib mesylate was previously known as STI-571

immune (i) relating to the body's response to antigens, whether by antibody production or T-cell responses (ii) able to mount a rapid and adequate response to an antigenic stimulus; usually indicative of a secondary response to a previously encountered antigen

immune complex a complex of **antigen** and **antibody**

immune complex disease a disease caused by deposition of **immune complexes** in tissues or on cells

immune deficiency inability to mount an adequate immune response

immune haemolytic anaemia a haemolytic anaemia mediated by **alloantibodies**, **autoantibodies**, drug-dependent autoantibodies or **immune complexes**

immune phenotype *see* **immunophenotype**

immune suppression suppression of immune responses by disease or by **immunosuppressive** therapy

immune system a system of molecules, cells and tissues involved in protection against infection, permitting innate and acquired immune responses

immune tolerance a state in which **autologous** antigens do not provoke an effective immune response

immunity the body's defence against foreign or abnormal material, e.g. invading micro-organisms; immune responses are either specific, being mediated by cells that can recognize antigens, or nonspecific, e.g. mediated by complement in the absence of specific immune responses

immunization the process by which immunity to various infections is promoted by exposure to altered or killed microorganisms or antigens derived from them

immunoblast a large transformed lymphocyte resulting from stimulation of a lymphocyte by an antigen or by a lectin such as phytohaemagglutinin; immunoblasts have a large central nucleolus and plentiful basophilic cytoplasm

immunoblastic lymphoma a large cell lymphoma with lymphoma cells resembling immunoblasts, in the **WHO classification** regarded as a subtype of diffuse large B-cell lymphoma (*see* Table 10, p. 137)

immunocytochemistry identification of **antigens** on cells by means of **antibodies**, the binding of which is recognized by means of a cytochemical reaction

immunocytoma a neoplasm of cells showing some degree of **plasma cell** differentiation; lymphoplasmacytoid lymphoma in the **WHO classification**

immunofixation a technique for characterizing **paraproteins** by means of **electrophoresis** followed by binding to a class-specific antibody (Fig. 47)

immunofluorescence a method of recognizing **antigens** by means of **antibodies** bound to **fluorochromes**

immunoglobulin a plasma or cell-bound glycoprotein with antibody activity, further categorized as immunoglobulin of five classes—G, A, M, E and D; each immunoglobulin molecule has a basic structure of two identical heavy chains and two identical light chains (Fig. 48)

immunoglobulin A an immunoglobulin with an α heavy chain, responsible for immunity at mucosal surfaces and present in secretions as a dimer with an additional secretory component that

Figure 47   Immunofixation.
Immunofixation to demonstrate the nature of a paraprotein in a patient with multiple myeloma. Serum protein electrophoresis shows a discrete band in the early γ region (arrow head, top). Immunofixation shows that the abnormal band reacts with anti-γ and ant-λ antisera and it therefore represents an IgGλ paraprotein. Antisera to α, μ and κ show only normal polyclonal immunoglobulins.

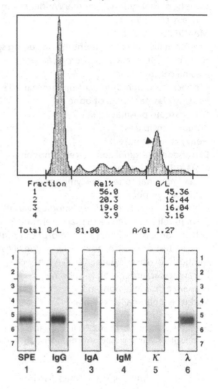

Fraction	Rel%	G/L
1	56.0	45.36
2	20.3	16.44
3	19.8	16.04
4	3.9	3.16

Total G/L   81.00   A/G: 1.27

SPE IgG IgA IgM κ λ
 1   2   3   4   5 6

protects against proteolysis; there are two subclasses (*see* Fig. 48)

immunoglobulin D an immunoglobulin with a δ heavy chain; as a cell surface molecule on B lymphocytes it binds antigens, probably leading to activation of the cell; as a plasma protein its physiological role is unknown

immunoglobulin E an immunoglobulin with an ε heavy chain, involved in defence against parasitic infections and in allergic reactions

immunoglobulin G an immunoglobulin with a γ heavy chain, of subtypes IgG1, IgG2, IgG3 and IgG4; responsible for **secondary immune responses** (*see* Fig. 48)

Figure 48   Immunoglobulin molecules.
The structure of immunoglobulin molecules of IgG,
IgA and IgM classes. The basic structure is of two
heavy (grey) and two light chains (black) with both
the light chains and the heavy chains having a
variable region, which gives antibody specificity,
and a constant region which conveys other
properties, such as binding to complement or to Fc
receptors on neutrophils and macrophages (a) the
IgG molecule has heavy chains with one variable
regions and three constant regions; the two heavy
chains are crosslinked and each light chain is
crosslinked to a heavy chain; (b) the IgA molecule
has a similar structure to the IgG molecule but is
present in secretions as a dimer with the two
monomers being joined by a J chain (crosshatched);
in addition, epithelial cells add a secretory
component (white); (c) the IgM is present in serum
as a pentamer; five identical subunits are joined to
each other and to a J chain. The heavy chain of the
IgM molecule differs from that of the IgG and IgA
molecules in that it has four rather than three
constant regions.

(a)

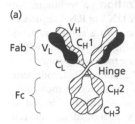

(b)

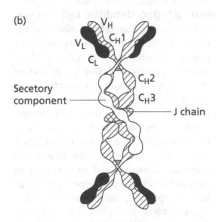

(c)

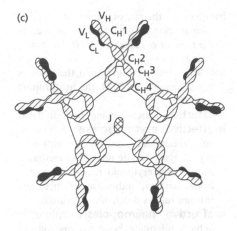

**immunoglobulin gene rearrange-
ment** the bringing together of non-
contiguous DNA sequences from the V, D
and J regions of the immunoglobulin heavy
chain locus or similarly the kappa locus
or the lambda locus (*see* Fig. 46, p. 135)

immunoglobulin heavy chain gene
a gene at the *IGH* locus encoding an
immunoglobulin heavy chain—γ, α μ, ε
or δ

immunoglobulin heavy chain locus
see IGH

immunoglobulin light chain the κ or
λ light chain of immunoglobulin

immunoglobulin M a pentomeric
immunoglobulin with μ heavy chains,
responsible for the **primary immune
response** (*see* Fig. 48)

immunoperoxidase technique a
technique for recognizing antibodies
which have bound to antigen, achieved
by linking the antibody to peroxidase
(direct immunoperoxidase technique) or
utilizing a peroxidase-conjugated anti-
immunoglobulin which binds to the first
antibody (indirect immunoperoxidase
technique)

immunophenotype the antigenic characteristics of a population of cells

immunophenotyping the recognition
of the antigenic profile of a population or
populations of cells (*see* Fig. 28, p. 104)

impedance a measurement of the flow
of electrical current between two electrodes
suspended in a conducting medium; an
alteration of impedance can be a consequence of the passage of a cell or other
particle between the electrodes

impedance counter an automated
counter using impedance technology to
count and size cells

incidence the rate of occurrence of a disease in a population, usually expressed as the number of cases per 100 000 of population per year

Indian a blood group system, the antigens being carried on **CD44**, the hyaluronate receptor

ineffective not achieving the desired end

ineffective erythropoiesis failure to achieve adequate bone marrow output of erythrocytes despite normal or increased numbers of erythroid precursors in the bone marrow, indicative of increased intramedullary death of erythroblasts

ineffective haemopoiesis failure to achieve adequate bone marrow output of erythrocytes, leucocytes and platelets despite normal or increased numbers of haemopoietic precursors in the bone marrow, indicative of increased intramedullary death of haemopoietic cells

infarct death of a tissue as a result of interruption of its blood supply

infectious mononucleosis glandular fever; an acute illness with fever, **pharyngitis**, **lymphadenopathy** and **atypical lymphocytes** in the peripheral blood. Caused by primary infection with the **Epstein–Barr virus**

inflammation non-specific changes in tissues as a response to infection or tissue damage

ING1 a gene, **I**nhibitor of **G**rowth **1**, gene map locus 13q34, encodes a widely expressed zinc finger nuclear protein which causes cell cycle arrest in G1; a candidate **tumour suppressor gene**, mutations have been found in squamous cell carcinomas of the head and neck

INK4a *see CDKN2A* and *ARF*

INK4b *see CDKN2B*

initiation (i) the process by which RNA **transcription** from a gene commences; (ii) the process by which protein **translation** from mRNA commences (*see* Fig. 74, p. 222)

initiation codon the three nucleotide codon (ATG) at the 5′ end of a gene which is essential to permit **initiation** of **transcription** of a gene, i.e. initiation of polypeptide synthesis

INK4a *see CDKN2A* and Table 5, p. 70

INK4b *see CDKN2B* and Table 5, p. 70

innate immunity naturally occurring immunity that is not permanently changed by encounter with an antigen, dependent on phagocytic cells, natural killer cells, inflammatory mediators, acute phase reactants and complement components

ins a cytogenetic abbreviation indicating an **insertion**

insertion either (i) the insertion of part of one chromosome into another chromosome or into another part of the same chromosome, detectable by conventional cytogenetic analysis and designated 'ins', or (ii) the insertion of a number of bases into a DNA molecule

in situ a method of studying a cell or a tissue without disrupting it so that positive or negative results can be related to individual cells

in situ hybridization a technique for detecting specific DNA or RNA sequences by hybridization with a complementary probe that is labelled, for example, with a fluorochrome or a radioactive isotope

integrin one of a family of heterodimeric transmembrane cell adhesion molecules, composed of non-covalently linked α and β subunits, that mediate cell–cell and cell–matrix interactions

interdigitating dendritic cell a tissue cell (including **Langerhans cells**) that becomes activated on **antigen** exposure and migrates to draining lymph nodes where it presents antigen to **helper T lymphocytes** in the context of major histocompatibility complex class II molecules

interferon one of a family of **cytokines** produced by various body cells, e.g. monocytes, fibroblasts and virus-infected cells, that are part of non-specific immune response to viruses and to cancer cells; they are categorized as type 1 (α and β) and as type 2 (γ); interferons are used in therapy, e.g. to treat chronic granulocytic leukaemia and hairy cell leukaemia

interferon-α one of two classes of cytokines synthesized by virus-infected cells that conveys, to other cells, resistance against viral infection

interferon-β one of two classes of cytokines synthesized by virus-infected cells that conveys, to other cells, resistance against viral infection

interferon-γ a cytokine synthesized by type 1 (Th1) **helper T cells** and **NK cells**, encoded by a gene on chromosome 6; γ interferon activates macrophage and neutrophil killing, stimulates NK cell function and enhances antigen-presentation by increasing expression of type II MHC molecules; it inhibits type 2 (Th2) helper T cells; a defect in γ-interferon or its receptor can cause an inherited susceptibility to mycobacterial infections

interferon regulatory factor (IRF) a family of transcription factors defined by a characteristic DNA-binding domain and the ability to bind to the interferon-stimulated response element; involved in cytokine signalling and the control of proliferation

interleukin a cytokine secreted by one type of leucocyte that has effects mainly on other leucocytes

interleukin-1 (IL1) a cytokine, also known as endogenous pyrogen, produced mainly by monocytes, that activates T cells and macrophages and mediates the acute phase response; there are 2 forms encoded by 2 separate genes at 2q14

interleukin-2 (IL2) an immunoregulatory lymphokine, encoded by *IL2*, produced by activated type 1 (Th1) helper T cells, which activates cytotoxic T cells, NK cells and macrophages

interleukin-2 receptor the multi-subunit IL2 receptor that is composed of various heterotrimeric and heterodimeric combinations of three different subunits, IL2Rα, also known as **CD25** (encoded by *IL2RA*), IL2Rβ, also known as CD122, (encoded by *IL2RB*) and IL2Rγ, also known as CD132 (encoded by *IL2RG*); the gamma chain is an indispensable component of the receptor and is also a component of other cytokine receptors (*see* **CD132**); αβγ trimers constitute the high affinity form of the receptor, βγ dimers the intermediate affinity form and αγ dimers the low affinity form; the α chain is not functional in IL2 internalization and signal transduction, but muta-

tions in it are associated with congenital immunodeficiency

interleukin-3 (IL3) a haemopoietic colony-stimulating factor, encoded by *IL3*, that is capable of supporting the proliferation of a broad range of haemopoietic cell types and also has neurotrophic activity

interleukin-4 (IL4) a lymphokine secreted by type 2 (Th2) helper T cells and activated B cells, encoded by *IL4*, which activates macrophages and B cells, promotes IgE class switching and has a role in mast cell sensitization, allergy and defence against nematodes; it stimulates the production of **eotaxin**—a chemokine involved in eosinophil recruitment; has an inhibitory effect on the growth of many leukaemic cell lines *in vitro*

interleukin-5 (IL5) a haemopoietic growth factor for B cells and eosinophils, secreted by type 2 (Th2) helper T cells, encoded by *IL5*

interleukin-6 (IL6) a cytokine with potent antiviral activity, which is also able to elicit an acute phase response; encoded by *IL6*; the aberrant production of IL6 by neoplastic cells is a contributory factor to the growth B-cell neoplasms, T-cell lymphomas and Kaposi's sarcoma; promoter polymorphisms in the *IL6* gene are associated with hypertriglyceridaemia and susceptibility to Kaposi's sarcoma in HIV-infected individuals, but there is no association with multiple myeloma.

interleukin-7 (IL7) a lymphokine capable of supporting the growth of pre-B cells *in vitro*, encoded by *IL7*

interleukin-8 (IL8) a cytokine secreted by several types of cell, including T cells and macrophages, in response to inflammatory stimuli, encoded by *IL8*; it is chemotactic for neutrophils, basophils and T cells and promotes angiogenesis; involved in the pathogenesis of viral bronchiolitis caused by the respiratory syncytial virus (RSV)—the level of IL8 appears to be correlated with disease severity

interleukin-9 (IL9) a cytokine with both myeloid and lymphoid stimulatory activity, encoded by *IL9*; it promotes IgE class switching; overproduced in Hodgkin's disease

interleukin-10 (IL10) an anti-inflammatory cytokine secreted by type 2 (Th2) helper T cells, which down regulates the immune response, inhibiting type I (Th1) helper T cells and inhibits allergic reactions, encoded by *IL10*; interleukin-10 limits HIV-1 replication *in vivo*; mutations in the *IL10* promoter have been associated with increased risk of HIV infection and once infected, rapid progression to AIDS

interleukin-11 (IL11) a widely expressed cytokine of unknown physiological function, encoded by *IL11*; acts synergistically with several other cytokines to stimulate cells of a variety of haemopoietic lineages; secreted by bone marrow stromal cells; stimulates the production of acute phase proteins

interleukin-12 (IL12) a dimeric cytokine, also known as natural killer cell stimulatory factor, composed of an alpha chain (p35 subunit encoded by *IL12A*) and a beta chain (p40 subunit encoded by *IL12B*); secreted by dendritic cells, macrophages and B cells; stimulates the production of interferon-γ by type 1 helper T cells and NK cells; mutations in *IL12B* or *IL12R* lead to inherited susceptibility to mycobacterial infections, including disseminated infection with BCG, and to susceptibility to *Salmonella enteritidis* infection

interleukin-13 (IL13) a cytokine secreted by activated type 2 (Th2) helper T cells, encoded by *IL13*, which stimulates the production of **eotaxin**, a chemokine involved in eosinophil recruitment; induces IgG4 and IgE synthesis by B cells; induces the pathophysiologic features of asthma, independently of IgE and eosinophils; polymorphisms in the *IL13* gene predispose to bronchial hyper-responsiveness and asthma susceptibility

interleukin-14 (IL14) a cytokine with B-cell stimulatory properties, gene map locus unknown

interleukin-15 (IL15) a cytokine which affects T-cell activation and proliferation

similarly to IL2, encoded by *IL15*; it appears to utilize the IL2 receptor

interleukin-16 (IL16) a proinflammatory cytokine which signals via CD4, inducing chemotactic and immunomodulatory responses in CD4+ T cells; encoded by *IL16*

interleukin-17 (IL17) a proinflammatory cytokine expressed by activated memory T cells, encoded by *IL17*; induces expression of **CD54** on B cells; archetypal member of a new family of proinflammatory cytokines (IL17 B–F)

interleukin-18 (IL18) a cytokine secreted by macrophages, encoded by *IL18*, which promotes interferon-γ secretion by T cells, suppresses IgE synthesis and augments NK cell responses

interleukin 19 (IL19) a cytokine closely related to and genetically linked with IL10 and IL20; regulates B-cell function; encoded by *IL19*

interleukin 20 (IL20) a cytokine closely related to and genetically linked with IL10 and IL19; encoded by *IL20*; IL20 receptors are found in the skin and are upregulated in psoriasis

intermediate filaments filaments with a diameter of 7–10 nm that form part of the cytoskeleton; they include keratin, desmin, vimentin, laminin, neurofilaments and glial fibrillary acidic protein

intermediate grade lymphoma a lymphoma with a degree of malignancy intermediate between low and high grade, recognized by the Working Formulation; includes **mantle cell lymphoma** which was previously sometimes designated 'lymphoma of intermediate differentiation'

interphase the stage when a cell is out of cycle (G0) (*see* Fig. 15, p. 72)

interstitial pertaining to the interstitium

interstitium the potential space between cells

intervening sequence (IVS) *see* **intron**

intracerebral within the brain

intracranial within the skull

intrasinusoidal within a sinusoid, e.g. within a bone marrow sinusoid

intravascular within blood vessels

intravenous within a vein (usually referring to a method of administering blood or blood components, fluids or drugs)

intrinsic contained within itself

intrinsic factor a factor secreted by the parietal cells of the stomach that combines with an extrinsic or dietary factor (**vitamin B₁₂**) to permit the absorption of vitamin B₁₂ in the small intestine

intrinsic factor antibodies antibodies directed at **intrinsic factor**, often present in the serum or the gastric juice of individuals with **pernicious anaemia**

intrinsic pathway a coagulation pathway for which all the factors necessary are already present in the blood, only contact with a foreign surface being required to initiate coagulation (*see* Fig. 17, p. 77)

intron a sequence of DNA in a gene which is not represented in processed messenger RNA or in the protein product (*see* Fig. 32, p. 111)

inv a cytogenetic abbreviation indicating an **inversion**

inversion (inv) the inversion of a segment of a chromosome

in vitro carried out or occurring outside a living body, literally 'in glass'

in vivo carried out or occurring in a living creature, literally 'in life'

ion an atom that has gained or lost one of its electrons so that it is not electrically balanced

IRF interferon regulatory factor

IRF1 a gene, Interferon Regulatory Factor 1, gene map locus 5q31.1, encodes an IRF transcription factor that upregulates several growth-suppressing genes; hemizygously lost in some patients with 5q–; mutations leading to variant proteins with reduced DNA-binding capacity have been observed in gastric and non-small cell lung carcinoma

IRF4 a gene, Interferon Regulatory Factor 4, also known as Multiple Myeloma oncogene 1—*MUM*, gene map locus 6p25, encodes an IRF transcription factor expressed only in lymphocytes; dysregulated by t(6;14)(p25;q32) in about 20% of patients with multiple myeloma.

iron Fe, a metal which is an essential constituent of **haemoglobin** and the muscle protein, myoglobin

iron-binding capacity the capacity of the serum to bind iron, dependent on the concentration of **transferrin** and other iron-binding proteins in the serum

iron deficiency a lack of adequate iron stores leading to some clinical or laboratory abnormality, e.g. anaemia or **glossitis**

iron deficiency anaemia anaemia caused by a lack of adequate supplies of iron

iron depletion absence of storage iron but without any associated haematological or clinical abnormality

iron-regulatory proteins proteins that interact with **iron-responsive elements** of genes; in the case of the **ferritin** genes and the **δ-aminolaevulinate synthase** gene, iron depletion leads to interaction and decreased translation of the gene; in the case of the **transferrin receptor** gene, iron depletion leads to interaction and increased translation of the gene

iron-responsive element a family of *cis*-acting non-coding mRNA structures located in the untranslated region of mRNA for **ferritins, δ-aminolaevulinate synthase** and **transferrin receptor**

iron stores iron stored in body macrophages in the form of **ferritin** and, particularly, **haemosiderin**

irradiation exposure to ionizing radiation

irregularly contracted cells erythrocytes lacking central pallor but, in contrast to spherocytes, being irregular in shape

IRTA1 a gene, Immunoglobulin superfamily Receptor Translocation-Associated gene 1, gene map locus 1q21, one of 5 related genes (*IRTA1-5*) clustered at this locus; encodes an inhibitory immunoglobulin superfamily receptor homologous to the Ig Fc receptor, normally expressed in perifollicular B cells but not in plasma cells; *IRTA1* is translocated to the *IGH* locus in t(1;14)(q21;q32) associated with less than 5% of cases of multiple myeloma, the fusion gene encoding a protein containing the signal peptide and first two amino acids of IRTA1 linked to the transmembrane and intracellular domains of the surface IgA receptor

IRTA2   a gene, Immunoglobulin superfamily Receptor Translocation-Associated gene 2, gene map locus 1q21, encodes an inhibitory immunoglobulin superfamily receptor homologous to the Ig Fc receptor, normally expressed in germinal centre centrocytes and a broad spectrum of perifollicular cells, which may include immunoblasts and memory cells but not centroblasts; dysregulated and overexpressed in Burkitt's lymphoma with 1q21 abnormalities, being the only member of the *IRTA* cluster to be expressed in this disorder—the mechanism for this is unclear

ISBT   International Society for Blood Transfusion

iso (or i)   a cytogenetic abbreviation indicating an **isochromosome**

isochromosome (i or iso)   a chromosome formed by duplication of either the short arm or the long arm of a chromosome

isoenzyme   a structurally different form of an enzyme present in different tissues of a single individual

isoniazid   a drug used to treat tuberculosis which can cause sideroblastic erythropoiesis

isotonic   having an osmolarity that is the same as that of normal body fluids

isotype   immunoglobulin molecules characterized by a specific type of heavy chain, e.g. immunoglobulin M rather than immunoglobulin A

isotype switching   change from secreting immunoglobulin M to secreting another class of immunoglobulin, e.g. IgG or IgA

ITGA2   the gene at 5q23-q31 encoding the integrin α2 chain; integrin $\alpha_2\beta_1$ (very late antigen-2, VLA-2) is platelet glycoprotein Ia/IIa (**CD49b/CD29**)

ITGA2B   the gene at 17q21.32 encoding the integrin α_{IIb} chain (**CD41a**), a component of platelet glycoprotein IIb/IIIa, mutation of which can lead to **Glanzmann's thrombasthenia**

ITGB2   the gene encoding **CD18**, the integrin β2 chain, mutation of which can cause **leucocyte adhesion deficiency**

ITGB3   the gene at 17q21.32 encoding the integrin β_3 chain (**CD61**), a component of platelet glycoprotein IIb/IIIa ($\alpha_{IIb}/\beta3$) and the vitronectin receptor ($\alpha_v/\beta3$); mutation of the gene can lead to **Glanzmann's thrombasthenia**

ITP   idiopathic thrombocytopenic purpura (now usually referred to as 'autoimmune thrombocytopenic purpura')

J

JAK janus kinase

JAK2 a gene, **Ja**nus **k**inase **2**, gene map locus 9p24, encodes a **janus kinase**; *JAK2* contributes to the *ETV6-JAK2* fusion gene in rare cases of acute lympho-blastic leukaemia and atypical chronic myeloid leukaemia, associated with either t(9;12)(p24;p13) or with a com-plex rearrangement with the same breakpoints

JAK3 a gene encoding a **janus kinase**, mutation of which can cause **severe combined immune deficiency**

Janus kinase (JAK) a family of non-receptor **tyrosine kinases** that are involved in intracellular signalling via a variety of cytokines; characterized by having two phosphotransferase domains

jejunum the proximal small intestine, between the duodenum and the ileum, the site of maximal **folic acid** absorption

Jk^a* and *Jk^b co-dominant alleles at the *HUT11* locus, encoding antigens of the Kidd blood group system (*see also* **Kidd** and *HUT11*)

Jk^a, Jk^b and Jk3 antigens of the Kidd blood group system (*see also* **Kidd** and *HUT11*)

Jordan's anomaly an inherited abnor-mality in which leucocytes of all types are vacuolated

jumping translocation translocation of part of a chromosome to multiple other partner chromosomes

JUN a transcription factor of the **leucine zipper family**

JUN a gene, gene map locus 1p32, that encodes a leucine zipper DNA-binding protein which is the cellular homologue of the transforming gene of avian sar-coma virus 17; JUN is a major compon-ent of the activator protein-1 (AP-1) transcription factor complex

juvenile chronic myeloid leukaemia a type of chronic myeloid leukaemia which occurs in infants, characterized by hepatosplenomegaly, lymphadenopathy, rash, anaemia, monocytosis and eleva-tion of haemoglobin F concentration, now usually designated **juvenile myelo-monocytic leukaemia**

juvenile myelomonocytic leukaemia an alternative designation of **juvenile chronic myeloid leukaemia**, the term recommended in the **WHO classification** (*see* Fig. 55, p. 168)

K

κ kappa, one of the two types of light chain found in about 60% of immunoglobulin molecules

κ the kappa immunoglobulin light chain gene, gene map locus 2p12; translocations involving this locus can lead to dysregulation of other genes, e.g. *MYC* or *BCL2*

Kaposi's sarcoma a sarcoma of endothelial cells which in common in AIDS; very rarely it infiltrates the bone marrow

karyogram an ordered array of chromosomes of a cell, usually a photograph with the pairs of chromosomes arranged in decreasing size (Fig. 49)

karyotype an abbreviated written description of the **karyogram** of a cell, clone or individual, conforming to certain conventions as to how abnormalities are described, e.g. a male with Klinefelter's syndrome would be described as having the karyotype 47,cXXY whereas a female with chronic granulocytic leukaemia would be expected to have a leukaemic clone with the karyotype 46,XY,t(9;22)(q34;q11)

karyotypic pertaining to a **karyotype**

Kawasaki's syndrome an acute febrile multisystem disease of children with cervical lymphadenopathy, changes in skin and mucous membranes and coronary arteritis

kb a **kilobase**

kD a **kilodalton**

Figure 49 A karyogram.
A karyogram of a patient with chronic granulocytic leukaemia showing cytogenetic evolution. The primary abnormality present was t(9;22)(q34;q11). A secondary abnormality has occurred, t(3;21)(q26;q22).

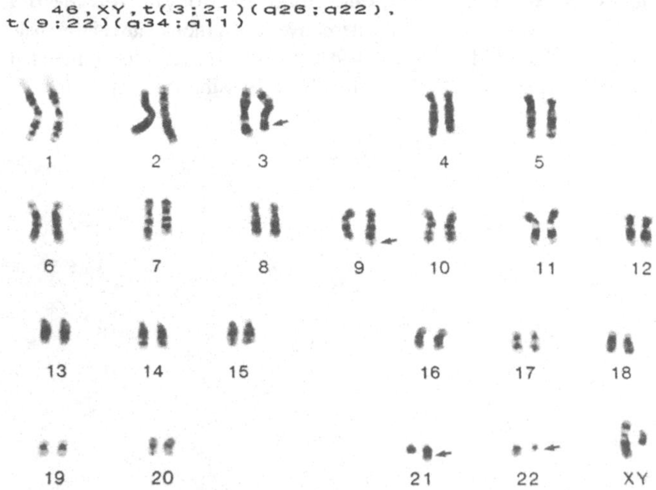

46,XY,t(3;21)(q26;q22),
t(9;22)(q34;q11)

Figure 50   A keratocyte.
A keratocyte showing two 'horns'.

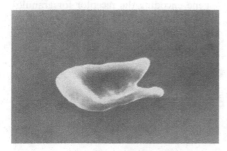

KEL   a locus at 7q33 where there are three closely linked sets of alleles encoding antigens of the Kell blood group system (**CD238**); the most important of the 25 known antigens and the genes encoding them are:
- K (*KEL1*) and k (*KEL2*)
- Kp^a (*KEL3*), Kp^b (*KEL4*) and Kp^c (*KEL21*)
- Js^a (*KEL6*) and Js^b (*KEL7*)

Kell   a red cell-specific blood group system, *see also* **KEL**

keratocyte   a cell with one or two pairs of spicules, symmetrically arranged (Fig. 50)

kernicterus   damage to the basal ganglia of the brain by a high concentration of bilirubin, e.g. in **haemolytic disease of the newborn**

Ki-1   a monoclonal antibody that recognizes the **CD30** cluster

Ki-1+ lymphoma   an earlier designation of **anaplastic large cell lymphoma**

Ki-67   a monoclonal antibody that identifies proliferating cells

KIAA0128   *see Septin 2*

Kidd   a blood group antigen system including the Jk^a and Jk^b antigens (*see also HUT11*)

Kiel classification   a lymphoma classification which was largely superseded by the REAL classification (*see* **Revised European–American Lymphoma classification**) and then by the **WHO classification**

killer cell   a lymphocyte which can kill another cell

kilobase (kb)   1000 **base pairs** of DNA

kilodalton (kD)   1000 **Daltons**

Kimura's disease   a chronic inflammatory disease of unknown aetiology, causing **lymphadenopathy** with reactive follicular hyperplasia and infiltration by eosinophils

kinase   an enzyme that transfers a phosphate group

KIP1   *see CDKN1B*

KIP2   *see CDKN1C*

KIT   a gene, gene map locus 4q11-34, encoding stem cell factor receptor, a receptor tyrosine kinase; KIT protein is recognized by **CD117** monoclonal antibodies; *KIT* is expressed on haemopoietic progenitors, megakaryocytes, mast cells and a subset of NK cells; it is often overexpressed in acute myeloid leukaemia and is usually mutated, leading to constitutive activation of KIT, in systemic mastocytosis; mutated in gastrointestinal stromal tumours, some germ cell tumours and some sino-nasal NK/T cell lymphoma.

Kleihauer test   a cytochemical stain for demonstrating erythrocytes, including fetal erythrocytes, with a high concentration of **haemoglobin F**

knockin mouse   an experimental animal from which, by means of manipulating and selecting embryonal stem cells, a specific gene has been 'knocked in' so that its function can be studied

knockout   mouse   an   experimental animal from which, by means of manipulating and selecting embryonal stem cells, a specific gene has been 'knocked out' and replaced by a disabled gene

Figure 51   Koilonychia.
Koilonychia in a patient with iron deficiency.

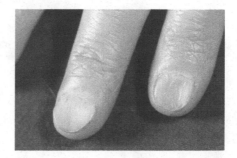

Knops a blood group system, the antigens being carried on **CD35**, a complement regulatory protein, the C3b/C4b receptor

koilonychia flat or spoon-shaped nails as a feature of iron deficiency (Fig. 51)

Kostmann's syndrome an inherited abnormality causing severe congenital neutropenia; a minority of case result from heterozygosity for a mutation in the gene encoding the receptor for granulocyte colony-stimulating factor (*G-CSFR*)

kwashiorkor a form of protein-calorie malnutrition

L

λ the Greek letter lambda, one of the types of light chain found in about 40% of immunoglobulin molecules

λ the lambda immunoglobulin light chain gene, gene map locus 22q11; translocations involving this locus can lead to dysregulation of other genes e.g. *MYC* or *BCL2*

L1, L2, L3 categories in the **FAB** classification of acute lymphoblastic leukaemia

labelling index the proportion of cells in which DNA synthesis is occurring, determined, for example, by incorporation of tritiated thymidine or bromodeoxyuridine

lactate dehydrogenase (LDH) an enzyme found in many body cells that catalyses the oxidation of L-lactate to pyruvate, elevated in haemolytic anaemia and in ineffective haemopoiesis

lactic acid the end product of anaerobic metabolism

lactoferrin an iron-binding protein found in neutrophils (and also milk and other body fluids) that retards bacterial proliferation

lactoferrin deficiency *see* **neutrophil specific granule deficiency**

LAF4 a gene, **L**ymphoid nuclear protein related to *AF4*, gene map locus 2q11.2-q12, encodes a lymphoid-restricted transcriptional activator that is a homologue of *AF4* and *AF5q31*; contributed to a fusion gene in a case of acute lymphoblastic leukaemia

LAK cell **lymphokine-activated killer cell**

lamellar bone bone with an orderly structure of concentric layers surrounding a central Haversian canal

Langerhans cell a cell of monocyte lineage, normally found in the skin and characterized by the presence of specific cytoplasmic granules designated Birbeck granules

Langerhans cell histiocytosis a group of neoplastic conditions of **Langerhans cells**, previously designated histiocytosis X, further categorized as **Letterer–Siwe disease, Hand–Schüller–Christian disease** and **eosinophilic granuloma**

Langerhans cell leukaemia an acute leukaemia of **Langerhans cell** lineage, occurring *de novo* or as the terminal phase of **Langerhans cell histiocytosis**

Langhans type giant cell a multinucleated giant cell of monocyte lineage characterized by peripherally placed nuclei

LAP **leucocyte alkaline phosphatase**

laparoscopy inspection of the abdominal cavity by means of a laparoscope inserted through a small incision

laparotomy surgical exploration of the abdomen for diagnostic or therapeutic purposes

LARG a gene, **L**eukaemia-**A**ssociated **Rh**o **G**uanine nucleotide exchange factor, also known as **Rh**o **G**uanine nucleotide **E**xchange **F**actor **12**, *RHGEF12*; gene map locus 11q23, encodes a guanine nucleotide exchange factor (GEF) with homology to BCR; contributed to a *MLL-LARG* fusion gene in a patient with acute myeloid leukaemia and a complex karyotype

large cell anaplastic lymphoma a large cell lymphoma of T lineage with cells showing strong **CD30** positivity and sometimes aberrant positivity for **epithelial membrane antigen**

large cell lymphoma a lymphoma of large lymphoid cells of T, B or NK lineage

large granular lymphocyte a large lymphocyte with plentiful cytoplasm and prominent azurophilic granules

large granular lymphocyte leukaemia a leukaemia of large granular lymphocytes of either T or NK lineage

large unstained cell (LUC) a term used to describe large, peroxidase-negative cells detected by Bayer automated instruments

larynx the part of the throat that contains the vocal cords

LAZ an alternative designation of *BCL6*

lazy leucocyte syndrome a syndrome of recurrent infections associated with defective response of neutrophils to chemotactic stimuli

LCAT lecithin-cholesterol acyl transferase

LCP1 a gene, Lymphocyte Cytosolic Protein 1, gene map locus 13q14.1, an IL2-responsive gene that encodes an actin-binding protein; contributes to the *LCP1-BCL6* fusion gene in B-lineage non-Hodgkin's lymphoma associated with t(3;13)(q27;q14); as a result of the translocation, the 5′ regulatory regions of the two genes are exchanged

Leach phenotype an inherited anomaly of the erythrocyte membrane associated with loss of the Gerbich antigens and elliptocytosis

LE cell a neutrophil with a round homogeneous inclusion representing altered nuclear material, characteristic of systemic lupus erythematosus, and demonstrated by incubating neutrophils with the patient's serum

lecithin-cholesterol acyl transferase deficiency (LCAT deficiency) an inherited metabolic disorder associated with increased target cell formation

lectin any protein other than an immunoglobulin that binds to a specific carbohydrate group, may be of plant, microbial or animal origin; may be used for identification of antigens (e.g. blood group antigens) or to stimulate cell growth and proliferation

Leder stain a histochemical stain to demonstrate chloroacetate esterase activity

LEDGF a gene, Lens Epithelium-Derived Growth Factor, gene map locus 9p22, encoding transcriptional coactivators, p52 and p75, which differ at their carboxy terminal ends; contributed to a *LEDGF-NUP98* fusion gene in a patient with *de novo* acute myeloid leukaemia; the fusion protein lacks the transactivating domain of LEDGF

left shift an increased proportion of immature cells of neutrophil lineage in either the peripheral blood or the bone marrow

Leishman–Donovan bodies the resting stage of *Leishmania donovani* observed in tissues including the bone marrow

leishmaniasis infection by the parasite *Leishmania donovani* or related species

Lennert's lymphoma an alternative designation of lymphoepithelioid lymphoma of the Kiel classification, included in the 'peripheral T-cell lymphoma, unspecified' category of the REAL classification and the WHO classification

lepirudin a recombinant form of hirudin, a thrombin inhibitor

Lermitte's syndrome tingling feelings spreading down the body when the head is bent forward, which may occur in vitamin B$_{12}$ deficiency and following irradiation for Hodgkin's disease

Letterer–Siwe disease a highly aggressive form of Langerhans cell histiocytosis occurring in infants

leucapheresis removal of white cells from the peripheral blood, usually either to relieve hyperviscosity or to obtain cells for peripheral blood stem cell transplantation

leucine rich repeat (LRR) a hydrophobic protein motif believed to participate in protein-protein interactions

leucine zipper a protein motif characterized by a leucine residue occurring every 7th base; required for homodimerization and heterodimerization

leucocyte a white blood cell, a term which includes all the mature peripheral blood cells of granulocyte, monocyte or lymphocyte lineage, i.e. neutrophils, eosinophils, basophils, lymphocytes and monocytes

leucocyte adhesion deficiency a genetically heterogeneous group of conditions in which there is defective adhesion of neutrophils to endothelium, leading to neutrophilia, a lack of extra-vascular neutrophils and susceptibility to infection: type 1 results from mutation in the *ITGB2* (integrin β2) gene, the gene encoding the β chain of the leucocyte integrins, which results in **CD18** deficiency; type 2 results from a defect in carbohydrate fucosylation so that endothelial sialyl-Lewis^x is not expressed and endothelium cannot bind E and P selectins (*see* **CD62E** and **CD62P**); a single case has also been reported in which there was deficiency in RAC2, the predominant GTPase in neutrophils

leucocyte alkaline phosphatase (LAP) the alkaline phosphatase isoenzyme in neutrophils; it should be noted that the term **'neutrophil alkaline phosphatase'** and the abbreviation **'NAP'** are to be preferred

leucocytosis an increased number of leucocytes in the peripheral blood

leucoerythroblastic anaemia anaemia with both erythroblasts and granulocyte precursors in the peripheral blood

leucopenia a reduced white cell count

leukaemia a myeloid or lymphoid neoplasm, characterized by circulating neoplastic cells but also encompassing similar cases in which there are neoplastic cells in the bone marrow but not in the peripheral blood

leukaemic reticuloendotheliosis an early designation of **hairy cell leukaemia**, not in current use

leukaemogenesis the mechanism of development of leukaemia

leukaemoid reaction a reactive condition which simulates or closely resembles leukaemia

Lewis blood group system a blood group system in which plasma glycosphingolipids, resulting from the expression of alleles at the *FUT1*, *FUT2*, *FUT3* and *ABO* loci, are adsorbed onto red cells (*see* Fig. 30, p. 108)

ligand a molecule that binds specifically to another molecule, e.g. **stem cell factor** is the ligand of **c-KIT** and **thrombopoietin** is the ligand of **MPL**

light chain the shorter polypeptide chain of a **heterodimer**; if not otherwise specified, the term applies to the light chain of the immunoglobulin molecule, each molecule having two heavy chains and two light chains; light chains may be kappa or lambda but in a given molecule are one or the other

light chain-associated amyloidosis amyloidosis occurring as a complication of a **plasma cell neoplasm**, either overt or occult, previously often designated 'primary amyloidosis' when the plasma cell neoplasm was occult

light chain deposition disease disease resulting from deposition of a monoclonal light chain in tissues, particularly in the kidneys

LIM domain a zinc-binding protein motif which provides an interface for protein interactions

linkage the presence of two or more genes sufficiently close to each other on a chromosome that they do not segregate independently

linkage disequilibrium the association of particular genes or other DNA sequences more frequently than would be expected by chance

lithium a drug used for treating depression that elevates the neutrophil count

LMAN1 a gene at 18q21.3-q22, encoding an intracellular mannose-specific protein that is involved in transport of early processed glycoproteins from endoplasmic reticulum to the Golgi apparatus; mutation can lead to **combined factor V and factor VIII deficiency**

locus (plural loci) the specific site on a chromosome where a **gene** and its **alleles** are located

LOD score a statistical test of linkage; the higher the LOD score the less the possibility that the association could occur by chance

log normal distribution having a **Gaussian** or bell-shaped distribution when the logarithm of the data is plotted as a histogram (*see* Fig. 45, p. 128)

LOH loss of heterozygosity

loiasis the disease resulting from infection by the filarial parasite, *Loa loa*

lomustine (CCNU)   an anti-cancer drug of the nitrosourea family

long term culture initiating cells (LTCIC)   cells that are able to give rise to long term cultures *in vitro*

loss of heterozygosity (LOH)   loss of one **allele** at a specific **locus**

low hyperdiploidy   having 47–50 chromosomes in a cell or clone

low molecular weight heparin   heparin that has been depolymerized so that the molecular weight is in the range of 4000 to 5000 daltons, e.g. **enoxaparin, dalteparin, tinzaparin, ardeparin**

LPP   a gene, LIM domain containing Preferred translocation Partner in lipoma, also known as Lipoma Preferred Partner, gene map locus 3q28, encodes a putative cell adhesion molecule that contains a **LIM domain**; contributed to *MLL-LPP* and *LPP-MLL* fusion genes in a patient with secondary M5 acute myeloid leukaemia with t(3;11)(q28;q23)

LTCIC   **long term culture initiating cells**

LU   the gene at 19q13.2 encoding the Lu^a and Lu^b antigens of the **Lutheran blood group system**

LUC   **large unstained cell**

lupus anticoagulant   an antibody that is an anticoagulant *in vitro* but is prothrombotic *in vivo*, occurs in **systemic lupus erythematosus** and in the **primary antiphospholipid syndrome; paraproteins** may also be lupus anticoagulants

Lutheran   a blood group system, Lutheran antigens (**CD239**) being encoded by the genes at the *LU* locus

LW   a locus at 19p13.3 encoding LW blood group antigens

LW   a blood group antigen system (**CD242**) encoded by genes at the *LW* locus

LYL1   a gene, Lymphoid Leukaemia gene, gene map locus 19p13, encodes a basic helix–loop–helix (bHLH) transcription factor closely related to TAL1, which is expressed in all haemopoietic cells except for T cells, dysregulated by proximity to the *TCRB* gene at 7q35 in T-lineage acute lymphoblastic leukaemia associated with t(7;19)(q35;p13)

lymph   a clear or opalescent fluid containing lymphocytes, which is transported

Figure 52   A lymphangiogram.
A lymphangiogram, showing images of lymph nodes which have trapped an oily radio-opaque dye that was injected into lymphatic vessels in the feet; the normal lymph nodes are small and have a fairly homogeneous texture whereas abnormal lymph nodes, identifiable below the left kidney, are large and heterogeneous in texture; an intravenous pyelogram has also been performed so that the renal pelvises and the ureters are outlined, showing that the left ureter is deviated around a group of abnormal lymph nodes; the patient had Hodgkin's disease.

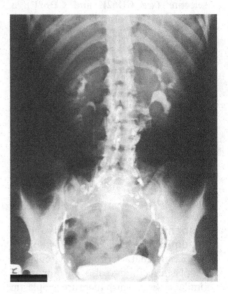

by lymphatics and ultimately drains into the blood stream through the thoracic duct

lymphadenopathy   enlargement of the lymph nodes

lymphangiogram   a radiological procedure for demonstrating lymph nodes by means of radio-opaque dye introduced into lymphatics on the dorsum of the feet (Fig. 52)

lymphatic   (i) relating to lymphocytes and lymph nodes (ii) an endothelium-lined vessel which transports lymph

lymph follicle   an organized nodule of mature B lymphocytes—smaller cells, designated follicle centre cells or **centrocytes**, and larger cells, designated **centroblasts**, in a lymph node or other tissue

lymph gland   a non-scientific term for **lymph node**

Table 11   WHO classification of T-cell and NK-cell neoplasms.

Precursor T-cell neoplasms
  Precursor T lymphoblastic leukaemia/lymphoblastic lymphoma
Mature T-cell and NK-cell neoplasms
  Leukaemic/disseminated
    T-cell prolymphocytic leukaemia
    T-cell large granular lymphocyte leukaemia
    Aggressive NK-cell leukaemia
    Adult T-cell leukaemia/lymphoma
  Cutaneous
    Mycosis fungoides
    Sezary syndrome
    Primary cutaneous anaplastic large cell lymphoma
    Lymphomatoid papulosis
  Other extra-nodal
    Extranodal NK/T-cell lymphoma, nasal type
    Enteropathy-type T-cell lymphoma
    Hepatosplenic T-cell lymphoma
    Subcutaneous panniculitis-like T-cell lymphoma
  Nodal
    Angioimmunoblastic T-cell lymphoma
    Peripheral T-cell lymphoma, unspecified
    Anaplastic large cell lymphoma
  Neoplasm of uncertain lineage and stage of differentiation
    Blastic NK-cell lymphoma

lymph node   an organized tissue composed mainly of T and B lymphocytes with some stromal cells and dendritic cells

lymphoblast   an immature cell of lymphoid lineage, having a high nucleocytoplasmic ratio, non-condensed chromatin and nucleoli (*see* Fig. 12, p. 29)

lymphoblastic   lymphoma   a lymphoma composed of **lymphoblasts**, occurring in a tissue other than the bone marrow

lymphocyte   a mature cell of lymphoid lineage

lymphocytic   pertaining to lymphocytes or to lymphoid cells

lymphocytopenia   a reduced lymphocyte count

lymphocytosis   an increased number of lymphocytes in the peripheral blood

lymphocytotoxin   also known as lymphotoxin and tumour necrosis factor β, a cytokine secreted by B cells and type 1 helper T cells, which promotes inflammation, encoded by a gene at 6p21

lymphoepithelioid lymphoma   Lennert's lymphoma, a T-cell lymphoma

with specific histological features including the presence of **epithelioid cells**, being recognized as a distinct entity in the **Kiel classification** and included in the 'peripheral T-cell lymphoma, unspecified' category of the **REAL classification** and the **WHO classification**

lymphogranulomatosis   a lymphoproliferative disorder, previously thought to be reactive but probably a low grade T-cell neoplasm

lymphoid   pertaining to lymphocytes or lymph nodes

lymphokine   any type of molecule, other than an immunoglobulin molecule, secreted by a lymphocyte and influencing the behaviour of other cells or tissues

lymphoma   a neoplasm of lymphocytes (T, B or natural killer cells); in contrast to lymphoid leukaemias, lymphomas involve predominantly tissues other than the bone marrow, rather than the bone marrow and blood; in the **WHO classification**, B-lineage and T-lineage lymphomas are designated as shown in Tables 10 (p. 137) and 11

lymphoma of intermediate differentiation an earlier designation of **mantle cell lymphoma**

lymphopenia *see* **lymphocytopenia**

lymphoplasmacytoid lymphoma a lymphoma in which some of the neoplastic cells show **plasma cell** differentiation

lymphoproliferative disorder a generic term including all lymphomas and also some disorders of undefined nature in which there is abnormal lymphoid proliferation of uncertain nature

lymphoproliferative T-cell deficiency with autoimmunity syndrome an immune deficiency syndrome resulting from mutation of the IL2 receptor gene at 10p14-15 with resultant **CD25** deficiency

lymphosarcoma an outmoded term for **non-Hodgkin's lymphoma**

Lyon hypothesis the hypothesis that one of the two X chromosomes in the cells of a normal female becomes inactive, this process occurring randomly so that, on average, each X chromosome is inactive in 50% of cells; it is hypothesized that the genetic inactivation of one chromosome permits X chromosomal dosage compensation—no matter how many X chromosomes a cell has only one remains

transcriptionally active. The inactive X chromosome is responsible for the neutrophil drumstick and in other cells may be detected as a Barr body, a condensation of chromatin below the nuclear membrane

lyonization the process by which one of the two X chromosomes in each normal female cell becomes genetically inactive; this process occurs during early embryonic life and is maintained in the progeny of that cell; it provides the basis of analysis of **X-linked polymorphisms** for presumptive establishment of monoclonality

lysis (i) destruction of a cell as a consequence of development of a hole in the plasma membrane, e.g. destruction of a red cell following antibody binding and complement fixation (ii) dissolution of a thrombus

lysosome a cellular organelle into which hydrolytic enzymes are secreted, responsible for the degradation of foreign material and cellular debris

lysozyme an enzyme secreted by monocytes and, to a lesser extent, neutrophils

lytic lesion an osteolytic lesion, generally detected radiologically which, if there is no associated **osteosclerosis**, is suggestive of **multiple myeloma**

M

μ   the Greek letter, mu (i) the heavy chain of immunoglobulin M (ii) the symbol for a micron (iii) the symbol for one millionth part of a unit, as in μg or μl

M   the designation of the phase of the cell cycle when mitosis occurs (*see* **cell cycle**)

M0, M1, M2, M3, M4, M5, M6, M7 categories in the **FAB** classification of acute myeloid leukaemia (*see* Table 3, p. 7)

MAC   the combined application of **M**orphology, **A**ntibody and **C**hromosome techniques to the study of individual cells

McLeod phenotype a syndrome of **acanthocytosis**, mild **haemolytic anaemia**, myopathy and cardiomyopathy resulting from deficiency of Kx protein and consequent weak expression or lack of expression of **Kell antigens**

macrocyte   a large erythrocyte

macrocytic anaemia an anaemia characterized by **macrocytosis**, e.g. in **megaloblastic anaemia** or the **myelodysplastic syndromes**

macrocytosis   having large erythrocytes

macroglobulinaemia an increased plasma concentration of macroglobulins, specifically IgM

macroglossia a large tongue, may be a feature of **amyloidosis**

macronormoblast an erythroblast which is larger than normal erythroblasts at the equivalent stage of development but which does not show the nucleocytoplasmic asynchrony which is characteristic of a megaloblast

macronormoblastic maturation erythroid maturation characterized by haemopoietic cells which are larger than normal but lack the nucleocytoplasmic asynchrony which is characteristic of **megaloblastic** haemopoiesis

macro-ovalocyte   an oval macrocyte

macrophage the end cell of the **monocyte** lineage, found mainly in tissues and, being **phagocytic**, important in protection against infection; neoplasms of macrophage and related lineages are designated in the **WHO classification** as shown in Table 6, p. 127

macrophage colony-stimulating factor (M-CSF) a haemopoietic growth factor, encoded by a gene at 1p13-21

macropolycyte a very large neutrophil, probably usually **tetraploid**

macrothrombocyte   a large platelet

macule   a skin lesion which is not raised

MAD   a gene, **Ma**x **D**imerization protein, gene map locus 2p13, archetypal member of a small family of transcriptional repressor proteins, which compete with MYC proteins for binding to **MAX**

MAF   a gene, avian **M**usculo**a**poneurotic **F**ibrosarcoma gene homologue, gene map locus 16q23, encodes a basic leucine zipper transcription factor; archetypal member of a family of such genes; *MAF* is dysregulated when brought into proximity to the *IGH* locus in 30–35% of patients with multiple myeloma and t(14;16)(q32;q23)

MAFB   a gene, avian **M**usculo**a**poneurotic **F**ibrosarcoma oncogene homologue **B**, gene map locus 20q11, encodes a MAF family basic region/leucine zipper transcription factor; *MAFB* is translocated and overexpressed when t(14;20)(q32;q11) brings it into proximity to the *IGH* locus in some cases of multiple myeloma

magnetic resonance imaging (MRI) or nuclear magnetic resonance imaging (NMR) an imaging technique using the inherent magnetic properties of body

Figure 53 A magnetic resonance imaging (MRI) scan.
A T2 weighted paracoronal magnetic resonance imaging (MRI) scan of the left shoulder; the humerus has an irregular articular outline and high and low signal bands in the subchondral region, typical of avascular necrosis; such lesions may be seen in patients with sickle cell disease.

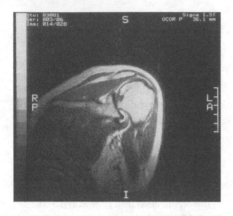

tissues containing free protons; paramagnetic molecules have their alignment changed by a combination of a strong magnetic field and radio frequency waves; as they regain their original position radio frequency waves are emitted which are then reconstructed into images (Fig. 53)

MAHA   microangiopathic   haemolytic anaemia

MAIPA   monoclonal   antibody-specific immobilization of platelet antigens

major   histocompatibility   complex (MHC)   a group of polymorphic proteins on the surface of cells, encoded by the HLA family of genes, which present modified antigen (as a short peptide in a surface groove) to T lymphocytes; molecules are divided into class I and class II; class I molecules (HLA-A, HLA-B and HLA-C) are concerned with recognition of antigens expressed on altered body cells and class II molecules (HLA-DP, HLA-DQ and HLA-DR) with the recognition of foreign antigens

MAL   a gene, T Lymphocyte Maturation-Associated protein, also known as *MKL1*, gene map locus 22q13, encodes a Golgi-associated membrane protein; *MAL* is over-expressed in primary mediastinal (thymic) B-cell lymphoma and contributes to the *OTT-MAL* fusion gene in infant M7 acute myeloid leukaemia associated with t(1;22)(p13;q13)

malabsorption   failure to absorb nutrients normally; haematological effects include deficiency of iron and vitamin B_{12} and folic acid and deficiency of vitamin K leading to coagulation defects

malaria   a disease resulting from infection by protozoan parasites of the Plasmodium genus

malignant   very injurious; in relation to neoplasms, aggressive and characterized by local invasion, distant spread (**metastasis**) and cytological differences from the equivalent normal tissues

malignant histiocytosis   a rare neoplasm of monocyte/macrophage lineage involving predominantly tissues other than the bone marrow; many patients reported to have had this condition have actually had a reactive haemophagocytic syndrome

malignant mastocytosis   an aggressive widespread **mast cell** neoplasm, more or less equivalent to aggressive systemic mastocytosis of the **WHO classification** (*see* Table 12)

malignant   melanoma   malignant tumour of cells analogous to melanocytes but not necessarily pigment-producing

malignant tertian malaria   malaria caused by *Plasmodium falciparum*

MALT   mucosa-associated lymphoid tissue

MALT-lymphoma   or   MALT-type lymphoma   a lymphoma of cells analogous to normal mucosa-associated lymphocytes

MALT   a   gene,   Mucosa-Associated Lymphoid Tissue lymphoma translocation gene 1, also known as *MLT*; gene map locus 18q21; encodes a cell surface adhesion molecule related to **CD22**, that is expressed strongly in blood, bone marrow, thymus and lymph node; contributes to the *AP12-MLT* fusion gene in MALT lymphoma associated with t(11;18)(q21;q21); in the presence of the API2-MLT fusion protein there is sequestration of BCL10 in the nucleus

Table 12   The WHO classification of mast cell disease (mastocytosis).

Cutaneous mastocytosis
Indolent systemic mastocytosis
Systemic mastocytosis with associated clinical, haematological an non-mast-cell lineage disease
Aggressive systemic mastocytosis
Mast cell leukaemia
Extracutaneous mastocytoma

mannose-binding lectin an **acute phase reactant**, synthesized by hepatocytes, that binds to bacteria, yeasts and some viruses and parasites, thereby activating mannose-associated proteases 1 and 2, which initiate the lectin pathway of complement activation (*see* **complement system** and Fig. 20, p. 81)

mannose-binding lectin deficiency an inherited condition in which mutation in the *MBL* gene leads to reduced plasma concentration of **mannose-binding lectin**, inability to activate the mannose-binding lectin complement pathway and recurrent pyogenic infections

mantle cell lymphoma a lymphoma of mature B cells analogous to lymphocytes in the **mantle zone** of a lymph node

mantle zone the circle of more darkly staining small lymphocytes that surrounds the paler germinal centre

mar a cytogenetic abbreviation indicating a **marker chromosome**

marasmus a form of protein-calorie malnutrition

marble bone disease *see* **osteopetrosis**

march haemoglobinuria haemolytic anaemia caused by mechanical trauma, e.g. from long marches on hard earth

marginal zone the zone between the red and white pulp of the spleen including the band of lymphocytes that surrounds the lymphoid follicles of the white pulp; the marginal zone lymphocytes are larger and paler than **mantle zone** lymphocytes

marginal zone lymphoma a lymphoma of mature B lymphocytes analogous to those in the marginal zone of lymphoid follicles; includes **MALT-type lymphoma**, **splenic marginal zone lymphoma** and **monocytoid B-cell lymphoma**

marker chromosome (mar) an abnormal chromosome that cannot be characterized by routine cytogenetic techniques

mast cell a tissue cell of myeloid lineage which is involved in immune responses and in inflammation

mast cell disease a WHO classification term for mast cell neoplasms, further categorized as shown in Table 12

mast cell leukaemia an acute leukaemia of **mast cell** lineage

mastocytosis an increase in mast cells, an alternative generic term encompassing all mast cell neoplasms used in the **WHO classification** being synonymous, in this context, with 'mast cell disease' (*see* Table 12)

matched unrelated donor (MUD) a bone marrow or haemopoietic stem cell donor who is unrelated to the recipient but has been matched for histocompatibility antigens (note: the term '**volunteer unrelated donor (VUD)**' is now preferred)

matrix metalloproteinases enzymes, with zinc at the active centre, that can cleave proteins of the extracellular matrix; they can be divided into four main groups—collagenases, gelatinases, stromeolysins and membrane-type metalloproteinases

maturation development of the features characterizing later cells of the same lineage

maturation arrest lack of maturing cells beyond a certain stage, e.g. arrest of granulopoiesis at the promyelocyte stage; usually indicates cell death at an inappropriate stage during maturation but an apparent maturation arrest can also result from immune destruction of maturing cells

Maurer's clefts linear inclusions in erythrocytes in *Plasmodium falciparum* malaria

MAX a gene, M̲YC-A̲ssociated factor X̲, gene map locus 14q23, encodes a helix–loop–helix leucine zipper protein which specifically heterodimerizes with **MYC** transcriptional activators and permits their binding to their cognate DNA binding sites (E-Boxes); also heterodimerizes with **MAD** family proteins (which encode transcriptional repressors) and allows them to bind E-boxes, thereby antagonizing the effects of MYC proteins

MAX a protein that forms heterodimers with **MYC** protein

May–Grünwald–Giemsa (MGG) a **Romanowsky** type stain used to stain blood and bone marrow films

May Hegglin anomaly an inherited anomaly with giant platelets and neutrophil inclusions resulting from a mutation in the non-muscle myosin heavy chain 9 gene (*NMMHC-A* or *MYH9*) at 22q11-13 (or 22q12.3-q13.2)

MBL the gene encoding **mannose-binding lectin**

McAb monoclonal antibody

MCH mean cell haemoglobin

MCHC mean cell haemoglobin concentration

M-CSF macrophage colony-stimulating factor

MCV mean cell volume

MDR multidrug resistance

MDS myelodysplastic syndrome or syndromes

MDS1 a gene, M̲yelod̲ysplasia S̲yndrome 1̲; gene map locus 3q26; this gene was previously thought to be an exon of *EVI1*, but is widely expressed both as a unique transcript and as a normal fusion transcript with EVI1; encodes a protein of unknown function; *MDS1* can contribute to an *AML1-MDS1* fusion oncogene in acute myeloid leukaemia, myelodysplastic syndromes and blast crisis of chronic granulocytic leukaemia associated with t(3;21)(q26;q22)

mean the average

mean cell haemoglobin (MCH) the average amount of haemoglobin in an individual's erythrocytes

mean cell haemoglobin concentration (MCHC) the average concentration of haemoglobin in an individual's erythrocytes

mean cell volume (MCV) the average size of an individual's erythrocytes

median the value that divides a population into two numerically equal halves

median disease-free survival the time when half of a studied population is still alive and free of relapse

median event-free survival the time when half of a studied population has neither died nor suffered relapse nor changed to alternative treatment

median overall survival the time when half of a studied population have died and half are still alive, synonymous with **median survival**

median survival the time when half of a studied population have died and half are still alive, synonymous with **median overall survival**

mediastinum the central part of the thoracic cavity, between the lungs

Medicines Act 1968 a UK Act of Parliament which provides the legal framework governing not only medicines but also the donation, testing, processing and issuing of blood components and products

Medicines Control Agency a UK organization that, among other duties, licences transfusion centres to prepare and provide blood components and products

medulla (i) the central part of a bone composed of an anastomosing network of trabecular or cancellous bone (ii) the central part of the kidney (iii) the central part of a lymph node (iv) the central part of the thymus

medullary cavity the spaces between the trabeculae of medullary bone occupied by fatty or haemopoietic marrow

MEFV the gene encoding pyrin or marenostrin, a protein expressed in myeloid cells and up-regulated during differentiation; strongly expressed in neutrophils and monocytes and thought to regulate phagocyte-induced inflammation; mutations in this gene can result in **familial Mediterranean fever**

megakaryoblast the earliest recognizable cell of **megakaryocyte** lineage

megakaryocyte a giant bone marrow cell, generally polyploid, of myeloid lineage which produces platelets by fragmentation of its own cytoplasm

megaloblast an erythroblast of larger than normal size showing retarded nuclear maturation in relation to cytoplasmic maturation

megaloblastic a term indicating abnormal haemopoiesis in which there is delayed nuclear development leading to large haemopoietic cells and erythrocytes, and dissociation between nuclear and cytoplasmic maturation (*see also* **giant metamyelocyte**)

megaloblastic anaemia anaemia with **megaloblastic** haemopoiesis

meiosis the process in which chromosomes of a cell replicate followed by two nuclear divisions so that the complement of chromosomes in the resultant cells is halved; the process by which germ cells are produced

MEL1 a gene, **PR D**omain-containing protein **16**, *PRDM16*, also known as *MDS1/EVI1*-Like gene **1**, gene map locus 1p36.6, encodes a PR **zinc finger** protein similar to MDS1, which is transcriptionally activated, probably by proximity to the ribophorin 1 gene, *RPN1*, at 3q21 in myelodysplastic syndrome and acute myeloid leukaemia associated with t(1;3)(p36;q21)

melaena black faeces, indicative of the presence of altered blood following haemorrhage into the upper gastrointestinal tract

melanocyte a pigmented skin cell found in the lower epidermis

melanoma a tumour of cells analogous to normal **melanocytes**; use of this term is often restricted to malignant tumours of melanocyte lineage

melphalan an alkylating agent used in the treatment of multiple myeloma and certain other tumours

memory cell a long-lived B cell or T cell that has already been exposed to an antigen and can participate in a secondary immune response following further exposure to the antigen

MEN an alternative name for *ELL*

meningeal leukaemia infiltration of leukaemic cells into the **meninges**

meninges the membranes covering the brain and spinal cord

meningitis inflammation of the **meninges**, often caused by bacterial or viral infection

menorrhagia heavy menstrual bleeding, may result from a haemostatic defect and may lead to **iron deficiency anaemia**

MER2 a gene at 11p15.5 that encodes antigens of the MER2 or RAPH blood group systems

M:E ratio myeloid:erythroid ratio

mercaptopurine an **antimetabolite** used in the maintenance treatment of acute lymphoblastic leukaemia

messenger ribonucleic acid (messenger RNA, mRNA) ribonucleic acid that is transcribed in the nucleus, on a DNA template, and moves to the cytoplasm, becoming attached to ribosomes and serving as a template for synthesis of proteins

metabolic acidosis acidosis other than that due to accumulation of carbonic acid

metabolic rate the rate of energy expenditure by the body

metabolism the aggregate of chemical process occurring in a living organism; includes anabolism, in which complex molecules and tissues are built up, and catabolism, in which tissues, cells and complex molecules are broken down

metachromatic staining uptake of a dye by a cell component with the dye then altering its colour

metamyelocyte a late, non-dividing cell in granulocyte maturation; it is derived from a myelocyte and matures to a band cell (*see* Fig. 25, p. 95)

metaphase the third of the five stages of **mitosis** in which the chromosomes become arranged around the equatorial plane of the **mitotic spindle** with their **centromeres** being attached to the spindle; the stage of nuclear division that is optimal for the examination of chromosomes (*see* Fig. 6, p. 14)

metarubricyte a name proposed for late erythroblasts

metastasis (i) the process by which a tumour spreads to distant parts of the body (ii) a deposit of tumour at a site distant from the primary tumour

metastatic able to metastasize or having metastasized

methaemalbumin a breakdown product of oxidized haemoglobin that has been bound to albumin; the Schumm's test detects methaemalbumin and a positive result gives evidence of intravascular haemolysis

methaemoglobin oxidized haemoglobin

methaemoglobinaemia an increased proportion of **methaemoglobin** in erythrocytes

methotrexate an **antimetabolite** that interferes with **folic acid** metabolism, used in the maintenance treatment of acute lymphoblastic leukaemia, in certain solid tumours and as an immunosuppressive agent

methylene blue a dye or stain which can be used as a component of a **Romanowsky** stain and also for staining **reticulocytes** and **Heinz bodies**; however, it should be noted that **new methylene blue** rather than methylene blue should be used for staining **haemoglobin H inclusions**

methylene tetrahydrofolate reductase an enzyme involved in **folic acid** metabolism; deficiency, resulting from homozygosity for a thermolabile variant, is present in 5% of the population and is associated with an increased risk of thrombosis

MGG May–Grünwald–Giemsa (stain)

MGUS **monoclonal gammopathy of undetermined significance**

MHC **major histocompatibility complex**

MIC the Morphologic-Immunophenotypic-Cytogenetic classification of leukaemias

MIC-M the Morphological-Immunophenotypic-Cytogenetic-Molecular genetic classification of leukaemias

microangiopathic haemolytic anaemia (MAHA) haemolytic anaemia caused by pathological processes, either endothelial damage or fibrin deposition, operating in small blood vessels

microarray analysis a method of assessing the RNA expression profile of a single tissue or cell line by means of synthetic oligonucleotides arrayed on a microchip

microcyte an abnormally small erythrocyte

microcytic anaemia anaemia characterized by **microcytosis**

microcytosis the presence of abnormally small erythrocytes

microfilaments 7 nm diameter filaments composed mainly of actin and actin-binding proteins that form part of the cytoskeleton of cells

microfilaria the stage of the life cycle of filaria which is identified by peripheral blood examination, the prelarval form of the parasite

microgram (μg) one millionth of a gram, 1×10^{-6} of a gram

microhaematocrit a haematocrit determination performed in a **capillary** tube

microlitre (μl) a millionth (10^{-6}) of a litre

micromegakaryocyte a megakaryocyte no more than 30 microns in diameter

micromole (μmol) a millionth (10^{-6}) of a mole

micron (μ) a millionth (10^{-6}) of a metre

microscope an instrument with a number of lenses for the visual examination of small objects

microscopic (i) very small (ii) pertaining to a microscope

microscopy examination by means of a **microscope**

microspherocyte a spherocyte which is smaller than a normal erythrocyte, formed by red cell fragmentation or by removal of parts of the erythrocyte membrane by splenic macrophages

microtubules polymers of tubulin, with a diameter of about 24 nm, that form part of the cytoskeleton; among other functions, they form the **mitotic spindle**

miliary tuberculosis disseminated tuberculosis with **granulomas** distributed through many organs

milligram (mg) one thousandth part (10^{-3}) of a gram

millilitre (ml) one thousandth part (10^{-3}) of a litre

millimole (mmol) one thousandth part (10^{-3}) of a mole

min a cytogenetic abbreviation for a **minute chromosome**

minimal residual disease (MRD) the presence of small numbers of neoplastic cells, detectable by techniques such as immunophenotyping or molecular genetic analysis, in bone marrow or blood samples in which no such cells are detectable by microscopic examination; minimal residual disease can be defined as the lowest level of residual disease detectable by available methods

minute chromosome (min) an **acentric** fragment of a chromosome, smaller than the width of a single **chromatid** (double minute chromosomes are acentric and atelomeric chromatin bodies composed of circular DNA)

miscarriage a spontaneous abortion

mis-sense mutation a mutation that results in the encoding of a different amino acid

mitochondrial pertaining to **mitochondria**

mitochondrial cytopathy an inherited disorder transmitted by genes on a circular mitochondrial chromosome, rather than by genes located on nuclear chromosomes

mitochondrion (plural mitochondria) a rod or oval-shaped organelle enclosed by two membranes with the inner membrane being folded into cristae which project into the matrix of the mitochondrion; the mitochondrion is the major site of energy production and has enzymes responsible for part of the haem synthesis pathway (*see* Fig. 34, p. 116)

mitogen an agent that promotes **mitosis**

mitomycin C an antitumour antibiotic which can cause **microangiopathic haemolytic anaemia**

mitosis the process of cell division in which chromosomes replicate before cell division; daughter cells therefore have the same complement of chromosomes as the parent cell (*see* Fig. 6, p. 14)

mitotic figure chromosomes visible during the process of **mitosis**

mitotic index the proportion of cells in **mitosis**

mitotic rate the rate at which cells enter **mitosis**

mitotic spindle the **microtubules** to which chromosomes attach during **metaphase**

mitozantrone an anti-cancer drug related to the anthracyclines, used in the treatment of lymphomas

MKL1 a gene, **M**ega**k**aryoblastic **L**eukaemia **1**, also known as *MAL*, gene map locus 22q13; encodes a nuclear protein containing a single SAP DNA-binding motif; *MKL1* contributes to *RBM15-MKL1* and *MKL1-RBM15* fusion genes in acute megakaryoblastic leukaemia of infants with t(1;22)(p13;q13); it is the *RBM15-MKL1* fusion gene (also known as *OTT-MAL*) which is likely to be oncogenic (*see also MAL, OTT*); the fusion protein retains all functional motifs encoded by each gene including an oligomerization domain in MKL1

MLF1 a gene, **M**yeloid **L**eukaemia **F**actor **1**, gene map locus 3q25.1, encodes a widely expressed protein of unknown function which has been observed in the cytoplasm and in the nucleus in discrete bodies; *MLF1* contributes to the *NPM-MLF1* fusion gene in acute myeloid leukaemia or myelodysplastic syndrome associated with t(3;5)(q25.1;q34)

MLL a gene, **M**ixed **L**ineage **L**eukaemia, also known as **M**yeloid-**L**ymphoid **L**eukaemia gene, *HRX, ALL-1* and *Htrx-1*, gene map locus 11q23, encodes a multidomain protein with some homology to the *Drosophila* transcriptional regulator, trithorax, which positively maintains the expression of multiple homeobox genes during development; *MLL* is fused to a great variety of other genes in acute myeloid leukaemia, acute lymphoblastic leukaemia and acute biphenotypic leukaemias; important functional domains include the AT hook (mediates DNA binding to AT-rich DNA sequences, phosphorylated in mitosis), subnuclear localization domains (SNLs, areas of high homology to trithorax), CxxC motifs (mediate interaction with transcriptional repressors), PHD **zinc fingers** (mediate interaction with nuclear cyclophilins), transactivation domain and **SET domains**; fusion proteins always retain the amino terminus of MLL (which carries the AT hook, SNL and CxxC motifs), and consistently lose the PHD, transactivation and SET domains, which are replaced by sequences of partner genes; *MLL* translocation breakpoints almost invariably lie within an 8.3 Kb breakpoint cluster region (bcr) which corresponds to a nuclear matrix attachment region and is susceptible to DNA cleavage in response to topoisomerase II inhibitors (e.g. etoposide) or apoptosis; there are at least 28 reported partner genes for *MLL* in leukaemia; fusion genes to which *MLL* contributes include:

- *MLL-AF1p* in t(1;11)(p32;q23)
- *MLL-AF1q* in t(1;11)(q21;q23)
- *MLL-LAF4* in t(2;11)(p15;p14)
- *MLL-LPP* and *LPP-MLL* in t(3;11)(q28;q23)
- *MLL-GMPS* in t(3;11)(q25;q23)
- *MLL-AF4* in t(4;11)(q21;q23)
- *MLL-GRAF* in t(5;11)(q31;q23)
- *MLL-AF5q31* in ins(5;11) (q31;q13q23)
- *MLL-AF6q21* in t(6;11)(q21;q23)
- *MLL-AF6q27* in t(6;11)(q27;q23)
- *MLL-AF9* in t(9;11)(p22;q23)
- *MLL-AF9q34* in t(9;11)(q34;q22)
- *MLL-ABI1* in t(10;11)(p11.2;q23)
- *MLL-AF10* in t(10;11)(p12;q23)
- *MLL-LARG* by interstitial deletion at 11q23
- *MLL-FBP17* in ins(11;9)(q23;q34) inv(11)(q13q23)
- *MLL-CALM* in inv(q14,2q23.1)
- *MLL-GPNH* in t(11;14)(q23;q24)
- *MLL-AF17* in t(11;17)(q23;q21)
- *MLL-RARA* in t(11;17)(q23;q12)
- *MLL-EEN* in t(11;19)(q23;p13)
- *MLL-ELL* in t(11;19)(q23;p13.1)
- *MLL-ENL* in t(11;19)(q23;p13.3)
- *MLL-CBP* in t(11;16)(q23;p13.3)
- *MLL-p300* in t(11;22)(q23;q13)
- *MLL-hCDCre* in t(11;22)(q23;q11.2)
- *MLL-AFX* in t(X;11)(q13;q23)
- *MLL-SEPTIN2* in two cases of AML with t(X;11;3;11) and ins(X;11)(q24;q23) respectively

MLL is also rearranged in acute myeloid leukaemia associated with t(8;11)(q24;q23) and t(10;11)(q22;q23); *MLL* is reduplicated in some patients

with acute myeloid leukaemia associated with trisomy 11 and in some with normal cytogenetics and is amplified in some patients with complex chromosomal rearrangements—in some of these patients *MLL* is found at multiple sites on the genome and in others the amplified gene has been located specifically in a ring chromosome, in a **homogeneously staining region** or in **double minute** chromosomes; duplication or amplification of a non-rearranged *MLL* gene is common in therapy-related myelodysplastic syndromes and acute myeloid leukaemia and is closely related to prior alkylating agents and to *TP53* mutations (which may be the cause of the duplication/amplification); partial amino terminal duplications of *MLL* due to genomic rearrangements have been reported in acute myeloid leukaemia and B-lineage acute lymphoblastic leukaemia, and carry a poor prognosis; deletions of exon 8 of *MLL* (encoding the first PHD domain) have been reported in T-lineage acute lymphoblastic leukaemia

MMSET a gene, **M**ultiple **M**yeloma **SET** domain, officially known as *WHSC1*—**W**olf-**H**irschhorn **S**yndrome **C**andidate gene **1**, gene map locus 4p16.3, encodes a **SET domain** protein; is involved, together with *FGFR3*, in a cryptic t(4;14)(p16.3;q32.2) translocation, which is present in about 20% of cases of multiple myeloma; the mechanism of dysregulation is proximity to an intronic enhancer on the der(4); Wolf–Hirschhorn syndrome is a congenital malformation syndrome associated with hemizygous deletions of 4p—it is unclear whether a single locus is involved in the phenotype —*WHSC1* is a candidate gene in the region

MN1 a gene, **M**eningioma **1**, gene map locus 22q12.3-qter, encodes a putative transcriptional activator, was initially cloned from a meningioma; *MN1* contributes to an *MN1-ETV6* fusion gene in acute myeloid leukaemia associated with t(12;22)(p13;q11); unusually for leukaemogenic fusion proteins involving *ETV6*, the MN1-ETV6 fusion protein lacks a functional ETV6 PNT (oligomerization) domain—the mechanism of transformation is unclear

MNS a red cell-specific blood group system, the relevant antigens being encoded by *GYPA* (M and N) and *GYPB* (S and s) and being expressed on glycophorins A and B respectively

molar solution a solution containing one **mole** per litre

mole the amount of a pure substance containing the same number of chemical units as there are atoms of carbon in exactly 12 grams of carbon^{12} (i.e. 6.023 × 10^{23}, Avogadro's number)

molecular genetic analysis analysis of DNA or RNA, analysis of genes

molecule the smallest unit of a chemical substance, formed from atoms

monoblast a blast cell of monocyte lineage, found in acute myelomonocytic leukaemia and acute monocytic/monoblastic leukaemia (FAB AML categories M4 and M5)

monoclonal relating to a single **clone**

monoclonal antibody (McAb) an antibody produced by a **clone** of lymphoid cells

monoclonal antibody-specific immobilization of platelet antigens (MAIPA) a test for anti-platelet antibodies

monoclonal gammopathy a neoplastic disorder in which a monoclonal immunoglobulin or part of an immunoglobulin in synthesized

monoclonal gammopathy of undetermined significance (MGUS) the presence of a serum **paraprotein** but without the criteria for a diagnosis of **multiple myeloma** being met, previously known as **benign monoclonal gammopathy**

monoclonal lymphocytes lymphocyte derived from a single precursor

monoclonal proliferation increased numbers of lymphoid (or other) cells belonging to a single clone, usually indicative of neoplasia

monocyte a mature cell of monocyte/macrophage lineage, derived from a promonocyte and maturing into a tissue macrophage

monocytic pertaining to monocytes

monocytopenia a low blood monocyte count

monocytosis an increase in the number of monocytes in the blood

monomer a molecule that combines with other similar molecules to form a **polymer**

mononuclear cell literally a cell with one nucleus but in practice this term is used to indicate a lymphocyte or a monocyte

monosomy the presence in a cell or a clone of cells of only a single copy of a chromosome of which there are normally two copies

monosomy 7 syndrome a myelodysplastic syndrome of infancy, now included in the category **juvenile myelomonocytic leukaemia** of the **WHO classification**

monozygotic arising from a single **zygote**, e.g. monozygotic twins

MORF a gene, **Mo**nocytic leukaemia zinc finger protein-**R**elated **F**actor; gene map locus 10q22; encodes a ubiquitously expressed histone acetylase related to *MOZ*; that contributed to *MORF-CBF* and *CBF-MORF* fusion genes in a child with M5 acute myeloid leukaemia

morphology the study of the appearance of cells or tissues of higher or lower organisms

Morquio's disease an inherited metabolic disorder, type IV mucopolysaccharidoses

mortality rate the rate of death, usually expressed as the number of deaths per 100 000 of population per year

morular cell a cell of **plasma cell** lineage containing multiple vacuoles, named because it is considered to resemble a mulberry; a **Mott cell**

mosaic an individual with two distinct cell lines arising from a single zygote

Mott cell a cell of plasma cell lineage containing multiple vacuoles, *see also* **morular cell**

mouse-rosette forming cell (MRFC) a lymphocyte able to form rosettes with mouse erythrocytes, an early test **for chronic lymphocytic leukaemia** used before monoclonal antibodies became available

MOZ a gene, **Mo**nocytic leukaemia **Z**inc finger, officially known as **Z**inc **F**inger protein **220** (*ZNF220*), gene map locus 8p11; leukaemogenesis mediated by

fusion gene products may be related to aberrant chromatin acetylation; *MOZ* fuses with:
- part of the *CBP* oncogene to form both *MOZ-CBP* and *CBP-MOZ* in M5 acute myeloid leukaemia associated with t(8;16)(p11;p13)
- part of the *TIF2* oncogene to form the *MOZ-TIF2* fusion gene in acute myeloid leukaemia associated with inv(8)(p11q13)
- part of the p300 gene to form both *MOZ-p300* and *p300-MOZ* fusion genes in M5 acute myeloid leukaemia associated with t(8;22)(p11;q13)

MPD myeloproliferative disorder

MPL a gene, **M**yelo**p**roliferative **L**eukaemia virus gene homologue, gene map locus 1p34, encodes the receptor for thrombopoietin, a truncated homologue of v-*mpl* which is an oncogene of a murine retrovirus; germline mutations in *MPL* are associated with congenital amegakaryocytic thrombocytopenia

MPO the gene at 17q23.1 encoding neutrophil **myeloperoxidase**

MPO **myeloperoxidase**

M-protein a largely disused term for a **paraprotein**

MRD **minimal residual disease**

MRFC **mouse-rosette forming cell**

MRI **magnetic resonance imaging**

mRNA **messenger ribonucleic acid**

MSF a gene, **M**LL **S**eptin-like **F**usion gene, gene map locus 17q25, encoding a protein of the septin family; *MSF* fused to *MLL* in a child who developed therapy-related acute myeloid leukaemia with t(11;17)(q23;q25)

MTCP1 a gene, **M**ature **T**-**C**ell **P**roliferation **1**, gene map locus Xq28, encodes two entirely different proteins, p8^MTCP1^ and p13^MTCP1^, which are generated by alternative splicing; p13^MTCP1^ has structural homology with *TCL-1*, which is more often involved in this type of leukaemia; p8MTCP1 is a cysteine-rich mitochondrial protein of uncertain function; *MTCP* is juxtaposed to the *TCRAD* (αδ) locus at 14q11 in some cases of T-prolymphocytic leukaemia with t(X;14)(q28;q11), leading to its overexpression; activation can also result

from proximity to the *TCRB* gene as a result of t(X;7)(q28;q35)

MTG8 an alternative designation of *ETO*

MTG16 a gene, **M**yeloid **T**ranslocation **G**ene on chromosome **16**, also known as **C**ore-**B**inding **F**actor, **A**lpha subunit **2**, **T**ranslocated to, **3**, *CBFA2T3*, gene map locus 16q24, a homologue of *MTG8 (ETO);* a widely expressed gene, it encodes 2 proteins which differ at their amino termini both of which carry 4 *nervy* zinc finger domains; *MTG16* is rearranged and translocated to the *CBFA2* locus in t(16;21)(q24;q22) associated with therapy-related acute myeloid leukaemia; analogous to the CBFA2/MTG8 (ETO) fusion protein, the CBFA2/MTG16 chimaera comprises the runt domain of CBFA2 fused to almost the entire coding region of MTG16

MTS1 *see CDKN2A*

MUC1 a gene, transmembrane **Mu**cin **1**, also known as **P**olymorphic **E**pithelial **M**ucin (*PEM*) and **P**eanut reactive **U**rinary **M**ucin (*PUM*), gene map locus 1q21, encodes an epithelium-specific mucin which is often overexpressed in carcinoma of the breast and is a target for the monoclonal antibodies HMFG-1, HMFG-2 and SM-3, used to detect solid tumour associated antigens; there is a series of tandem repeats which constitutes much of the coding region of the gene, with marked allelic variation due to variation in their number—consequently, *MUC1* is a locus used for VNTR (variable number of tandem repeats) analysis; *MUC1* is rearranged and over-expressed in B-cell non-Hodgkin's lymphoma associated with t(1;14)(q21;q32), as a result of being brought into proximity to the *IGH* enhancer; also overexpressed in epithelial tumours

mucin a mucopolysaccharide secreted by mucous glands

mucopolysaccharidoses a group of inherited metabolic disorders in which there is abnormal accumulation of mucopolysaccharides

mucosa mucous membrane, lining of the gastrointestinal, respiratory and genitourinary tracts

mucosa-associated lymphoid tissue (MALT) lymphoid tissue associated with mucous membranes such as the pharynx, larynx, bronchi and small intestine

mucous membrane mucosa, the lining of the gastrointestinal, respiratory and genitourinary tracts

MUD matched unrelated donor (note: **volunteer unrelated donor (VUD)** is now the preferred terminology)

multidrug resistance (MDR) genetically-based resistance of cells to the actions of multiple anti-cancer drugs

multiple myeloma a disseminated **plasma cell neoplasm** affecting predominantly the bone marrow, most cases being characterized by synthesis of a monoclonal immunoglobulin, a **Bence Jones protein** or both (Fig. 54); in the **WHO classification** it is designated 'plasma cell myeloma'

multiplex PCR a PCR reaction using a number of pairs of primers so that a number of DNA segments can be amplified simultaneously

multipotent myeloid stem cell a haemopoietic stem cell capable of giving rise to all myeloid lineages, also know as the **common myeloid progenitor**

MUM1 see *IRF4*

MUM2/3 see *IRTA1* and *IRTA2*

murine relating to the mouse

mutagen an agent capable of causing mutation

mutagenic a description of an agent that can cause mutation

mutation a structural alteration in the DNA of a cell, either a **germ cell** or a **somatic cell**, which can be transmitted to the fertilized gamete or to the progeny of the somatic cell

MYB a gene, avian <u>My</u>elo<u>b</u>lastosis viral oncogene homologue, gene map locus 6q22, encodes a transcriptional activator protein, c-MYB, with sequence-specific DNA-binding activity, that is expressed in haemopoietic precursor cells; archetypal member of a small family of related genes including *a-MYB* (at 8q22, expressed in germ cells and breast tissue) and *b-MYB* (at 20q13.1, ubiquitously expressed); the c-MYB protein plays a key role in cell cycle control in haemopoi-

Figure 54 Multiple myeloma.
Laboratory investigations in multiple myeloma. Scanning densitometry of an electrophoretic strip (top) showing two bands in the early γ region (arrow) and late γ region (arrowheads) respectively. The corresponding electrophoretic strip is shown in the left lane (bottom). Immunofixation shows a single band identifiable with anti-γ (lane 2) and two bands identifiable with anti-λ (lane 6); the patient therefore has an IgGλ paraprotein and a λ Bence Jones protein in the serum. Serum Bence Jones protein is seen in the serum in patients with multiple myeloma and renal failure.

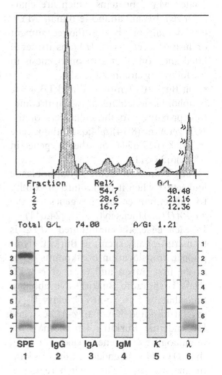

etic cells, its expression declining as they differentiate; the first intron of *MYB* contains two interferon-responsive regulatory elements; c-MYB protein is overexpressed in oestrogen-receptor positive breast cancer; b-MYB is constitutively phosphorylated by **cyclin A1** in cases of acute myeloid leukaemia that overexpress *CCNA1*

MYC a gene, avian <u>My</u>elo<u>c</u>ytomatosis viral oncogene homologue, gene map locus 8q24.12, encodes three widely expressed basic helix–loop–helix-leucine zipper transcription factors derived from

alternative translational start sites on the same mRNA (known as 62KD *c*-MYC, 64KD *c*-MYC and S-MYC); all three proteins are inactive as monomers or homodimers and heterodimerize with MAX to bind target DNA sequences known as E-boxes; they are involved in the activation of genes involved in cellular proliferation and the inhibition of growth inhibitory genes; *c*-MYC is the archetypal member of a family of related MYC proteins which are characterized by an amino-terminal 'MYC box' domain involved in the recruitment of histone acetylases; *MYC* is dysregulated and contributes to oncogenesis in the following circumstances:
• in Burkitt's lymphoma and L3 acute lymphoblastic leukaemia when it comes into proximity to the enhancers of the *IGH* gene in t(8;14)(q24;q32), the κ gene in t(2;8)(p12;q24) or the λ gene in t(8;22)(q24;q11)
• in T-lineage acute lymphoblastic leukaemia when it comes into proximity to the enhancer of the genes of the *TCRAD* (αδ) locus in t(8;14)(q24;q11)
In each case, the unmutated *MYC* is transcriptionally silent; in Burkitt's lymphoma, translocation breakpoints occur in the first intron and exon of *c-MYC* (class I, sporadic Burkitt's lymphoma), immediately 5′ to *c-MYC* (class II) or several hundred Kb 5′ to *c-MYC* (class III, endemic Burkitt's lymphoma); the immunoglobulin gene breakpoint is in the VDJ region in endemic Burkitt's lymphoma, but in a class switch region in sporadic and HIV-associated Burkitt's lymphoma; most translocated *MYC* genes carry additional point mutations or small deletions, typically at the boundary of intron 1 and exon 1 and result from somatic hypermutation (*see* Fig. 46, p. 135); *MYC* is amplified, uncommonly, in acute myeloid leukaemia

Mycobacterium a genus of microorganisms including those that cause tuberculosis and leprosy

mycophenolate mofetil an immunosuppressive drug that can cause neutropenia, hypolobulation of neutrophils and detached nuclear fragments in cells of neutrophil lineage

Mycoplasma a genus of microorganisms that are smaller than bacteria, including *Mycoplasma pneumoniae* which can cause atypical pneumonia, often with an associated **cold agglutinin**

mycosis fungoides a cutaneous T-cell neoplasm with formation of cutaneous tumours composed of lymphoma cells

myeloblast the earliest morphologically recognizable cell of the granulocyte lineages (*see* Fig. 25, p. 95)

myelocyte an intermediate cell in granulocyte maturation, derived from a promyelocyte and undergoing two cycles of mitosis before maturing into a metamyelocyte (*see* Fig. 25, p. 95)

myelodysplasia morphologically abnormal myeloid maturation

myelodysplastic syndrome or syndromes (MDS) a group of related neoplastic disorders that have in common that haemopoiesis is morphologically dysplastic and functionally ineffective; MDS may evolve into AML; in the WHO classification designated as shown in Table 13 (*see also* Fig. 55, p. 168)

myelofibrosis fibrosis of the bone marrow; this term is best restricted to a bone marrow that shows collagen deposition, not merely increased reticulin; the latter is better referred to as 'reticulin fibrosis' or 'increased reticulin deposition'

myelogenous pertaining to bone marrow haemopoietic cells

myeloid (i) pertaining to the bone marrow (ii) pertaining to granulocyte–monocyte lineages

myeloid:erythroid ratio (M:E ratio) the ratio of cells of granulocyte–monocyte lineage to cells of erythroid lineage in the bone marrow

myeloid metaplasia the occurrence of haemopoiesis at extramedullary sites; myelofibrosis with myeloid metaplasia is an alternative designation of **idiopathic myelofibrosis**

myelokathexis an inherited disorder in which neutrophils have long filaments separating lobes

Table 13 The WHO classification of myelodysplastic syndromes (MDS)*.

Disease	Peripheral blood findings	Bone marrow findings
Refractory anaemia (RA)	Anaemia, blasts rarely seen and always less than 1%	Dysplasia confined to erythroid lineage, < 5% blasts, < 15% ringed sideroblasts
Refractory anaemia with ringed sideroblasts (RARS)	Anaemia, no blasts	Dysplasia confined to erythroid lineage, < 5% blasts, ≥ 15% ringed sideroblasts
Refractory cytopenia with multilineage dysplasia (RCMD)†	Cytopenias (bicytopenia or pancytopenia), no or rare blasts, no Auer rods, < 1 × 10⁹/l monocytes	Dysplasia in ≥ 10% of the cells of two or more myeloid cell lineages, < 5% blasts, < 15% ringed sideroblasts, no Auer rods
Refractory cytopenia with multilineage dysplasia and ringed sideroblasts (RCMD-RS)†	Cytopenias (bicytopenia or pancytopenia), no or rare blasts, no Auer rods, < 1 × 10⁹/l monocytes	Dysplasia in ≥ 10% of the cells of two or more myeloid cell lineages, < 5% blasts, ≥ 15% ringed sideroblasts, no Auer rods
Refractory anaemia with excess blasts 1 (RAEB-1)†	Cytopenias, < 5% blasts, no Auer rods, < 1 × 10⁹/l monocytes	Unilineage or multilineage dysplasia, 5–9% blasts, no Auer rods
Refractory anaemia with excess blasts 2 (RAEB-2)†	Cytopenias, 5–19% blasts, Auer rods sometimes present, < 1 × 10⁹/l monocytes	Unilineage or multilineage dysplasia, 10–19% blasts, Auer rods sometimes present
Myelodysplastic syndrome-unclassified (MDS-U)†	Cytopenias, no or rare blasts, no Auer rods	Unilineage dysplasia, < 5% blasts. No Auer rods
MDS associated with isolated del(5q)	Anaemia, platelet count usual normal or elevated, < 5% blasts	Megakaryocytes in normal or increased numbers but with hypolobated nuclei, < 5% blasts, no Auer rods

$$\text{subscripts as shown; superscripts denote } 10^9/l$$

* Reproduced from Bain BJ, *Leukaemia Diagnosis*, 3rd edn, Blackwell Publishing, Oxford, 2003.
† If cases are therapy-related, this should be specified and it should be further specified whether cases are alkylating agent-related (the majority) or topoisomerase II-interactive drug-related (a small minority).

myeloma a tumour composed of cells of plasma cell lineage (*see* **multiple myeloma**)

myelomatosis an alternative designation of **multiple myeloma**

myeloperoxidase the peroxidase isoenzyme in cells of granulocyte and monocyte lineages, neutrophil myeloperoxidase being encoded by the *MPO* gene

myeloperoxidase deficiency a deficiency of neutrophil **myeloperoxidase**, resulting from a mutation in the *MPO* gene; deficiency is usually asymptomatic but in people with diabetes mellitus can lead to disseminated **candidiasis**

myelophthisic anaemia a little used term for **leucoerythroblastic anaemia**

myeloproliferative disorder (MPD) a neoplastic conditions in which there is expansion of at least one myeloid lineage with retention of normal maturation so that increased numbers of mature end cells are produced (Table 14) (*see also* Fig. 55)

myeloproliferative-myelodysplastic disorder a WHO category of haematological neoplasms encompassing cases with both myeloproliferative and myelodysplastic features (Fig. 55)

Figure 55   the relationship between the myelodysplastic and myeloproliferative disorders.
A diagrammatic representation, based on the WHO classification, showing the myeloproliferative disorders, the myelodysplastic syndromes and the 'overlap' myelodysplastic/myeloproliferative disorders.

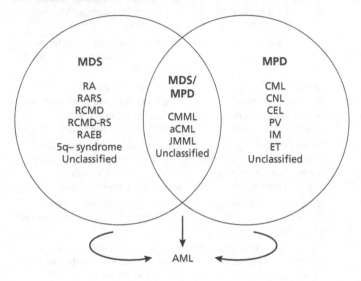

Table 14   The WHO classification of the chronic myeloproliferative disorders.

Chronic myelogenous leukaemia, Philadelphia chromosome positive (t(9;22)(q34;q11), *BCR-ABL* fusion)
Chronic neutrophilic leukaemia
Chronic eosinophilic leukaemia/hypereosinophilic syndrome
Chronic idiopathic myelofibrosis
Polycythaemia vera
Essential thrombocythaemia
Myeloproliferative disorders, unclassifiable

myelosclerosis an alternative designation of **myelofibrosis**

myelosuppression inhibition of haemopoiesis

myeov a gene, My̱eloma o̱verexpressed gene, gene map locus 11.q13, encodes a putative RNA-binding protein with a hydrophobic carboxy terminal tail characteristic of cytoplasmically exposed membrane proteins; overexpressed, together with *cyclin D1*, in a subset of cell lines with t(11;14)(q13;q32) derived from patients with multiple myeloma

MYH11 a gene, My̱osin H̱eavy chain gene **11**, also known as *SMMHC—*

Smooth Muscle Myosin Heavy Chain gene, gene map locus 16p13.13; part of *MYH11* fuses with part of *CBFB* at 16q22 in M4Eo acute myeloid leukaemia associated with inv(16)(p13q22) and t(16;16)(p13;q22)

myocardial infarction infarction of cardiac muscle, usually resulting from **coronary occlusion**; haematological effects include **neutrophilia** and an increase in the **erythrocyte sedimentation rate**

myxoedema hypothyroidism; haematological effects include anaemia, macrocytosis and the presence of **acanthocytes**

N

NAD nicotine adenine dinucleotide

NADP nicotine adenine dinucleotide phosphate

naïve lymphocyte a T or B lymphocyte that has not yet encountered **antigen**

nanogram one thousandth millionth of a gram, 1×10^{-9} of a gram

NAP neutrophil alkaline phosphatase

NAP score a summation of the grading of **neutrophil alkaline phosphatase** activity in 100 neutrophils

naphthol AS acetate esterase (NASA) a **non-specific esterase** activity characteristic on the monocyte lineage

naphthol AS-D acetate esterase (NASDA) a **non-specific esterase** activity characteristic of the monocyte lineage

naphthol AS-D chloroacetate esterase (chloroacetate esterase, CAE) esterase activity specific for neutrophils (and mast cells)

NASA esterase naphthol AS acetate esterase

NASDA esterase naphthol AS-D acetate esterase

National External Quality Assurance Scheme (NEQAS) a UK based national quality assurance scheme for pathology laboratories

National Institute of Clinical Excellence (NICE) a body set up to assess new treatments, compile clinical guidelines and facilitate introduction of cost effective treatments (UK)

natural killer cell (NK cell) a lymphocyte which has **Fc receptors** and can kill cells by **antibody-dependent cellular cytotoxicity** (ADCC) but is also capable of direct killing of cells, e.g. virus-infected cells or tumour cells, without a requirement for the presence of an antibody directed at cellular antigens; the latter NK activity is usually overruled by a killer-inhibitory receptor that recognizes MHC type I molecules on normal body cells

natural killer cell leukaemia a leukaemia of cells analogous to **natural killer** cells, which may or may not retain natural killer function

naturally occurring antibody a blood group antibody that develops without exposure to the corresponding red cell antigen

naturally occurring anticoagulants a collective name for **protein C, protein S, antithrombin** and **tissue factor pathway inhibitor** (Fig. 56)

NBS1 a gene at 8q21, **N**ijmegen **B**reakage **S**yndrome **1**, that is mutated in the **Nijmegen breakage syndrome**; encodes a **forkhead** domain protein, nibrin, which is part of the 'BRCA1-associated genome surveillance complex', involved in the detection and repair of abnormal DNA structures

NCCLS National Committee for Clinical Laboratory Standards (USA)

NCF1 a gene at 7q11.23 encoding **N**eutrophil **C**ytosolic **F**actor **1** (p47—*phox*), mutation of which can lead to **chronic granulomatous disease**

NCF2 a gene at 1q25 encoding **N**eutrophil **C**ytosolic **F**actor **2** (p67—*phox*), mutation of which can lead to **chronic granulomatous disease**

NCI National Cancer Institute (USA)

neonatal alloimmune thrombocytopenia intrauterine or neonatal thrombocytopenia resulting from transplacental passage of maternal platelet alloantibodies

Figure 56 Naturally occurring anticoagulants.
The naturally occurring anticoagulants and inhibitors of coagulation. Positive effects are shown by an arrow and negative effects by a crossed arrow. Plasma contains two naturally occurring anticoagulants, antithrombin (AT) and tissue factor pathway inhibitor (TFPI). AT inhibits all the serine proteases of the coagulation network— XIIa, XIa, IXa, Xa and IIa (thrombin); its action is greatly enhanced by heparin or by heparin-related molecules on the surface of cells. TFPI, both that present in plasma and that released by activated platelets, inhibits tissue factor (TF), VIIIa and Va. The generation of thrombin leads to activation of other naturally occurring anticoagulants. Thrombin binds to thrombomodulin, a receptor on endothelial cells, and the complex activates protein C (PC) to activated protein C (APC), which is a serine protease capable of destroying factors VIIIa and Va. The action of APC is enhanced by protein S (PS), which binds PC to the platelet surface. AT and TFPI are both synthesized in endothelial cells.

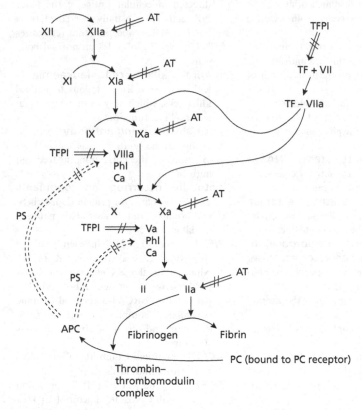

neoplasia the process by which neoplasms develop

neoplasm literally a 'new growth' or tumour; in modern usage proliferation of a population of cells derived from a genetically altered precursor cell leading to formation of a solid tumour, such as a carcinoma, or to leukaemia or a related condition

neoplastic pertaining to a **neoplasm**

nephritis inflammation of the kidneys

nephrotic syndrome fluid retention and oedema as a consequence of hypoalbuminaemia caused by heavy proteinuria

NEQAS National External Quality Assurance Scheme

neuroblastoma a malignant tumour of neuroendocrine origin occurring mainly in children

neurofibromatosis an inherited condition characterized by multiple neurofibromas· and small areas of skin pigmentation (café au lait spots); there is an increased incidence of **juvenile myelomonocytic leukaemia** (including **monosomy 7 syndrome**) (*see also* **NF1**)

neuronal lipofuscinosis (Batten's disease) an inherited metabolic disorder which may be a cause of vacuolated bone marrow macrophages

neutropenia reduced numbers of neutrophils in the blood

neutrophil a granulocyte with neutrophilic granules, i.e. with granules which are neither strongly acidophilic nor strongly basophilic but take up both components of the stain

neutrophil alkaline phosphatase (NAP) the isoenzyme of alkaline phosphate that is present in a neutrophil

neutrophil elastase a protease which is one of the major constituents of azurophilic granules of neutrophils and is expressed more weakly in the granules of monocytes and macrophages, encoded by the *ELA* gene at 19p13.3; monoclonal antibodies to neutrophil elastase can be used to identify maturing cells of neutrophil lineage

neutrophilia increased numbers of neutrophils in the blood

neutrophilic leukaemia a chronic Philadelphia-negative leukaemia in which the major cell in the blood is a mature neutrophil

neutrophil leucocytosis increased numbers of neutrophils in the blood

neutrophil specific granule deficiency an inherited defect of neutrophil function in which there are bilobed or poorly lobulated neutrophils that are deficient in at least one primary granule protein and all secondary and tertiary granule proteins, resulting from mutation in the *ClEBPε* gene; eosinophil granules also lack specific proteins

new methylene blue a dye or stain which can be used in a **Romanowsky stain** and also to stain **reticulocytes, Heinz bodies** and **haemoglobin H inclusions**

NEXIN1 a gene, also known as Protease Nexin 1 (*PN1*) and Protease Inhibitor 7 (*PI7*); gene map locus 2q33–q35; encodes a member of the Serpin superfamily, an important physiological regulator of thrombin in tissues; PN1 forms 1:1 (stoichiometric) complexes with thrombin which are removed by cellular endocytosis

NF1 a gene, Neurofibromatosis, type 1 also known as neurofibromin, gene map locus 17q11, a candidate tumour suppressor gene, encodes a ubiquitously expressed **GTPase**-activating protein (GAP), which accelerates the hydrolysis of **GTP** by **RAS**, thereby inactivating it—loss of *NF1* can lead to increased RAS activity; alternative splicing of *NF1* gives rise to at least four isoforms; mutations of *NF1* cause neurofibromatosis type 1, in which there is a propensity to the development of juvenile myelomonocytic leukaemia (often associated with loss of the normal allele) and acute myeloid leukaemia; acquired mutations of *NF1* are also associated with an increased rate of occurrence of juvenile myelomonocytic leukaemia; mutations are also sometimes present in myelodysplastic syndrome

NFκB1 a gene, Nuclear Factor κ (kappa) B, subunit 1, gene map locus 4q23-q24, encodes two widely expressed transcription factors, p50 and p105, that are activated by a wide range of inflammatory signals; NFκB proteins normally complex with **REL** proteins; in the quiescent state, the NFκB/REL complex is sequestered in the cytoplasm by the inhibitory proteins IκB1 and IκB2; inflammatory cytokines promote IκB degradation by inducing their phosphorylation, thereby allowing the NFκB/REL complex to enter the nucleus and induce transcription (*see also TAX*)

NFκB2 a gene, Nuclear Factor κ (kappa)-B, subunit 2, also known as *LYT10*, gene map locus 10q24; see also *NFκB1*; encoding p52 and p100 members of the REL/NFκB family of transcription factors; *NFκB2* is involved in t(10;14)(q24;q32) which is found in less than 1% of cases of diffuse large B-cell lymphoma but in a somewhat higher percentage of low grade B-cell lymphoma.

NICE National Institute of Clinical Excellence

nicotine adenine dinucleotide (NAD) and nicotine adenine dinucleotide phosphate (NADP) coenzymes that act as electron and hydrogen carriers in some oxidation-reduction reactions

NIDDM non-insulin dependent diabetes mellitus

Niemann–Pick disease an inherited metabolic disorder of which foamy macrophages in the bone marrow are one feature

night sweats heavy nocturnal sweating, characteristic of lymphoma, particularly Hodgkin's disease, but not pathognomonic

NIH National Institutes of Health (USA)

Nijmegen breakage syndrome an autosomal recessive chromosomal instability syndrome characterized by microcephaly, mental retardation, café au lait spots, growth retardation, immunodeficiency and cancer predisposition, resulting from mutation in the *NBS1* gene; associated with an increased incidence of B-lineage neoplasms and a lesser increase in T-lineage neoplasms

nitrogen mustard one of the earliest cytotoxic drugs, related to mustard gas and previously used in the treatment of Hodgkin's disease

nitrosourea a group of anti-cancer drugs, including BCNU and CCNU, used in treating lymphomas and solid tumours

nitrous oxide an anaesthetic gas; heavy exposure can cause megaloblastic haemopoiesis as a consequence of inactivation of **vitamin B$_{12}$**

NK cell natural killer cell

NMR nuclear magnetic resonance (imaging)

nomogram a diagram representing the relationship between variables in a given system, e.g. the relationship of surface area to height and weight (*see* Fig. 71, p. 212) or between pounds and kilograms

non-Hodgkin's lymphoma (NHL) any lymphoma other than Hodgkin's disease (*see* Tables 10 and 11, pp. 137 and 153)

non-insulin dependent diabetes mellitus a form of **diabetes mellitus** with onset usually in middle or old age, which can be controlled by diet and oral hypoglycaemic agents

non-random chromosomal abnormality (i) a chromosomal abnormality present in a population of cells; as defined by the International System of Nomenclature a non-random (or clonal) abnormality is present if at least two cells show the same structural abnormality or additional chromosome or if at least three cells show the same chromosomal loss (ii) a recurring chromosomal abnormality, often associated with a specific neoplasm

non-reciprocal translocation a translocation in which a segment of one chromosome moves to another chromosome but there is no reciprocal transfer

non-secretor *see FUT1*

non-secretory myeloma multiple myeloma in which there is no **paraprotein** in the serum nor any **Bence Jones protein** in the urine

nonsense mutation a mutation that converts a codon from one encoding an amino acid to one that does not encode an amino acid and therefore functions as a stop codon

normal distribution having a Gaussian or bell-shaped distribution when plotted as a histogram (*see* Fig. 45, p. 128)

normal range the range of results of a specific laboratory test expected in a healthy population (*see also* **reference range**)

normoblast an erythroblast showing normoblastic maturation

normoblastic maturation erythroid maturation in which the nucleus and cytoplasm mature synchronously

normochromic normally staining (of a red cell)

normocytic of normal size (of a red cell)

Northern blot a modification of a **Southern blot**, a technique for separating RNA molecules according to size, for subsequent 'blotting' onto a membrane and hybridization: the name is a play on words

NPM1 a gene, **N**ucleo**p**hos**m**in/nucleoplasmin family, member **1**, gene map locus 5q34-35, encodes a nucleolar phosphoprotein whose levels increase in normal cells when they are mitotically

stimulated; it is involved in the assembly of ribosomal proteins into ribosomes and is associated with unduplicated centrosomes, and is dissociated from them by **CDK2/cyclin** E-mediated phosphorylation; part of *NPM* fuses with:
* part of the *RARA* gene to form *NPM-RARA* in t(5;17)(q32;q21) associated with M3-like acute myeloid leukaemia; the fusion protein exhibits both positive and negative transcriptional properties
* part of the *MLF1* oncogene to form an *NPM-MLF1* fusion gene in acute myeloid leukaemia or myelodysplastic syndrome associated with t(3;5)(q25.1;q34)
* part of the *ALK* oncogene to form an *NPM-ALK* fusion gene in T-lineage anaplastic large cell lymphoma associated with t(2;5)(p23;q35); it can then shuttle NPM-ALK to the nucleus

NSD1 a gene, **N**uclear receptor-binding **S**u-var, enhancer of zeste, and trithorax **D**omain protein **1**, also known as SET domain protein 1, gene map locus 5q35, encodes a widely expressed **SET domain** protein; two transcripts are made from the gene, one of which is only seen in haemopoietic cells; *NSD1* contributes to *NUP-NSD1* and *NSD1-NUP98* fusion genes in childhood acute myeloid leukaemia associated with t(5;11)(q35;p15.5)

nuclear magnetic resonance imaging (NMR) *see* **magnetic resonance imaging (MRI)**

nuclear membrane the lipid bilayer that encloses the nucleus

nucleated red blood cell (NRBC) the term often used to designate **erythroblasts** in the circulating blood

nucleolus a unique region of the nucleus created by the **transcription** of rRNA

nucleoside a purine or pyrimidine base bonded to a pentose sugar (*see also* **nucleotide**)

nucleoside analogue drugs which are analogues of **nucleosides**, including a group of anti-cancer drugs (fludarabine, pentostatin and cladribine) and also certain drugs used in treating **HIV** infection

nucleotide the basic unit of DNA and RNA: a nucleotide is composed of a

nitrogenous base (a heterocyclic ring containing nitrogen and carbon atoms), a 5-carbon ring-shaped sugar molecule (a pentose) which, in the case of DNA is deoxyribose and in the case of RNA is ribose, and a phosphate group; a base linked to the pentose group is designated a **nucleoside**, which when phosphorylated at the 3' position of the pentose group is designated a nucleotide; the nitrogenous bases fall into two classes; purines have fused five and six member rings and pyrimidines have six member rings

nucleus that part of a cell, which includes chromosomal DNA and nuclear proteins such as histones, enclosed in a nuclear membrane

NuMA a gene, **Nu**clear **M**itotic **A**pparatus, gene map locus 11q13; encodes a nuclear protein that localizes to the spindle apparatus during mitosis; contributes to the *NuMA-RARα* fusion gene in M3-like acute myeloid leukaemia associated with t(11;17)(q13;q21)

NUP98 a gene, **Nu**cleo**p**orin **98**, gene map locus 11p15; encodes a component of the nuclear pore complex which regulates nucleocytoplasmic transport of protein and RNA; belongs to a subgroup of nucleoporins that contain FG (phenylalanine-glycine) repeats which are docking sites for nuclear transport receptors; *NUP98* contributes to:
* the *NUP98-PMX1* fusion gene in therapy-related acute myeloid leukaemia and blast crisis of chronic granulocytic leukaemia associated with t(1;11)(q23;p15)
* the *NUP98-HOXD13* gene and the *NUP-FN1* gene in therapy-related and *de novo* acute myeloid leukaemia associated with t(2;11)(q31;p15)
* the *NUP98-RAP1GDS1* gene in T-lineage acute lymphoblastic leukaemia associated with t(4;11)(q21;p15)
* the *NUP-NSD1* and *NSD1-NUP98* fusion genes in childhood acute myeloid leukaemia associated with t(5;11)(q35;p15.5)
* the *NUP98-HOXA9* fusion gene in myelodysplastic syndrome and acute myeloid leukaemia associated with t(7;11)(p15;p15)

• the *NUP98-HOXA11* fusion gene in a patient with Ph-negative chronic myeloid leukaemia progressing rapidly to acute myeloid leukaemia

• the *NUP98-FGFR1* fusion gene in acute myeloid leukaemia associated with t(8;11)(p11;p15)

• a fusion gene with *LEDGF* in a patient with *de novo* acute myeloid leukaemia associated with t(9;11)(p22;p15)

• the *NUP98-DDX10* gene in inv(11)(p15q22) associated with *de novo* and therapy-related acute myeloid leukaemia and myelodysplastic syndromes

• the *NUP98-TOP1* gene in therapy-related acute myeloid leukaemia or myelodysplastic syndrome associated with t(11;20)(p15;q11)

In all cases, chimaeric proteins involving NUP98 carry the amino terminal FG repeats of NUP98 fused to the carboxy terminus of the partner protein; the FG repeats enable

NUP214   *see CAN*

O

O_2 oxygen

oat cell carcinoma   a previous designation of small cell carcinoma of the lung

occult   hidden, as in 'occult neoplasm'

Oct2   a transcription factor for immunoglobulin genes which is expressed in the neoplastic cells of nodular lymphocyte predominant Hodgkin's disease but not in the neoplastic cells of classical Hodgkin's disease

oedema   an increase of interstitial (or intra-alveolar) fluid

OK   a blood group system, antigens being encoded by polymorphic variants of the *BSG* gene at 19p13.3

oligoclonal   a description of lymphocytes, plasma cell or both belonging to a small number of clones

oligonucleotide   a short chemically produced sequence of nucleotides, often complementary to a sequence of cellular DNA or RNA and therefore suitable for use as a probe or as a PCR **primer**

oliguria   marked reduction in urine production

Omenn's syndrome   combined immunodeficiency with absence of circulating B cells and presence of activated oligoclonal T cells, which infiltrate the skin and intestine, resulting from a mutation of the *RAG1* or *RAG2* genes; clinical features often include erythroderma, lymphadenopathy, hepatomegaly, splenomegaly and an increased incidence of life-threatening infections.

OMIM   Online Mendelian Inheritance in Man, website http://www.ncbi.nlm.nih.gov/omim/

onchocerciasis   a disease resulting from infection by the parasite *Onchocerca volvulus*

oncogene   a transduced, cancer-inducing gene in the genome of a transforming virus; most oncogenes have cellular counterparts, termed **proto-oncogenes** which have normal physiological functions, but which may be either dysregulated or structurally modified and contribute to **oncogenesis** in various tumours; the term 'oncogene' is often used to refer not only to these proto-oncogenes but also to any gene that contributes to the development, maintenance or further evolution of a neoplastic condition

oncogenesis   the process of development of a tumour or other neoplasm

oncoprotein   a protein encoded by an **proto-oncogene** that causes or contributes to the malignant phenotype of a neoplastic cell

open reading frame   a series of triplet codes that can be read as a genetic message

ophthalmic   pertaining to the eye

ophthalmology   the branch of medicine dealing with the eye

ophthalmoscope   a device for examining the interior of the eye

opportunistic infection   an infection that occurs as a result of reduced host defences, e.g. in a patient with a lymphoproliferative disorder or AIDS or during the administration of anti-cancer chemotherapy, often caused by an organism that in the normal host is generally non-pathogenic

opsonin   a protein, such as **immunoglobulin** or an activated **complement component**, that coats a foreign particle, such as a bacterium, and by so doing makes **phagocytosis** more likely

opsonization   the binding of an **opsonin** to a bacterium or other foreign particle

optic pertaining to vision

optic atrophy atrophy of the optic nerve, the end stage of **optic neuropathy**, may be a feature of **vitamin B$_{12}$ deficiency**

optic disc the pale area at the back of the eye where the optic nerve enters the eye

optic nerve one of the two cranial nerves arising in the retina and conducting impulses to the optic cortex of the brain

optic neuropathy degeneration of the neurones of the **optic nerve**, may be a feature of **vitamin B$_{12}$ deficiency**

oral pertaining to the mouth

Oraya fever a disease occurring in South America, resulting from infection by *Bartonella bacilliformis* and having **haemolytic anaemia** as one of its features

organ an arrangement of tissues into a compact organized structure with specific functions

organelle one of a group of highly organized membrane-enclosed structures within the cytoplasm, each with its own specific function, e.g. **mitochondrion, Golgi apparatus, endoplasmic reticulum, lysosome, peroxisome**

organic pertaining to substances containing carbon from living or once living sources

organism a living animal or plant or any size from a microbe to man

organomegaly enlargement of organs; in haematological jargon 'no organomegaly' usually indicates no enlargement of the abdominal organs such as the liver and spleen

osmolarity a measure of the concentration of solutes in a solution

osmosis the movement of a solvent such as water through a semipermeable membrane from a less to a more concentrated solution

osmotic fragility curve a graphical representation of the results of an **osmotic fragility test** (Fig. 57)

osmotic fragility test a test of the resistance of red cells suspended in hypotonic solutions to lysis

osmotic pressure the pressure exerted on a semipermeable membrane by a solution containing solutes that cannot cross the membrane

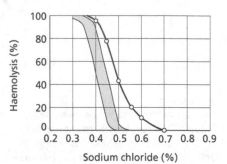

Figure 57   An osmotic fragility curve. An osmotic fragility curve showing that erythrocytes from a patient with hereditary spherocytosis lyse more readily than normal cells in a hypo-osmolar solution.

osteitis fibrosa cystica a disorder of bone resulting from a combination of **hyperparathyroidism** and **osteomalacia**

osteoarthritis a degenerative rather than inflammatory arthritis

osteoblast a bone-forming cell of mesenchymal but not haemopoietic origin

osteoclast a generally multinucleate bone-destroying cell of monocyte lineage

osteocyte a bone cell found in small cavities within bone, derived from an **osteoblast** that has been enclosed in bone

osteogenesis imperfecta an inherited disorder of bone resulting from a defect in collagen synthesis and leading to thinning of the cortex and bony trabeculae

osteoid non-calcified bone

osteomalacia a disorder of bone, resulting from vitamin D deficiency, in which there is defective mineralization

osteomyelitis infection of bone

osteomyelosclerosis an advanced stage of **idiopathic myelofibrosis** in which there is **osteosclerosis** as well as bone marrow fibrosis

osteopetrosis marble bone disease, a congenital form of **osteosclerosis**, resulting from a defect in osteoclast numbers or function, which leads to bone marrow failure

osteoporosis a reduction of bone density due to thinning of the cortex and medullary trabeculae

osteosclerosis thickening of bony trabeculae

OTT a gene, <u>O</u>ne <u>T</u>wenty <u>T</u>wo, gene map locus 1p12, also known as <u>R</u>NA-<u>B</u>inding <u>M</u>otif protein <u>15</u>, *RBM15*; encodes a ribonucleoprotein; *OTT* is a homologue of the *Drosophila* gene *spen* (split ends); its function in man is unclear; *OTT* contributes to the *OTT-MAL* fusion gene (also known as *RBM15-MKL1* fusion gene) in infant M7 acute myeloid leukaemia associated with t(1;22)(p13;q13) (*see also RBM15* and *MKL1*)

ovalocyte an oval red cell

ovalocytosis an inherited abnormality of the erythrocyte membrane in which cells are oval in shape

overall survival survival, regardless of whether there has been disease relapse or the need to change to alternative treatment (*see also* **disease-free survival, event-free survival**)

overt obvious, readily apparent

ovum (plural ova) a germ cell produced in the ovary of a female

oxalosis an inherited metabolic disorder leading to deposition of oxalic acid crystals in tissues including the bone marrow

oximeter a device or instrument for measuring the oxygen saturation of blood

oxygen (O_2) a tasteless, colourless gas that is essential for metabolism and therefore for life; transferred to the blood stream from the inspired air in the alveoli of the lungs and transported to tissues by haemoglobin

oxyhaemoglobin haemoglobin combined with O_2

P

3 prime (3′) the end of a gene where transcription terminates

5 prime (5′) the end of a gene where transcription commences

8p11 syndrome a myeloproliferative/ lymphoproliferative stem cell disorder resulting from one of a number of translocations that involved the *FGFR1* gene, characterized by a myeloproliferative disorder with eosinophilia, T-lineage lymphoblastic lymphoma and evolution to acute myeloid leukaemia

^{32}P a radio-active isotope of phosphorus, used in the treatment of **myeloproliferative disorders**

p (i) the short arm of a chromosome, from the French *petit* (ii) an abbreviation for protein, e.g. p53, the protein encoded by the *TP53* tumour suppressor gene

p+ a chromosome with material added to the short arm

p− a chromosome with loss of material from the short arm

P a blood group system with the great majority of individuals expressing the P_1 antigen; P_1-negative (p) individuals are resistant to parvovirus B19 infection; the P_1 antigen is an indirect, carbohydrate-defined product of the *P* gene at 22q11.2-qter; autoanti-P is a biphasic haemolysin causing **paroxysmal cold haemoglobinuria**

p15 a protein that negatively regulates cell proliferation by inhibiting cyclin–cyclin-dependent kinase 4 complexes, encoded by the *CDKN2B* gene (also known as *INK4b*) at 9p21 (*see also* Table 5, p. 70)

p16 a protein that negatively regulates cell proliferation, encoded by the *CDKN2A* gene (also known as *INK4a*, *MTS1* and *CDKN2*) which is located at

9p21 in tandem with *INK4b* (*see also* Table 5, p. 70)

p18 the protein encoded by *CDKN2C*

p19 the protein encoded by *CDKN2D*

p21^{RAS} the product of the *RAS* gene

p21^{WAF} a protein that negatively regulates cell proliferation, encoded by the *CDKN1A* gene

p27 the protein encoded by *CDKN1B*

p51 a homologue of p53

p50 the partial pressure of oxygen at which haemoglobin is half saturated

p53 a 53 kD protein encoded by the tumour suppressor gene *TP53*; p53 is a transcription factor that upregulates *CDKN1A* (encoding p21$^{Cip1/Waf1}$) and therefore arrests the **cell cycle** temporarily at **G1/S**, thus allowing time for detection and repair of damaged DNA; in addition, p53 increases **BAX** expression, thus promoting **apoptosis** of damaged cells

p57 the protein encoded by *CDKN1C*

p73 a homologue of p53

p300 the provisional name for a gene, E1A-binding protein, 300-kD; gene map locus 22q13; encodes a *bromodomain* containing transcriptional adaptor protein which is very similar in function to **CBP**; contributes to:

• the *MLL-p300* fusion gene in acute myeloid leukaemia associated with t(11;22)(q23;q13);

• contributes to the *MOZ-p300* and *p300-MOZ* fusion genes in M5 acute myeloid leukaemia associated with t(8;22)(p11;q13)

packed cell volume (PCV) the proportion of a column of centrifuged anticoagulated blood which is occupied by erythrocytes or an equivalent measurement determined by an automated instrument

'packed film' jargon for a thick blood film, characteristic of **polycythaemia**

'packed marrow' jargon for a heavy uniform infiltration of the bone marrow by neoplastic, usually lymphoma, cells

PAFAH2 a gene, Platelet-Activating Factor Acetylhydrolase 2, gene map locus 11q23, encodes a widely expressed cytoplasmic protein; dysregulated by proximity to the *IGH* locus in t(11;14)(q23;q32) associated with B-cell malignancy

Paget's disease, Paget's disease of bone an acquired disorder of bone in which the normal lamellar pattern of mature bone is lost, the bone showing a mosaic pattern in histological sections

PAI-1 plasminogen activator inhibitor 1

PAI-2 plasminogen activator inhibitor 2

paired box a DNA-binding domain present in a family of transcription factors (PAX proteins); several members of this family also contain homeodomains

palliative treatment treatment intended to relieve symptoms

pallidin a red cell membrane protein, previously known as band 4.2, encoded by the *EPB42* gene at 15q15 (*see* Fig. 64, p. 199)

pancreas an abdominal organ with both endocrine and exocrine functions, secreting insulin and digestive enzymes

pancreatitis inflammation of the pancreas

pancytopenia reduction in the white cell count, the red cell count (and haemoglobin concentration) and the platelet count

P$_{aO2}$ partial pressure of oxygen in arterial blood

papilloedema swelling of the **optic disc**

Pappenheimer bodies iron-containing inclusions in erythrocytes, as seen on a **Romanowsky stain**

papule a small raised skin lesion

paracentric a term to describe a chromosomal inversion which involves the long arm or the short arm but not both

paracortex adjacent to the cortex, e.g. the part of a lymph node immediately below the cortex, occupied mainly by T lymphocytes

paracrine a hormonal pathway characterized by the production of a biologically active substance that passes by diffusion to a nearby cell where it initiates a response

paraprotein an abnormal **monoclonal** immunoglobulin produced by a neoplastic clone of cells, either a complete **immunoglobulin** molecule or a monoclonal **heavy chain** or **light chain**

parasitaemia the presence of **parasites** in the blood

parasite an organism which lives in or on another creature, causing some damage to its host

parasthesiae abnormal sensations such as tingling, numbness, 'pins and needles'; can be indicative of **peripheral neuropathy** and be a feature of **vitamin B$_{12}$ deficiency** or caused by chemotherapy with **vinca alkaloids**

paratrabecular adjacent to a bony spicule, characteristic site of bone marrow infiltration in follicular lymphoma

parietal cell a stomach cell secreting hydrochloric acid and **intrinsic factor**

parietal cell antibodies autoantibodies directed at parietal cells, a feature of **pernicious anaemia** (present in 90–95% of patients) and atrophic gastritis (present in 60% of patients) but also present not infrequently in apparently healthy elderly people

paroxysmal cold haemoglobinuria (PCH) an acquired haemolytic anaemia characterized by biphasic antibody-mediated haemolysis; an antibody, usually anti-P, designated a **Donath–Landsteiner antibody**, is bound to the cell in the cold and with rewarming there is complement-induced lysis

paroxysmal nocturnal haemoglobinuria (PNH) an acquired haemolytic anaemia characterized by intermittent **haemolysis**, and often **pancytopenia**, consequent on a clonal genetic disorder with a mutation in a *PIG-A* gene

partial pressure of oxygen that part of the total blood gas pressure exerted by oxygen

partial remission (PR) regression of a disease but with clinical or pathological evidence of residual disease

partial thromboplastin time the time for clotting to occur if a partial thromboplastin, acting as a platelet substitute in the **intrinsic pathway** of coagulation, is added to plasma (*see also* **activated partial thromboplastin time**) which has now replaced the (non-activated) partial thromboplastin time

parvovirus B19 a very small double-stranded DNA virus which is the cause of erythema infectiosum or fifth disease; parvovirus is capable of causing **pure red cell aplasia** (with anaemia generally occurring only when the red cell survival is shortened) and, less often, **neutropenia** or **thrombocytopenia**; infection during pregnancy can lead to severe fetal anaemia and **hydrops fetalis**

PAS **periodic acid-Schiff stain**

pathogen a micro-organism capable of causing disease

pathogenesis the process by which a disease develops

pathogenic capable of causing disease

pathognomonic an abnormality which is diagnostic of a certain condition, i.e. that permits no other diagnosis

pathology the study of disease

Paul–Bunnell test a test for the **heterophile antibody** characteristic of **infectious mononucleosis**

Pautrier's abscess or microabscess a focal accumulation of T lymphocytes within the epidermis, a feature of cutaneous T-cell lymphoma

PAX3 <u>Pa</u>ired bo<u>x</u> gene <u>3</u>, gene map locus 2q35, encodes a paired box transcription factor which also has a **homeodomain**; germline mutations in this gene are seen in the dysmorphic disorder Waardenburg's syndrome type I; *PAX3* contributes to the fusion gene, *PAX3-FKHR*, in t(2;13)(q35)(q14) associated with alveolar rhabdomyosarcoma

PAX5 a gene, <u>Pa</u>ired bo<u>x</u> gene <u>5</u>, gene map locus 9p13, also known as <u>B</u>-cell lineage-<u>S</u>pecific <u>A</u>ctivator <u>P</u>rotein, *BSAP*; gene map locus 9p13, encodes a **paired box** transcription factor expressed at early stages of B-cell differentiation, but which also regulates isotype switching; *PAX5*:

- is dysregulated by proximity to the *IGH* enhancer in t(9;14)(p13;q32) found in about 50% of cases of lymphoplasmacytoid lymphoma
- was dysregulated by replacement of its promoter by the *IGH* switch Sμ promoter in a splenic marginal zone lymphoma associated with t(2;9;14)(p12;p13;q32)
- is dysregulated by proximity to *IGH* in t(9;14)(p13;q32) in B-cell non-Hodgkin's lymphoma
- contributed to a *PAX5-ETV6/TEL* fusion gene in a case of acute lymphoblastic leukaemia

PAX7 a gene, <u>Pa</u>ired bo<u>x</u> gene <u>7</u>, also known as *HUP1*, gene map locus 1p36.2, encodes a **paired box** transcription factor which also has a **homeodomain**; contributes to the *PAX7-FKHR* fusion gene, in t(1;13)(p36;q14) associated with alveolar rhabdomyosarcoma

PB **peripheral blood**

PBSCT **peripheral blood stem cell transplantation**

PBX1 a gene, <u>Pre-B</u>-cell leukaemia transcription factor <u>1</u>, gene map locus 1q23, encodes a ubiquitously expressed non-cluster (class II) homeobox transcription factor; archetypal member of a family of **homeobox genes** that modulate the activity of other homeobox genes by forming heterodimeric complexes with them, the complexes having high binding activity on a subset of potential DNA recognition sites; these complexes can be inhibitory or activating; *PBX1* contributes to the *E2A-PBX1* fusion gene in B-lineage acute lymphoblastic leukaemia associated with t(1;19)(q23;p13)

PcAb **polyclonal antibody**

PCH **paroxysmal cold haemoglobinuria**

PCR **polymerase chain reaction**

PCR-SSOP **polymerase chain reaction–sequence-specific oligonucleotide probing**

PCR-SSP **polymerase chain reaction–sequence-specific priming**

PCV **packed cell volume**

PDGFRB a gene, <u>P</u>latelet-<u>D</u>erived <u>G</u>rowth <u>F</u>actor <u>R</u>eceptor <u>B</u>eta, gene map locus 5q33, encodes the beta chain of the PDGF receptor β, also known

as **CD140b**, a dimeric receptor tyrosine kinase, at 5q33 which contributes to:
- the *ETV6-PDGFRB* fusion gene in chronic myelomonocytic leukaemia with eosinophilia associated with t(5;12)(q33;p13);
- the *H4(10S170)-PDGFRB* gene in atypical chronic myeloid leukaemia associated with t(5;10)(q33;q22);
- the *HIP1-PDGFRB* fusion gene in chronic myelomonocytic leukaemia associated with t(5;7)(q33;q11.2);
- *Rabaptin5-PDGFRB* fusion gene in a patient with CMML

in each case, the fusion protein encodes a constitutively activated tyrosine kinase receptor

Pearson's syndrome a **mitochondrial cytopathy**, resulting from deletion of mitochondrial DNA, characterized haematologically by neutropenia, sideroblastic erythropoiesis and vacuolation of haemopoietic cells; non-haematological manifestation may include exocrine pancreatic deficiency, metabolic acidosis, renal disease, liver failure and diabetes mellitus

pegylation attachment of a polyethlyene glycol (PEG) polymer group to a protein, such as thrombopoietin, interferon or granulocyte colony-stimulating factor, in order to decrease plasma clearance and increase efficacy

Pel–Ebstein fever a periodic fever, characteristic of **Hodgkin's disease**

Pelger–Huët anomaly an inherited anomaly in which neutrophils are hypolobulated but functionally normal (Fig. 58)

pencil cell a particularly long thin ellipocyte, typical of iron deficiency anaemia but not pathognomonic

penetrance the expression of a gene, a gene either being expressed or not

penicilliosis infection by fungi of the genus Penicillium, e.g. by *Penicillium marneffei*

pentose shunt a metabolic pathway which gives cells the ability to resist oxidant damage (Fig. 59)

pentostatin a **nucleoside analogue** used in treating hairy cell leukaemia

Figure 58 Pelger–Huët anomaly. A diagram contrasting a normal segmented neutrophil and band form with two neutrophils showing the Pelger–Huët anomaly.

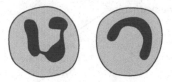

Normal neutrophil and neutrophil band form

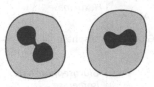

Neutrophils in Pelger–Huët anomaly

peptic ulceration ulceration of the stomach or duodenum induced by gastric secretions

percentile one hundredth part of a statistical distribution; a conventional 95% reference range extends between the 2.5 and the 97.5 percentiles

PERF1 the gene, <u>Perf</u>orin, gene map locus 10q22, encoding **perforin**; germ-line mutation in this gene is the cause of **familial haemophagocytic lymphohistiocytosis type 2**

perforin a protein secreted by cytotoxic T cells and NK cells that is inserted into the membrane of a target cell, creating a pore through which cytotoxic enzymes, granzymes, can enter with resultant activation of **caspases** and **apoptosis**

pericentric a term to describe a chromosomal inversion that has breakpoints on either side of the centromere so that the centromeric parts of both long and short arms are involved in the inversion

periodic acid-Schiff stain (PAS stain) a cytochemical stain for complex carbohydrates including glycogen

Figure 59 The pentose shunt.
A diagram showing the pentose shunt and related metabolic pathways.

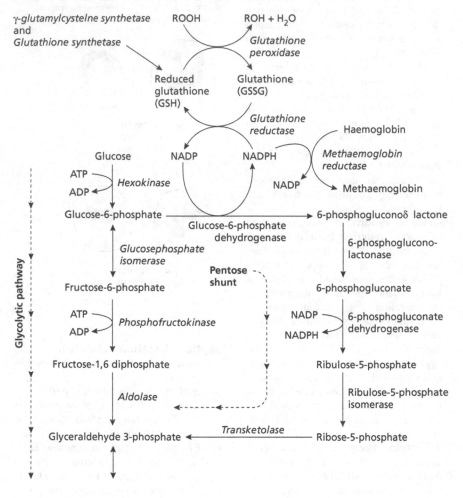

periosteum the connective tissue cells covering the surface of a bone

peripheral blood (PB) the blood circulating through arteries and veins

peripheral blood stem cell transplantation (PBSCT) transplantation of haemopoietic stem cells harvested from the peripheral blood

peripheral neuropathy degeneration of the peripheral nerves, may be caused by **vitamin B$_{12}$ deficiency** or be associated with the presence of a **paraprotein**

peripheral T-cell lymphoma all T-lineage lymphomas except those composed of lymphoblasts

peripheral vascular disease narrowing of the arteries to the limbs, usually caused by atheroma

Perls' stain a Prussian blue stain, used to identify iron in the form of **haemosiderin**

permeabilization the process by which a cell is made permeable to antibodies so that intracellular antigens can be recognized

pernicious injurious, destructive, fatal

pernicious anaemia an autoimmune disease characterized by gastric atrophy, inadequate gastric secretion of **intrinsic factor**, **vitamin B₁₂ deficiency** and **megaloblastic anaemia**; other features may include **peripheral neuropathy, optic atrophy** and **subacute combined degeneration of the spinal cord**; pernicious anaemia is part of a spectrum of autoimmune diseases that includes diabetes mellitus, autoimmune thyroid disease and **vitiligo**; since vitamin B₁₂ became available for treatment this anaemia is no longer 'pernicious'

peroxisomes organelles containing oxidative enzymes and responsible for detoxification

pertussis whooping cough, the illness resulting from *Bordetella pertussis* infection; the major haematological feature is lymphocytosis

PET pre-eclamptic toxaemia

petechiae pin-point skin haemorrhages, a form of **purpura**

PET scan positron emission tomography scan

Peyer's patches a focal accumulation of lymphocytes in the small intestine, part of the **mucosa-associated lymphoid tissue (MALT)**

PFGE pulsed field gel electrophoresis

pH an abbreviation of 'potential hydrogen', an expression of the H+ ion concentration; water has a pH of 7.0 and is considered chemically neutral; acids have a pH below 7.0 and alkalis a pH above 7.0

Ph the Philadelphia chromosome; it should be noted that the preferred abbreviation is now Ph not Ph[1]

phagocyte a cell capable of ingesting and destroying micro-organisms and cellular debris, e.g. a neutrophil or a macrophage

phagocytic pertaining to **phagocytosis**, able to carry out phagocytosis

phagocytosis the ingestion of a cell or inert material by a phagocytic cell such as a neutrophil or monocyte; a specialized form of **endocytosis**

phagolysosome the cytoplasmic vacuole that results from fusion of a **phagosome** with the cytoplasmic granules of a neutrophil or monocyte

phagosome the cytoplasmic vacuole that results from **phagocytosis**

pharyngitis inflammation of the pharynx

pharynx the throat

phenotype the appearance of something, cf. **genotype**

Philadelphia chromosome (Ph chromosome) a 22q– chromosome formed as a result of t(9;22)(q34;q11)

phlebotomy removal of blood from a vein for therapeutic or diagnostic purposes

phosphofructokinase an erythrocyte enzyme in the glycolytic pathway (*see* Fig. 33, p. 113)

phosphoglyceratekinase an erythrocyte enzyme in the glycolytic pathway (*see* Fig. 33, p. 113)

phosphoinositides (PIs) phosphatidylinositol phospholipids, a group of lipid second messenger molecules

phototherapy a method of treating neonatal **hyperbilirubinaemia** by exposure of the baby to ultraviolet light

Phox homology (PX) domain a **phosphoinositide** (PI)-binding protein motif which plays a critical role in the intracellular localization of a variety of cell-signalling proteins

phytohaemagglutinin a plant lectin able to stimulate T lymphocyte to proliferate

pica a craving to eat unusual substances, e.g. ice or clay; can be a feature of **iron deficiency**

Pickwickian syndrome polycythaemia consequent on **hypoventilation** and **hypoxia** in severe obesity

picogram 1×10^{-12} of a gram

PIFT platelet immunofluorescence test

PIG-A a gene at Xp22.1 (glycosyl**p**hos**p**hatidyl**i**nositol-**g**lycan complementation class **A**), encoding one of the four genes necessary for synthesis of **glycosylphosphatidylinositol (GPI)**; mutated in **paroxysmal nocturnal haemoglobinuria**

PIK3CA a gene, **P**hosphatidyl**i**nositol-**3** **K**inase p110 **Ca**talytic **A**lpha subunit, gene map locus 3q26-27, encodes the catalytic subunit of phosphatidylinositol-3 kinase, that is amplified and overexpressed in several gynaecological malignancies

PKB see *AKT1*

PKLR a gene at 1q21 encoding liver and red cell **pyruvate kinase**; mutation may lead to **pyruvate kinase deficiency** and consequent chronic **haemolytic anaemia**

plaque a skin lesion that is elevated but flat

plasma the fluid part of blood; plasma for laboratory tests is prevented from clotting by the addition of either an anticoagulant or a chelating agent that binds calcium

plasma cell the end cell of the B-lymphocyte lineage; an antibody-secreting cell

plasma cell dyscrasia any plasma cell neoplasm, including **multiple myeloma, monoclonal gammopathy of undetermined significance, light-chain-associated amyloidosis**

plasma cell leukaemia a leukaemia of cells analogous to normal **plasma cells**, occurring either *de novo* or as the terminal phase of **multiple myeloma**

plasmacytoma a tumour composed of neoplastic **plasma cells**

plasmacytosis increased numbers of **plasma cells** in the blood or bone marrow

plasma membrane the lipid bilayer which encloses a cell

plasmapheresis removal of plasma from the circulating blood by connection of the patient's blood stream to a specialized centrifuge, usually performed as part of plasma exchange therapy but occasionally used to obtain plasma for transfusion; the plasma removed is replaced by an isotonic solution

plasma protein the proteins in plasma, classified according to their electrophoretic mobilities and chemical characteristics as albumin, α, β and γ globulins and fibrinogen

plasma volume the total volume of plasma in the circulating blood, can be measured by isotopic dilution techniques

plasmid a circular autonomously replicating extrachromosomal DNA molecule

plasmin an specific enzyme capable of degrading **fibrin** (*see* Fig. 27, p. 103)

plasminogen a plasma protein that is converted to **plasmin** (*see* Fig. 27, p. 103);

deficiency, which is very rare, is associated with increased risk of thrombosis

plasminogen activator a serine protease, synthesized by vascular endothelial cells, that activates **plasminogen**; deficiency, which is very rare, is associated with an increased risk of thrombosis

plasminogen activator inhibitor 1 (PAI-1) a **serpin**, a plasma protein that inhibits **plasminogen activator**; mutations of the gene, which are very rare, can lead to increased levels, which are associated with an increased risk of thrombosis

plasminogen activator inhibitor 2 (PAI-2) a serpin, an intracellular and extracellular inhibitor of **plasminogen activator**, expressed in monocytes, endothelial cells and other cells

platelet a fragment of megakaryocyte cytoplasm which circulates in the blood and participates in **haemostasis**

platelet glycoprotein (Gp) surface membrane antigen of platelets but may also be expressed on other cells

platelet glycoprotein Ia/IIa (GpIa/IIa) a platelet glycoprotein that mediates collagen adhesion; carries HPA-5 and HPA-13w antigens

platelet glycoprotein Ib/IX/V (Gp Ib/IX/V) a platelet glycoprotein that binds **von Willebrand's factor** and mediates adhesion to damaged endothelium; there is lack of expression in **Bernard–Soulier syndrome**; GpIbα carries HPA-2 antigens and GpIbβ carries HPA-12w antigens (*see* Table 9, p. 131)

platelet glycoprotein IIb/IIIa (Gp IIb/IIIa) a platelet glycoprotein that binds fibrinogen, fibronectin and vitronectin and has an important role in platelet aggregation; there is lack of expression in **Glanzmann's thrombasthenia**; GpIIb carries HPA-3 and HPA-9w antigens; GpIIIa caries HPA-1, HPA-4, HPA-6, HPA-7w, HPA-8w, HPA-10w and HPA-11w antigens (*see* Table 9, p. 131)

platelet glycoprotein IV CD36, carries the Vis antigen which has not yet been assigned an HPA number

platelet glycoprotein VI a platelet glycoprotein required for collagen-induced aggregation

platelet immunofluorescence test (PIFT) a test for anti-platelet antibodies

platelet peroxidase the isoenzyme of peroxidase that is present in megakaryocytes and platelets

plateletpheresis removal of platelets form the circulating blood, usually to obtain platelets for transfusion but occasionally to remove platelets from a patient with thrombocytosis

platelet-poor plasma plasma from which the majority of platelets have been removed by centrifugation, used for coagulation tests

platelet-rich plasma plasma from which platelets have not been removed, used for platelet aggregation studies

platelet-type von Willebrand's disease an autosomal dominant form of von Willebrand's disease in which a gain-of-function mutation of *GPIBA*, the gene encoding platelet glycoprotein Ib, leads to increased binding of von Willebrand factor by platelets, platelet aggregation, thrombocytopenia and reduced concentration of plasma von Willebrand's factor

pleckstrin homology (PH) domain a phosphoinositide (PI)-binding protein motif involved in intracellular signalling, cytoskeletal organization and regulation of intracellular membrane transport

pleomorphic varying considerably in size, shape and other characteristics

pleomorphism showing considerable variation on size, shape and other characteristics

pleura the thin layer of cells covering the surface of the lungs and the internal surface of the thoracic cage

pleural effusion the accumulation of fluid in the pleural space

Plummer–Vinson syndrome oesophageal webs associated with iron deficiency anaemia

pluripotent stem cell a stem cell capable of giving rise to both lymphoid and myeloid lineages, the common lymphoid–myeloid progenitor cell

PLZF a gene, Promyelocytic Leukaemia Zinc Finger gene, also known as Zinc Finger protein 145, *ZNF145*, gene map locus11q23.1, that encodes a zinc finger transcriptional repressor of the BTB/POZ family, normally expressed in primitive haemopoietic cells; transcriptional repression is mediated via the amino terminal **POZ domain**; *PLZF* contributes to the *PLZF-RARA* fusion gene in t(11;17)(q23;q21) associated with M3-like acute myeloid leukaemia

PML nuclear body (POD) a multiprotein nuclear organelle where transcriptional regulatory proteins are assembled and modified in response to cellular signals; POD structure and function is disrupted in acute promyelocytic leukaemia

PML a gene, Promyelocytic Leukaemia; gene map locus 15q22, encodes a **RING finger** protein which is a component of multiprotein nuclear organelles known as PML nuclear bodies or PODs; PODs are structures where transcriptional regulatory proteins are assembled and modified in response to cellular signals; PML complexed in PODs can act as a transcriptional repressor or activator; contributes to a *PML-RARA* fusion gene in t(15;17)(q22;q21) associated with M3 and M3 variant acute myeloid leukaemia (acute promyelocytic leukaemia); in M3 AML, PML is dispersed from PODs into hundreds of tiny structures throughout the cytoplasm and nucleus (microparticulate pattern); normal PODs reappear on treatment with all-*trans*-retinoic acid; *PML-RARA* exerts a dominant negative effect on wild type *RARα* function

PMX1 a gene, Paired Mesoderm Homeobox, also known as *PHOX1*, gene map locus 1q23, encodes a non-cluster (class II) homeobox protein expressed in cardiac, skeletal, and smooth muscle tissues in adults; contributes to the *NUP98-PMX1* fusion gene in acute myeloid leukaemia and blast crisis of chronic granulocytic leukaemia associated with t(1;11)(q23;p15); the fusion protein localizes to the nucleus and may function as a transcription factor

PNH paroxysmal nocturnal haemoglobinuria

Po$_2$ partial pressure of oxygen

POD PML nuclear body

POEMS syndrome a syndrome resulting from a plasma cell neoplasm and characterized by Polyneuropathy, Organomegaly (hepatomegaly, splenomegaly, lymphadenopathy), Endocrinopathy, M-protein and Skin changes

poikilocyte an erythrocyte of abnormal shape

poikilocytosis the presence of **poikilocytes** in the blood; increased variability in the shape of erythrocytes

point mutation the substitution of a single base in a DNA molecule that may result in (i) no change in the amino acid encoded (ii) encoding of a different amino acid (iii) conversion of a coding codon to a stop codon (iv) conversion of a stop codon to a coding codon (v) interference with splicing

polyarteritis nodosa an inflammatory disorder of blood vessels

polychromasia the presence of a blue tinge in the cytoplasm of erythrocytes, indicative of a young red cell

polychromatic cell an erythrocyte with a blue tinge to the cytoplasm, indicating that it is a young red cell

polychromatic macrocyte a **polychromatic cell** that is larger than normal erythrocytes

polyclonal a description of lymphocytes, plasma cells or both belonging to many **clones**

polyclonal antibody (PcAb) an antibody derived from polyclonal lymphocytes, e.g. produced by immunization of an animal, also known as an antiserum

polyclonal gammopathy an increased concentration of polyclonal immunoglobulins

polycythaemia an increased red cell count, haemoglobin concentration and packed cell volume

polycythaemia rubra vera a myeloproliferative disorder mainly affecting erythropoiesis; the **WHO classification** prefers the designation 'polycythaemia vera'

polycythaemia vera *see* **polycythaemia rubra vera**

polymer a compound formed by the linking together of like or unlike **monomers**

polymerase chain reaction (PCR) an enzymatic method for the exponential amplification of target DNA *in vitro* using a thermostable DNA-dependent **DNA polymerase**, target-specific oligonucleotide **primers** and cyclical reaction conditions that allow the repeated denaturation of nascent products (double-stranded DNA being converted to single-stranded DNA) and re-annealing of primers (Fig. 60)

polymerase chain reaction–sequence-specific oligonucleotide probing (PCR-SSOP) a PCR technique using generic primers that will amplify all alleles of interest followed by the application of probes specific for each **allele**, used for HLA typing

polymerase chain reaction–sequence-specific priming (PCR-SSP) a PCR technique using **primers** that will amplify only a specific **allele**, used for HLA and HPA typing

polymerization formation of a **polymer**, e.g. the polymerization of haemoglobin S at low oxygen tensions

polymorph jargon for a neutrophil

polymorphism the presence in a population of two variants of a gene so that the frequency of the least common is at least 1%, e.g. β^S is polymorphic in West African populations

polymorphonuclear leucocyte strictly any granulocyte but the term is more often applied only to neutrophil granulocytes

polymyalgia rheumatica an inflammatory condition of muscles with a characteristically high **erythrocyte sedimentation rate**

polypeptide a chain of amino acids linked by peptide bonds

polyploid having multiple sets of chromosomes, e.g. normal megakaryocytes are polyploid as are some neoplastic cells

porphyria a disease resulting from abnormal tissue accumulation of porphyrins

porphyria cutanea tarda an inherited or acquired condition characterized by skin fragility and formation of bullae in sun-exposed areas; familial cases may result from mutation in the *URO-D* gene,

Figure 60   The polymerase chain reaction (PCR).
The first four rounds of a polymerase chain reaction (PCR) are shown. The reaction mixture contains template, oligonucleotide DNA primers specific for the target sequence to be amplified, reaction buffer and a thermostable DNA polymerase enzyme. The starting template (either double stranded DNA or a DNA/RNA hybrid [reverse-transcription PCR]) is heat denatured and allowed to cool so that the first oligonucleotide can bind to (anneal to) its target sequence; it is then warmed to the optimum temperature for polymerase activity; the thermostable polymerase generates nascent DNA complementary to the sequence 3′ to the primer. Subsequent denaturation and annealing allows for further polymerization, this time nascent DNA can also act as a template. The initial products are heterogeneous in size but eventually a product of a size defined by the distance between the primers will predominate.

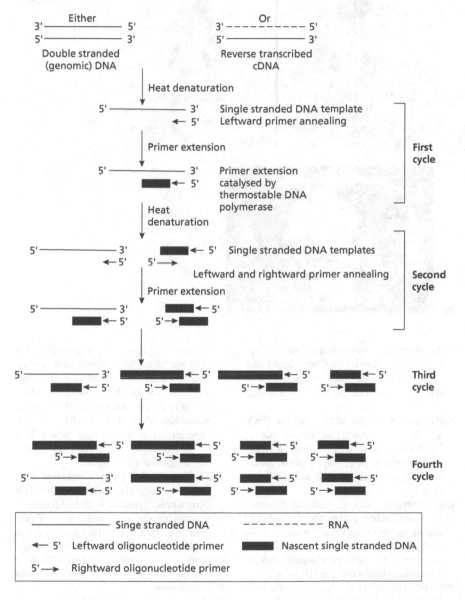

Figure 61   Positron emission tomography.
Imaging in a patient with Hodgkin's disease: (a) a positron emission tomography (PET) scan showing a increased signal in the chest (isotope concentrated in the kidneys and bladder is normal); (b) CT scan showing that the increased signal is the result of a mass of lymph nodes behind the heart.

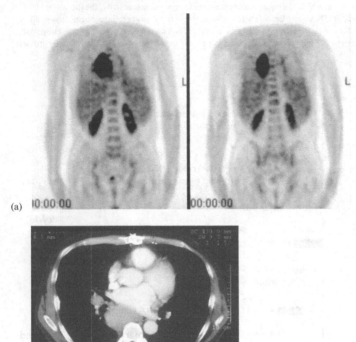

(a)

(b)

encoding uroporphyrinogen decarboxylase; enzyme activity may be reduced and the disease precipitated by **haemochromatosis**, alcohol excess, oestrogen intake or hepatitis C infection

positron emission tomography (PET scan) an imaging technique using ^{18}F-fluorodeoxyglucose position emission tomography to detect glycolysis in metabolically active tissue such as lymphoma (Fig. 61)

post-partum occurring after childbirth

post-transfusion purpura **thrombocytopenic purpura** occurring usually 7–10 days after a blood transfusion as a result of the development of **alloantibodies** to the **human platelet antigen** HPA-1a

power the ability of an experiment or a clinical trial to detect a real difference between alternatives—expressed, for example, as an 80% chance that accrual of a given number of patients to a clinical trial will be able to demonstrate a 5% difference in **median survival** with a **probability** level of $P = 0.05$; trials or experiments of inadequate power lead to the likelihood of a β **error**, i.e. that a real difference will be missed

POZ domain a highly conserved zinc finger domain, also known as the BTB (**B**ric a brac, **T**ramtrack, **B**road complex) domain, present on a wide range of proteins, e.g. **PZLF** and **BCL6**, which can mediate dimerization, transcriptional repression by the recruitment of histone deacetylases, and nuclear microspeckled localization

PPD **purified protein derivative**

PPP platelet-poor plasma

PR partial remission

PRAD1 an alternative designation of *BCL1*

pRB the protein encoded by the **tumour suppressor gene**, *TP53*

pre-B cell (i) a lymphoid cell of B lineage with cytoplasmic μ chain but lacking surface membrane immunoglobulin (as defined by **EGIL**) or (ii) any B-cell **precursor**

precursor a cell which precedes another and gives rise to it by a process of proliferation and maturation

pre-eclamptic toxaemia (PET) **pregnancy-associated hypertension** but without epileptiform convulsions (which would indicate eclampsia rather than preeclampsia), may be associated with a **microangiopathic haemolytic anaemia**

preleukaemia the phase before leukaemia develops when a preleukaemic disorder may be recognizable, more or less synonymous with '**myelodysplastic syndrome**'

preleukaemic predisposing to or preceding leukaemia

pre-partum occurring during pregnancy, before delivery

prevalence the number of cases of a condition present in a community at any one time, often expressed as the number per 100 000 of population

primary occurring of itself, not caused by any external influence, occurring first

primary acquired sideroblastic anaemia an alternative designation of **refractory anaemia with ring sideroblasts**, a FAB category of **myelodysplastic syndrome**

primary amyloidosis light chain-associated amyloidosis; the term, which is now less used, was mainly applied to cases without an overt **plasma cell neoplasm**

primary antiphospholipid syndrome a clinical syndrome with a thrombotic tendency and recurrent miscarriages caused by the presence of a **lupus anticoagulant** but without the features necessary for a diagnosis of **systemic lupus erythematosus**

primary granules the azurophilic granules that appear at the **promyelocyte** stage of granulocyte maturation

primary immune response the immunological response which occurs on first exposure to an **antigen**

primary karyotypic abnormality the initial chromosomal abnormality occurring in a clone of cells and present at disease onset, e.g. t(9;22) in **chronic granulocytic leukaemia**

primary mediastinal B-cell lymphoma a large B-cell lymphoma of the mediastinum, probably originating in thymic B cells

primary proliferative polycythaemia an alternative designation of **polycythaemia rubra vera**

primary thrombocythaemia an alternative designation of **essential thrombocythaemia**

primary tumour a tumour at the site where it initially developed

primed *in situ* hybridization (PRINS) a technique for identifying specific chromosomes by means of **primers**, which are annealed to target α satellite chromosome-specific repetitive DNA sequences followed by *in situ* primer extension using Taq DNA polymerase and incorporating fluorochrome-labelled dUTP

primer a short oligonucleotide sequence that provides the starting point for producing a complementary strand of DNA or RNA under the influence of **DNA polymerase** or **reverse transcriptase**

PRINS primed *in situ* hybridization

proband index case

pro-B cell an immature lymphoid cell of B lineage that does not express CD10 or cytoplasmic or surface membrane immunoglobulin

probe a labelled oligonucleotide that can be used to identify a complementary sequence of DNA or RNA

PROC the gene at 2q13-q14, <u>Pro</u>tein **C**, that encodes **protein** C, mutation of which can lead to **protein C deficiency**

Product liability the liability of a manufacturer—including manufacturers, suppliers and keepers of blood products—under the terms of the UK Consumer Protection Act 1987 for harm resulting from any defect in a product

proerythroblast the earliest morphologically recognizable cell in the erythroid lineage (*see* Fig. 25, p. 95)

prophase the first stage of **mitosis** in which the chromosomes condense and become visible within the nucleus (*see* Fig. 6, p. 14)

prometaphase the second of the five stages of **mitosis** in which the two chromatids of each chromosome become visible

progenitor cell an early precursor cell capable of giving rise to later cells

prognosis the likely outcome of an illness

prognostic pertaining to **prognosis**

proliferation the process of cell growth and division leading to expansion of a population of cells

proliferation centre a focal accumulation of larger nucleolated lymphocytes in a lymph node in chronic lymphocytic leukaemia or small lymphocytic lymphoma

prolymphocyte an abnormal lymphoid cell which is larger than a normal lymphocyte and has plentiful cytoplasm and a large prominent nucleolus; the characteristic cell of B and T-lineage prolymphocytic leukaemia (*see* Fig. 14, p. 31)

promonocyte a monocyte precursor derived from a monoblast and giving rise to monocytes

promoter a sequence of DNA at the 5′ end of a gene which is essential for initiation of **transcription** (*see* Fig. 73, p. 221)

promyelocyte an immature cell of granulocytic lineage, derived from a myeloblast and giving rise to myelocytes (*see* Fig. 25, p. 95)

properdin a protein in the **alternative complement pathway**

prophylactic intended to prevent disease; however 'prophylactic cranial irradiation' in **acute lymphoblastic leukaemia** is, strictly speaking, treatment of **occult** disease rather than prophylactic treatment

prophylaxis prevention of disease or protection against disease

propositus index case

proptosis protrusion of an eye

prorubriblast an alternative designation of a proerythroblast

prorubricyte an alternative designation of an **early erythroblast**

PROS1 the gene at 3p11.1-q11.2, Protein S, that encodes **protein S**, mutation of which can lead to **protein S deficiency**

prostate-specific antigen an antigen expressed by prostatic cancer cells and sometimes by cells of large bowel adenocarcinoma

prostate-specific acid phosphatase an antigen expressed by prostatic cancer cells

protamine sulphate a **heparin** antagonist

protease an enzyme that breaks down protein, *see also* **proteinase**

protease inhibitors a group of drugs used to treat **HIV** infection

proteasome a **ubiquitin**-dependent multicatalytic cytoplasmic complex, which is the main non-lysosomal mechanism for the degradation or processing of intracellular proteins—both damaged cellular proteins and short-lived regulatory proteins—which are then either further degraded in the **cytosol** to amino acids or are transferred into the **endoplasmic reticulum**

proteasome inhibitor an inhibitor of the **proteasome**; proteasome inhibitors lead to cell cycle arrest and **apoptosis** and have therapeutic potential in haematological neoplasms

protein a three-dimensional structure formed by folding of a polypeptide chain

proteinase an enzyme that breaks down protein, *see also* **protease**

proteinase 3 a **protease** which is one of the constituents of azurophilic granules of neutrophils, also known as myeloblastin

protein C a **vitamin K**-dependent **naturally occurring anticoagulant**, encoded by the *PROC* gene; after activation by the thrombin–thrombomodulin complex on the surface of endothelial cells, and with **protein S** and non-activated **factor V** as cofactors, activated protein C inactivates factors Va and VIIIa; activated protein C is a serine protease; in heterozygotes (3 per 1000 prevalence in the general population), deficiency leads to **thrombophilia**, particularly if **factor V Leiden** is co-inherited; homozygotes are prone to neonatal **purpura fulminans** (*see* Fig. 56, p. 170)

protein–calorie malnutrition a lack of both protein and total calories leading to the clinical presentations of **marasmus** and **kwashiorkor**

protein S a **vitamin K**-dependent **naturally occurring anticoagulant**, encoded by the *PROS1* gene; the major part of circulating protein S is bound to **C4b-binding protein**, with the bound protein S possibly having a role in localizing complement regulatory activity to certain cell surfaces; free protein S is a cofactor of activated **protein C**; protein S also has a protein C-independent anticoagulant effect, interacting with factor Va, Xa and phospholipid to inhibit thrombin generation; heterozygous protein S deficiency (i.e. deficiency of free protein S with or without deficiency of total protein S) leads to **thrombophilia** while homozygotes are prone to neonatal **purpura fulminans**

proteinuria the presence of protein in the urine

protein Z a **vitamin K**-dependent **naturally occurring anticoagulant**, encoded by the *PZ* gene, which binds to factor Xa, in association with phospholipid, and serves as a cofactor for its inactivation by protein-Z dependent protease inhibitor

proteoglycan a post-translationally modified protein in which a **glycosaminoglycan** chain is covalently linked to an amino acid residue

proteomics the quantification of and the functional analysis of all the proteins encoded by an organism's genome (*see also* **structural proteomics**)

prothrombin a coagulation factor, also known as factor II, encoded by the *F2* gene; it is activated by factor Xa in the presence of factor V and phospholipid; on activation, it is known as **thrombin** (*see* Figs 17 and 18, pp. 77 and 78); a common polymorphism in the 3'-untranslated region of the *F2* gene (20210→A) leads to an increased plasma prothrombin concentration and an increased probability of thrombosis

prothrombin deficiency an inherited, **autosomal recessive**, deficiency of prothrombin, resulting from mutation in the *F2* gene

prothrombin time (PT) a test of the **extrinsic pathway** of coagulation

protocadherin a subfamily of the 'non-classical' **cadherins**, encoded by 3 clusters of genes at 5q31

proto-oncogene a cellular equivalent of an **oncogene** of a **transforming virus**

PRP **platelet rich plasma**

Prussian blue a stain for iron, the basis of the **Perls' stain**

pseudo- false

pseudodiploid a **karyotype** with 46 chromosomes but with structural or other abnormalities, e.g. coexisting monosomy 7 and trisomy 8 would give a pseudodiploid karyotype as would the occurrence of a **translocation**

pseudo-Gaucher cells storage cells resembling **Gaucher's cells** but not resulting from **Gaucher's disease**

pseudogene a DNA sequence that resembles a gene but lacks genetic function

pseudolymphoma a term previously used to designate a chronic unexplained proliferation of B lymphocytes which is now considered to represent a low grade B-cell neoplasm

pseudo-Pelger–Huët anomaly acquired Pelger–Huët anomaly

pseudopolycythaemia apparent polycythaemia, consequent on reduction of the plasma volume, less appropriately referred to as 'stress polycythaemia'

PT **prothrombin time**

PU.1 a transcription factor, which is expressed by neoplastic cells in nodular lymphocyte predominant Hodgkin's disease but not by neoplastic cells of classical Hodgkin's disease or T-cell-rich B-cell lymphoma

pulmonary pertaining to the lungs

pulmonary embolism the process of embolization of the lungs

pulmonary embolus a blood clot which has become detached from a peripheral vein or from the right side of the heart and has travelled to the lungs

pulsed field gel electrophoresis (PFGE) an electrophoretic technique for separating large proteins by periodically altering the direction of the electric field through which they are migrating

PUO pyrexia of unknown origin

pure red cell aplasia a lack of erythroid cells beyond the **proerythroblast** stage but with no significant abnormality of other lineages

purified protein derivative (PPD) a blood product composed mainly of albumin

purine one of the two types of nitrogenous base found in nucleic acids; purines (adenine and guanine) have a double ring structure; *see also* **pyrimidine**

purpura subcutaneous or submucosal haemorrhage, classified as **ecchymoses** and **petechiae**

purpura fulminans extensive **purpura** and skin **necrosis** resulting from **thrombosis**; may be a consequence of severe deficiency of **protein S**, **protein C** or (rarely) **antithrombin** or may result from meningococcaemia or **disseminated intravascular coagulation**

P value the statistical probability attached to a certain observation, e.g.

$P < 0.05$ means that the probability of the observation occurring by chance is less than 1 in 20

pyknosis the process by which a nucleus becomes dense and homogeneous prior to cell death

pyrexia fever

pyrexia of unknown origin (PUO) fever of which the cause is unknown

pyrimidine one of the two types of nitrogenous base found in nucleic acids; pyrimidines (cytosine, thymine and uracil) have a single ring structure; *see also* **purine**

pyrimidine 5′ nucleotidase an erythrocyte enzyme involved in **nucleotide** metabolism; deficiency leads to haemolytic anaemia with prominent basophilic stippling

pyropoikilocytosis *see* **hereditary pyropoikilocytosis**

pyruvate kinase an enzyme in the **glycolytic pathway** which catalyses the conversion of phosphoenolpyruvate to pyruvate, encoded by the *PKLR* gene at 1q21; the *PKLR* gene encodes both liver and red cell pyruvate kinase by means of two tissue-specific promoters (*see* Fig. 33, p. 113)

Q

5q– syndrome a specific subtype of **myelodysplastic syndrome**, defined in the **WHO classification** as having 5q– as an isolated abnormality and blast cells less than 5% in both blood and bone marrow

q the long arm of a chromosome

q+ a chromosome with addition of material to its long arm

q– a chromosome with loss of material from its long arm

Q-banding a technique for producing a banded pattern on chromosomes by staining with quinacrine

Q fever a disease resulting from a rickettsial infection (by *Coxiella burnetti*)

R

r a cytogenetic abbreviation for a **ring chromosome**

RA refractory anaemia

Rabaptin-5 a gene, gene map locus 17q13, that encodes a protein which is an important regulator of early endosomal transport through interaction with the RAS family **GTPases**, Rab5 and Rab4; it contributed to a *Rabaptin5-PDGFRB* fusion gene in a patient with chronic myelomonocytic leukaemia; the fusion protein oligomerizes on account of the coiled-coil domains of rabaptin-5 leading to constitutive activation of the tyrosine kinase moiety of PDGFRB

RAC1 a gene, <u>RA</u>S-related <u>C</u>3 botulinum toxin substrate <u>1</u>, gene map locus 12q13.12, encodes a small GTP-binding protein; a member of the Rho family of **RAS**-like signalling molecules; RAC1 is a key regulator of cadherin-mediated cell–cell adhesion; it has inherent low level **GTPase** activity which is augmented by the **BCR** protein

radiation α or β particles or γ rays; γ rays are also known as X-rays

radioactive giving off radiation as the result of disintegration of the nucleus

radioactive isotope a form of an element which is **radioactive** but otherwise has very similar qualities to other forms of the element, often used in diagnosis and treatment

radiograph an image produced by means of **X-rays** passing through a part of the body to expose part of a photographic film, popularly known as an X-ray (Fig. 62)

radioimmunoassay (RIA) a laboratory technique for determining the concentration of an antigen or antibody in the serum by means of a radio-labelled reagent

Figure 62 A radiograph of the skull. A radiograph of the skull showing lytic lesions in a patient with multiple myeloma.

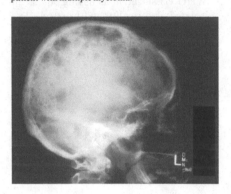

radiotherapy the treatment of disease, particularly neoplastic disease, by means of X-rays or gamma rays

RAEB refractory anaemia with excess of blasts

RAEB-T refractory anaemia with excess of blasts in transformation

RAG1 and ***RAG2*** two <u>R</u>ecombination <u>A</u>ctivating <u>G</u>enes which mediate the process of V(D)J recombination leading to the assembly of antigen-receptor genes encoding **immunoglobulin** and **T-cell receptors**; mutation leads to **severe combined immunodeficiency** (SCID) and **Omenn's syndrome**

RAMP a gene, <u>R</u>earranged in an <u>A</u>typical <u>M</u>yelo<u>p</u>roliferative disorder, an alternative designation of ***ZNF198***

random occurring by chance

random chromosomal abnormality a chromosomal abnormality occurring in a single cell or not meeting the criteria for definition of a clonal abnormality

randomized trial a comparison of two or more forms of therapy in which treatment is assigned randomly; *see also* **double blind**

RAP1GDS1 a gene, **G**TPase-GDP **D**issociation **S**timulator **1**, gene map locus 4q21, encodes a stimulatory GDP/GTP guanine nucleotide exchange factor (GEF) with **GTPase** activity; contributes to a *NUP98-RAP1GDS1* fusion gene fusion gene in t(4;11)(q21;p15) associated with 3% of adult cases of T-lineage acute lymphoblastic leukaemia; the chimaeric protein, which consists of the FG repeat-rich region of NUP98 fused to the entire coding region of RAP1GDS1, is found in both the cytoplasm and the nucleus.

RARA a gene, **R**etinoic **A**cid **R**eceptor **A**lpha, gene map locus 17q12, encodes a transcriptional regulator which is a nuclear receptor for **all-*trans* retinoic acid (ATRA)** and 9-cis retinoic acid (cRA); it belongs to a subfamily of the nuclear receptor group of ligand-activated transcription factors that also includes RARβ and RARγ; each *RAR* encodes 2 isoforms which differ at their amino termini; RARs bind to specific DNA sequences called retinoic acid response elements (RAREs), but only when heterodimerized to an **RXR** (α, β or γ); in the absence of ligand the RXR/RAR complex acts as a transcriptional repressor by recruiting histone deacetylases, but in the presence of retinoids the complex acts as an activator; *RARA* contributes to:

• a *PML-RARA* fusion gene in t(15;17)(q22;q21) associated with M3 and M3 variant acute myeloid leukaemia

• a *PLZF-RARA* fusion gene in t(11;17)(q23;q21) associated with M3-like acute myeloid leukaemia

• a *NuMA-RARA* fusion gene in t(11;17)(q13;q21) in rare cases of M3-like acute myeloid leukaemia

• a *NPM-RARA* fusion gene in t(5;17)(q32;q21) associated with rare cases of M3-like acute myeloid leukaemia

• a *STAT5b-RARA* fusion gene described in one patient with der(17) and M1 acute myeloid leukaemia

• a *MLL-RARA* fusion gene in M5 acute myeloid leukaemia with t(11;17)(q23;q12)

RARS refractory anaemia with ring sideroblasts

RAS a family of genes, **Ra**t **S**arcoma viral oncogene homologue, encoding three related p21^{RAS} proteins, H-RAS (gene map locus 11p15.5), K-RAS (gene map locus 12p12.1) and N-RAS (gene map locus 1p13.2); archetypal members of a larger superfamily of at least 100 related small GTP-binding proteins which function as simple 'on/off' molecular switches, activated by GTP binding and inactivated by hydrolysis of GTP to GDP; have low-level intrinsic GTPase function which is augmented by GTPase activating proteins (GAPs), which lead to their activation; *RASGRP4* encodes a myeloid specific **GEF** for RAS proteins; small GTP-binding proteins regulate diverse functions such as receptor mediated signalling and cytoskeletal organization; *N-RAS* and *K-RAS* mutations are common as second events in many cancers including multiple myeloma, acute lymphoblastic leukaemia (20–30% of cases) and myeloid neoplasms (20–30% of cases of acute myeloid leukaemia, 15–20% of myelodysplastic syndromes—particularly in those with a poor prognosis—and chronic myeloid leukaemia, 20% of atypical chronic myeloid leukaemia); *K-RAS* is often mutated in carcinoma (e.g. 90% of pancreatic carcinomas and 60% of colonic carcinomas) whereas *N-RAS* is characteristically mutated in myeloid neoplasms; drugs designed to interfere with the oncogenicity of RAS-encoded proteins are under development

RB1 a gene, **R**etinoblastoma **1**, gene map locus 13q14, encodes the ubiquitously expressed archetypal member of a family of proteins that link signals controlling the cell cycle to the nuclear transcriptional apparatus; a candidate tumour suppressor gene; RB1 inhibits the progression from G1 to S phase of the **cell cycle**; the inhibition of the **E2F** transcription factor by RB1 is key to this growth-suppressing action; RB1 is phosphorylated by **cyclin D/CDK4** and once phosphorylated is unable to interact with E2F; wildtype p53 suppresses transcription of *RB1*; implicated in familial retinoblastoma and possibly in the progression of chronic lymphocytic leukaemia (although another gene at 13q14 may be more relevant), acute myeloid leukaemia and acute lymphoblastic leukaemia; deleted in about 50% of patients with T-cell prolymphocytic leukaemia but other sequences at 13q14 are more often deleted; deleted in some patients with multiple myeloma; loss or mutation of *RB1* occurs in up to 30% of patients with blast crisis of chronic granulocytic leukaemia

RBC   red blood cell count

RBM15   a gene, **R**NA-**B**inding **M**otif protein **15**, gene map locus 1p12, also known as *OTT*, has homology to *Drosophila spen* and encodes a protein that interacts with RAS and E2F; it contributes to *RBM15-MKL1* and *MKL1-RBM15* fusion genes in acute megakaryoblastic leukaemia of infants with t(1;22)(p13;q13); it is the *RBM15-MKL1* fusion gene which is likely to be oncogenic; the chimaeric protein generated by this fusion contains all putative functional motifs encoded by each gene

RBTN1   a gene, **R**hom**b**o**t**i**n**-**1**, also known as **LIM** domain **O**nly **1** (*LMO1*) and **T**-cell **T**ranslocation **G**ene 1 (*TTG1*), gene map locus 11p15, encodes a **LIM domain** transcriptional regulator which is a nuclear partner of **SCL** and which is important in T-cell development; *RBTN1* is dysregulated, possibly by proximity to the *TCRAD* (αδ) locus, in T-lineage acute lymphoblastic leukaemia associated with t(11;14)(p15;q11)

RBTN2   a gene, **R**hom**b**o**t**i**n**-**2**, also known as **LIM** domain **O**nly **2** (*LMO2*) and **T**-cell **T**ranslocation **G**ene 2 (*TTG2*); gene map locus 11p13; encodes a **LIM domain** transcriptional regulator which is a nuclear partner of **SCL** and which is important in haemopoiesis and vasculogenesis; *RBT2* is dysregulated by:
• proximity to the *TCRB* gene in T-lineage acute lymphoblastic leukaemia associated with t(7;11)(q35;p13)
• by proximity to the *TCRAD* (αδ) locus in T-lineage acute lymphoblastic leukaemia associated with t(11;14)(p13;q11)

RCK   a gene, also known as **D**E**A**D/H bo**x** **6** (DDX6) and RNA helicase p54, gene

map locus 11q23.3, encodes an RNA helicase which contains the evolutionarily conserved Asp-Glu-Ala-Asp (DEAD) box sequence (*see also* **DEAD box** and **DDX10**); dysregulated by proximity to the *IGH* locus in t(11;14)(q23;q32) associated with B-cell malignancy

RDW   red cell distribution width

reactive   an abnormality that is a response to another primary disease or pathological process

REAL   classification   the Revised **European–American Lymphoma classification**

real time PCR (RQ-PCR)   a semiquantitative PCR technique in which estimation of the rate of generation of the product during the exponential phase permits quantification of the amount of the target DNA originally present (Fig. 63); RQ-PCR techniques include **Taq-Man** and Dye intercalation

rearrangement   the process by which the structure of a chromosome or a gene is altered by means of breaking and rejoining of sequences of DNA in one or more chromosomes; rearrangement may be a normal process, in antigen recognition by lymphoid cells, or a pathological process which, in some circumstances, leads to neoplastic transformation of a cell and clonal proliferation

receptor tyrosine kinase (RTK)   a transmembrane protein with an extracellular ligand-binding domain, a transmembrane domain and an intracellular domain that, on activation of the protein, can phosphorylate tyrosine residues on substrate proteins

recessive   a mode of inheritance in which a characteristic or a disease occurs in **homozygotes** or compound heterozygotes but not in simple **heterozygotes**

reciprocal translocation   a translocation in which segments of chromosome are exchanged between two (or more) chromosomes (*see also* **balanced translocation** and **unbalanced translocation**)

recombinant coagulation factors   coagulation factors, e.g. factor VIII, factor IX or factor VIIa, produced by inserting a human gene into a mam-

Figure 63   Real-time Polymerase Chain Reaction (RQ-PCR).
There are a number of techniques available which make a PCR semi-quantitative. These depend on the kinetics
of PCR and include intercalating dye technology and Taqman™ RQ-PCR.
(a) Kinetics of PCR—as long as the reaction substrates or the activity of the enzyme are not limiting, the amount
of product that is generated in a PCR, which can be measured by a fluorescence method, doubles after every
cycle. Each product molecule is itself able to act as a template in the next round of amplification. Depending on
the amount of template at the start, the efficiency with which the primers anneal and the activity of the enzyme,
after a certain number of cycles in any PCR, the amount of product generated per cycle increases in a linear
fashion (the exponential phase). It is during this phase that real time PCR systems are able to quantify and
compare the amounts of products made in different reactions. Eventually the amount of new product generated
per cycle decreases to zero (plateau phase). This occurs when either enzyme or substrates become limiting.
(b) Intercalating dye technology—an intercalating dye, e.g. SybrGreen™, fluoresces only when it binds to
double stranded DNA. Fluorescence is proportional to the amount of double stranded DNA (PCR product).
(c) (*overleaf*) Taqman™ technology—the PCR is carried out using a thermostable polymerase with 'proof-
reading' (5′ to 3′ exonuclease) activity. An oligonucleotide probe complementary to a short stretch of the DNA
to be amplified is added to the reaction. The probe has a fluorescent 'reporter' group (R) and a 'quencher'
(Q) covalently bound to its ends. The physical proximity of the Q group to the R group in the intact molecule
suppresses the fluorescence of the latter. If the probe hybridizes to the template during the extension phase
of the PCR, then it will be degraded by the exonuclease activity of the enzyme. This separates the reporter and
quencher and allows the reporter to fluoresce. Fluorescence is proportional to the amount of free reporter which
in turn depends upon the amount of specific amplified product to which the probe can hybridize.

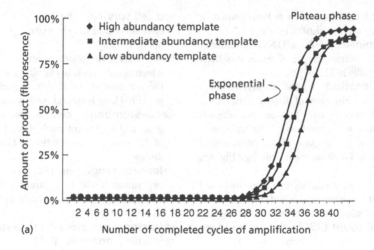

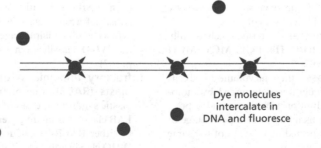

(*Continued*)

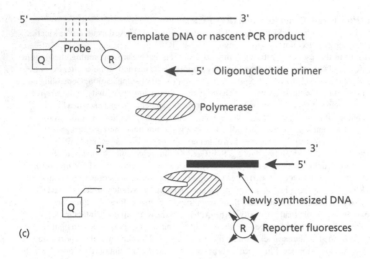

5'——————————————3'
Template DNA or nascent PCR product

Q Probe R

◄———— 5' Oligonucleotide primer

Polymerase

5'——————————————3'

◄——— 5'

Q

Newly synthesized DNA

R Reporter fluoresces

(c)

malian cell line which is then grown in culture on an industrial scale

recombinant DNA   a DNA molecule in which rearrangement of genes has been artificially induced

recombination   (i) the occurrence of a new combination of linked genes as a result of cross-over between **homologous chromosomes** at **meiosis** (ii) the rearrangement of the regions of an immunoglobulin or T-cell receptor gene (*see* Fig. 46, p. 135)

red cell   an erythrocyte, a non-nucleated cell of the peripheral blood the main function of which is the transport of oxygen

red cell count (RBC)   the number of red cells in a defined volume of blood

red cell distribution width (RDW)   an estimate of anisocytosis produced by automated full blood counters

red cell indices   a term which usually indicates: **RBC, Hb, PCV, MCV, MCH** and **MCHC**

red cell mass   the total volume of red cells in the circulation, determined by radioisotopic dilution techniques and expressed either as ml/kg or as a percentage of what is expected in a person of the same height and weight

red cell membrane   the lipid bilayer with many specialized molecules bearing antigenic determinants which encloses the red cell (Fig. 64)

red cell survival   the time for which red cells survive in the circulation, normally about 120 days

red marrow   haemopoietic marrow which is red in colour, in adults found in the vertebra, sternum, ribs, clavicles and proximal long bones (cf. **yellow marrow**)

Reed–Sternberg cell   a binucleated giant cell with giant nucleoli that is part of the neoplastic population in **Hodgkin's disease**

reference range   the range of laboratory values found in a carefully defined reference population, usually expressed as a 95% range

refractory   not responsive to treatment

refractory anaemia (RA)   one of the myelodysplastic syndromes; cases of RA in the **FAB** classification are assigned to either **refractory anaemia** or **refractory cytopenia with multilineage dysplasia** in the **WHO classification** (*see* Table 13, p. 167)

refractory anaemia with excess of blasts (RAEB)   one of the myelodysplastic syndromes; cases of RAEB in the **FAB** classification are generally assigned to either **RAEB-I** or of **RAEB-II** in the **WHO classification** (*see* Table 13, p. 167)

refractory anaemia with excess of blasts in transformation (RAEB-T)   one of the myelodysplastic syndromes, according to the **FAB classification**; in the

Figure 64 The red cell membrane.
A diagram illustrating the structure of the red cell membrane; protein or glycoprotein molecules project from or pass through the lipid bilayer that encloses the cell. The transmembrane molecules (band 3 and glycophorin C) are linked to molecules of the cytoskeleton, which maintains the shape and yet permits the flexibility of the cell.

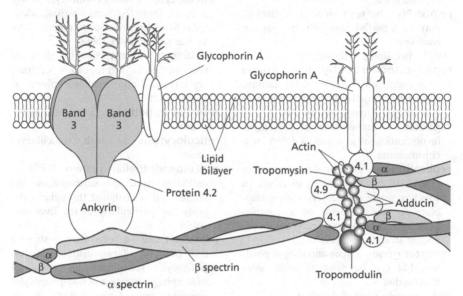

WHO classification these patients are classified as acute myeloid leukaemia if they have more than 20% of blast cells in the peripheral blood or bone marrow or are classified as myelodysplastic syndrome, RAEB-II if they have Auer rods but fewer blasts (*see* Table 13, p. 167)

refractory anaemia with ring sideroblasts (RARS) one of the myelodysplastic syndromes; cases classified as RARS in the **FAB** classification are classified, in the **WHO classification** as either RARS or refractory anaemia with multilineage dysplasia and ring sideroblasts (*see* Table 13, p. 167)

refractory cytopenia a FAB category of the myelodysplastic syndrome, referring to cases with either **neutropenia** or **thrombocytopenia** that do not meet the criteria for any other category of MDS

rejection the immunological process leading to destruction of engrafted tissue

REL a gene, avian Reticuloendotheliosis viral oncogene homologue, gene map locus 2p13-p12; encodes c-REL, one of three related proteins, the others being encoded by *RELA* (gene map locus 11q12-q13), and *RELB* (gene map locus 19q13.32), which heterodimerize with either **NFκB1** or **NFκB2** to form NFκB transcription factors which recognise specific DNA-binding sites (κB sites); in addition c-REL and RELA, but not RELB, can form homodimers; the term NFκB is often used for the NFκB1p50-RELA heterodimer, which is the major REL complex in most cells; NFκB is constitutively activated in Hodgkin and Reed–Sternberg cells and this may relate to duplication of 2p; *REL* is amplified in mediastinal large B-cell lymphoma.

REL a domain homologous to retroviral v-rel that characterizes a family of **transcription factors** including **BCL3**

relapse the recurrence of a disease

relapsing fever illness caused by Borrelia species, characterized by an intermittent fever

relative risk the odds ratio, the ratio of the likelihood of a disease in a group exposed to a particular hereditary or environmental influence to the risk in a group not so exposed; an odds ratio of 2 would indicate that the likelihood of the disease was increased twofold in the exposed group

remission the regression of a disease, may be a **partial remission** or **complete remission**

renal pertaining to the kidney

renal osteodystrophy bone disease consequent on chronic renal failure, caused by a combination of vitamin D deficiency and hyperparathyroidism

replicate to make copies of oneself, as in replication of a strand of DNA or a chromosome

replication the process of making copies of oneself, e.g. the copying of DNA, in which a single strand serves as a template for the synthesis of a complementary strand, thus recreating the double-stranded molecule

reporter gene a gene encoding a product that can be detected easily after **transfection**

RES reticuloendothelial system

respiratory burst a burst of metabolic activity in phagocytes which leads to the sequential reduction of oxygen to produce toxic oxygen metabolites such as hydrogen peroxide, hydroxyl radicals and singlet oxygen

restriction endonuclease an enzyme capable of cleaving DNA only at specific internal sites determined by DNA sequence

restriction enzyme *see* **restriction endonuclease**

restriction fragment a fragment of DNA produced by cleavage by a **restriction endonuclease**

restriction fragment length polymorphism (RFLP) variation between homologous chromosomes with regard to the length of DNA fragments produced by application of a specific **restriction endonuclease**; can be used for the demonstration of **heterozygosity** and for studies of **clonality** or for demonstration of a specific gene that removes or creates a specific cleavage site

reticular agenesis an inherited disorder when all leucocytes are lacking

reticulin a fibrillar protein which forms part of the bone marrow stroma, identified by its argyrophilia (uptake of silver)

reticulocyte a young erythrocyte, newly released form the bone marrow, identified by its uptake of certain vital stains such as **new methylene blue**

reticulocyte count quantification of **reticulocytes** as a proportion of total erythrocytes or in a defined volume of blood

reticulocytopenia a low reticulocyte count

reticulocytosis a high reticulocyte count

reticuloendothelial system (RES) a collective name for **macrophages** and related cells distributed throughout the body but particularly in the liver and spleen

reticulum cell a bone marrow stromal cell, probably of two distinct lineages, phagocytic reticulum cells being of macrophage lineage and non-phagocytic reticulum cells of mesenchymal origin, probably being related to fibroblasts and the adventitial cells of sinusoids

reticulum cell sarcoma an outmoded term for large cell lymphoma

retinoblastoma a malignant tumour of the retina

retrovirus a group of RNA viruses containing **reverse transcriptase** in the virion, includes the oncogenic human virus, **HTLV-I**, and also a number of viruses causing leukaemia in various animals

reverse transcriptase an enzyme which permits the synthesis of cDNA from an RNA template, RNA-dependent DNA polymerase; it is encoded by genes of RNA viruses and is used experimentally in the **reverse transcriptase polymerase chain reaction (RT-PCR)**

reverse transcriptase-polymerase chain reaction (RT-PCR) a technique for amplifying DNA that had first been synthesized from an RNA template by means of **reverse transcriptase**

RFLP restriction fragment length polymorphism

Rh a complex system of at least 45 blood group antigens (**CD240CE, CD240D,**

Table 15 Rh genotypes, phenotypes and shorthand notations or describing the genotype.

Rh antigens expressed	Phenotype	Most likely genotype among Caucasians (alternative practical terminologies)		Most likely genotype among Caucasians (genes described according to current terminology)
CDce	CcDee	CDe/cde	R^1r	D + Ce/d + ce
CDe	CCDee	CDe/CDe	R^1R^1	D + Ce/D + Ce
cDEe	ccDEe	cDE/cde	R^2r	D + cE/d + ce
cDE	ccDEE	cDE/cDE	R^2R^2	D + cE/D + cE
CcDEe	CcDEe	CDe/cDE	R^1R^2	D + Ce/D + cE
cDe	ccDee	cDe/cde	R^0r	D + ce/d + ce
ce	ccee	cde/cde	rr	d + ce/d + ce
Cce	Ccee	Cde/cde	r'r	d + Ce/d + ce
cEe	ccEe	cdE/cde	r''r	d + cE/d + ce
CcEe	CcEe	Cde/cdE	r'r''	d + Ce/d + cE

CD240DCE, CD241), expressed only on red cells, previously known as the Rhesus blood group system (Table 15)

rhabdomyosarcoma a malignant tumour of muscle cells

RHCE a gene at 1p36.2-p34 which has four main alleles, *CE, Ce, cc* and *cE*, encoding C + E, C + e, c + e and c + E

RHD a gene at 1p36.2-p34 encoding the Rh D antigen, a non-glycosylated transmembrane protein: reduced expression leads to a D^U phenotype; a partial D phenotype is one in which some epitopes of the D antigen are lacking; homozygous deletion of the *RHD* gene and certain mutations of the gene lead to the dd phenotype

Rhesus *see* **Rh**

rheumatoid arthritis a chronic inflammatory arthritis, autoimmune in nature; haematological features include anaemia, which may be normocytic and normochromic or microcytic and hypochromic, an elevated **erythrocyte sedimentation rate** and, sometimes, **Felty's syndrome**

rheumatoid factor an autoantibody, usually IgM, directed at IgG, present in the serum in **rheumatoid arthritis**

RH locus a locus at 1p36.2-p34 with two highly homologous very closely linked genes, *RHD* and *RHCE*

Rh-negative lacking the Rh D antigen —dd

Rh-null the failure to express any Rh antigens; this can result from null alleles at the *RH* locus or from homozygosity for an X chromosome regulator gene

RhoH *see* ***TTF***

Rh-positive having the Rh D antigen

RIA **radioimmunoassay**

ribonucleic acid (RNA) a polynucleotide in which the nitrogenous bases are adenine, guanine, cytosine and uracil and the sugar is ribose; RNA is produced in the nucleus and in mitochondria from DNA templates

ribosomal lamellar complex an organelle composed of concentric layers of membranes to which ribosomes are attached, characteristic of hairy cell leukaemia

ribosomal RNA (rRNA) RNA that, together with protein, constitutes the ribosomes

ribosome a cytoplasmic structure on which proteins are translated from messenger RNA; ribosomes may be free within the cytosol or form part of the rough endoplasmic reticulum

ribozyme an RNA molecule that can cleave single-stranded RNA

Richter's syndrome a high grade large cell transformation of chronic lymphocytic leukaemia

right shift increased segmentation of neutrophils

ring chromosome (r) an abnormal chromosome in the shape of a ring

Figure 65   RNA processing.

Newly transcribed (nascent) RNA must undergo several enzymatic modifications (processing) before it is exported from the nucleus as messenger RNA (mRNA). For simplicity, the steps in this process are depicted as occurring after transcription, but it is known that they occur during transcription itself (*see* Figure 73, p. 221). These modifications to nascent RNA (pre mRNA) comprise (i) Addition of a cap structure to the 5′ end of the RNA which occurs after about 30 nucleotides have been added. The triphosphate of the first base is hydrolyzed to a diphosphate; then the GMP moiety from a GTP substrate is joined by a 5′–5′ triphosphate bond to the first nucleotide of the nascent RNA. The transferred GMP is then methylated at the N7 position to give a mature cap. The cap is recognized by proteins that export mRNAs into the cytoplasm. (ii, iii) Excision of introns and splicing together of exons occurs as nascent RNA is synthesised, and is catalysed by a structure called the spliceosome, composed of proteins and small nucleolar RNAs (snRNA). The 5′ exon/intron border (/) has the consensus sequence AG/GURAGU and the 3′ intron/exon border is YAG/RNNN (R = A or G, Y = U or C, N = A,G,C or U), in addition, all introns have a 'branchpoint' sequence about 100 bp from their 3′ ends containing a CURAY motif. Splicing occurs in two steps; the 2′OH of the branchpoint adenosine attacks the phosphodiester bond at the 5′ exon/intron boundary, freeing the 5′ exon and creating a panhandle ('lariat') structure comprising the intron and downstream exon; subsequently the 3′OH of the freed exon cleaves the downstream intron/exon border. (iv) Polyadenylation of the 3′ end of the nascent transcript is the final step in RNA processing and occurs in the mRNAs of all genes except histones. It involves the addition of about 250 adenosine residues and is triggered by a hexamer motif I (the polyadenylation signal) in the 3′UTR—AAUAAA. The polyadenylation signal and other sequence motifs in the 3′UTR are necessary for transcriptional termination. They permit the enzymatic cleavage of the nascent transcript, leading to its release from the RNA polymerase complex. This in turn allows the polymerase itself to leave the template.

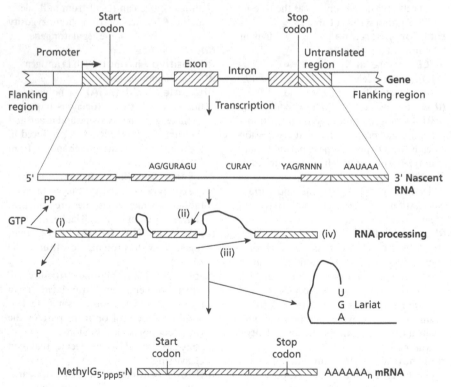

RING finger Really Interesting New Gene, a zinc-binding protein motif generally found close to an amino or carboxy terminus and present in over 200 proteins including **PML**, **BRCA1** and ubiquitination enzymes; plays a key role in the ubiquitination of other proteins prior to their proteolysis (*see also* **ubiquitin** and **ubiquitination**)

ring sideroblast or ringed sideroblast an erythroblast with a ring of **siderotic granules** surrounding its nucleus

ristocetin an antibiotic used in testing for **von Willebrand's disease**; ristocetin induces **platelet aggregation** in the presence of **von Willebrand's factor**

ristocetin cofactor assay a quantification of the ability of plasma to support ristocetin-induced platelet aggregation, indicative of the concentration of **von Willebrand's factor** in the plasma

RNA ribonucleic acid

RNAi RNA interference

RNA interference (RNAi) a process whereby introduction of double stranded RNA into a cell inhibits gene expression in a sequence-dependent fashion

RNA processing the process by which newly synthesized RNA is modified (Fig. 65)

Robertsonian translocation a translocation resulting in fusion of the long arms of two **acrocentric chromosomes** at the **centromere**, the short arms being lost

Romanowsky stain a stain composed of a mixture of **old methylene blue** and **eosin**, initially devised by a nineteenth-century parasitologist for staining malaria parasites; by extension, a stain based on Romanowsky's principle of mixing acidic and basic dyes; both **May–Grünwald–Giemsa** and **Wright's stain** are Romanowsky stains

rough endoplasmic reticulum **endoplasmic reticulum** to which many **ribosomes** are attached, giving it a granular or 'rough' appearance; the rough endoplasmic reticulum is a site of protein synthesis

rouleau (plural rouleaux) red cells stacked up like a pile of coins, indicative of an increased concentration of immunoglobulins or other plasma proteins, particularly high molecular weight plasma proteins

RPL2 see *EAP*

RPN1 the Ribophorin gene, gene map locus 3q21, encodes a ubiquitously expressed ribosomal protein; the enhancers of *RPN1* are responsible for:

• dysregulation of *EVI1* in acute myeloid leukaemia associated with inv(3)(q21q26) and t(3;3)(q21;q26)

• dysregulation of the *MEL1* gene in acute myeloid leukaemia and myelodysplastic syndrome associated with t(1;3)(p36;q21)

RPS19 a gene encoding a ribosomal structural protein, mutations of which cause some cases of **Diamond–Blackfan syndrome**

RQ-PCR real time polymerase chain reaction

rRNA ribosomal RNA

RTK receptor tyrosine kinase

RT-PCR reverse transcriptase polymerase chain reaction

rubella a viral infection; German measles

RUNX1 see *AML1* and Fig. 22, p. 83

RUNX2 the approved name for *AML3/CBFA2* (*see* **CBF** and Fig. 22, p. 83)

RUNX3 the approved name for *AML2/CBFA3* (*see* **CBF** and Fig. 22, p. 83)

Russell body a large round cytoplasmic inclusion composed of **immunoglobulin** in the cytoplasm of a **plasma cell**

R$_x$FISH cross-species **fluorescence** *in situ* **hybridization**

RXRs genes encoding Retinoid X Receptors; a family of three retinoid receptors (α, β or γ; gene map loci 9q34.3, 6p21.3 and 1q22-q23 respectively) that have low ligand affinities, bind only the 9-cis isomer of retinoic acid and cannot autonomously induce transcription on binding; they function as promiscuous heterodimerization partners for many nuclear receptors, e.g. the vitamin D receptor, retinoic acid receptors (RARs) and the peroxisome proliferator-activated receptors (PPARs).

S

S the designation of the phase of the cell cycle when synthesis of DNA occurs (*see* **cell cycle**)

SACD **subacute combined degeneration of the spinal cord**

saline pertaining to salt, usually sodium chloride

saline solution a solution of sodium chloride

Sanfilippo syndrome an inherited metabolic disorder, one of the muco-polysaccharidoses

SAP an alternative name for the *SH2D1A* gene (*see* **X-linked lymphoproliferative disease**)

SAP domain a motif present in proteins that recruit other proteins, involved in transcription and RNA processing, to the matrix attachment regions of chromatin

sarcoidosis a granulomatous disorder of unknown nature

sarcoma a malignant neoplasm of soft tissue cells such as **osteocytes** or **fibroblasts**

SBB **Sudan black B**

SC an abbreviation sometimes used to indicate the presence of haemoglobin S and haemoglobin C but not recommended because of its ambiguity

SC a gene at 1p36.2-p34 encoding the Scianna blood group antigens

scanning electron microscopy (SEM) an electron microscopy technique that produces an apparently three-dimensional image (*see* Figs 4, 24, 43 and 69, pp. 5, 91, 125 and 208 respectively)

scanning densitometry a process of optically scanning an electrophoretic strip to quantitate the proteins present, applicable to serum protein electrophoresis (Fig. 66) and haemoglobin electrophoresis

Figure 66 Scanning densitometry. The application of scanning densitometry to quantitating serum proteins from an electrophoretic strip: (a) normal showing, from right to left, albumin and α1, α2, β and γ globulins; (b) a sample from a patient with multiple myeloma showing a paraprotein in the γ region and a reduction of normal polyclonal immunoglobulins; (c) a sample from a second patient with multiple myeloma showing a large amount of a λ Bence Jones protein in the β region (arrowhead) and an IgGλ paraprotein in the γ region (short arrow); the nature of the bands was determined by immunofixation.

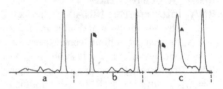

SCF **stem cell factor**

SCF a gene at 12q22-24, encoding **stem cell factor**

Schilling test a test of absorption of vitamin B_{12}, with and without intrinsic factor, performed using vitamin B_{12} labelled with a radioactive isotope

schistocyte an erythrocyte fragment

Schuffner's dots cytoplasmic inclusions in erythrocytes parasitized by *Plasmodium vivax* or *Plasmodium ovale*

SCID **severe combined immunodeficiency**

SCL an alternative designation of *TAL1*

scurvy the disease resulting from deficiency of vitamin C or ascorbic acid, can cause anaemia and mucocutaneous haemorrhage

SD **standard deviation**

Se an allele of *FUT2*, conveys **secretor** status

se an allele of *FUT2*, conveys **non-secretor** status if homozygous

sea-blue histiocyte a storage cell containing ceroid or lipofuscin which can occur in inherited metabolic disorders and also in various acquired conditions

sea-blue histiocytosis ceroid-lipofuscinosis, a group of inherited metabolic disorders

Sebastian syndrome a giant platelet syndrome with thrombocytopenia and neutrophil inclusions, resulting from a mutation in the non-muscle myosin heavy chain 9 gene (*NMMHC-A* or *MYH9*) at 22q11-13 (or 22q12.3-q13.2)

secondary (i) having an external cause (ii) jargon for a metastasis (iii) developing later

secondary granules the specific granules of neutrophils, eosinophils and basophils

secondary immune response the immune response on a second or subsequent exposure to an antigen

secondary karyotypic abnormality a chromosomal abnormality occurring during the subsequent evolution of an abnormal clone that already shows a **primary karyotypic abnormality** (*see* Fig. 49, p. 146)

secondary leukaemia (i) leukaemia secondary to exposure to anti-cancer chemotherapy or irradiation, usually acute myeloid leukaemia but occasionally acute lymphoblastic leukaemia or acute biphenotypic leukaemia, also known as **therapy-related leukaemia** (ii) more broadly, leukaemia following exposure to mutagenic agents or occurring during the course of another haematological disorder

secondary myelodysplastic syndrome a myelodysplastic syndrome secondary to exposure to anti-cancer chemotherapy or irradiation

secondary polycythaemia polycythaemia secondary to another disease or an environmental factor

secretor an individual who has ABH antigens in saliva and other body fluids as a result of expression of the *Se* allele of the *FUT2* gene; secretors are *SeSe* or *Sese* whereas non-secretors are *sese*; non-secretors cannot synthesize Le^b antigen (*see FUT1*)

sedimentation rate the erythrocyte sedimentation rate

segmented neutrophil a mature neutrophil with a nucleus divided into lobes or segments

selectin one of a family of three cell adhesion molecules, E-, L- and P-selectin (**CD62E, CD62L** and **CD62P**)

SEM scanning electron microscopy

semipermeable membrane a membrane that can be crossed by solvent but not solute

sensitivity the capacity of a test to detect the presence of an abnormality

sepsis infection

septicaemia an acute illness associated with bacteraemia

SEPTIN 2 a gene, also known as *KIAA00128*, the homologue of mouse *septin 6*, gene map locus Xq22, encoding a **GTPase**; *SEPTIN2* contributed to a *MLL-SEPTIN 2* fusion gene in two infants with acute myeloid leukaemia associated respectively with t(X;11;3;11) and ins(X;11)(q24;q23)

sequencing analysis of the sequence of bases in a DNA molecule

serous atropy gelatinous transformation, deposition of increased ground substance or acid mucopolysaccharide in the bone marrow

serpin one of a family of intracellular and extracellular serine protease inhibitors including **antithrombin, antiplasmin, plasminogen activator inhibitor** 1 and 2, α_1 antitrypsin, **C1 inhibitor**

serum (plural sera) the liquid part of blood that remains after clotting has led to the removal of fibrinogen

serum protein electrophoresis the separation of the proteins of serum into albumin and α, β and γ immunoglobulins by **electrophoresis** (Fig. 67) (*see also* Fig. 66)

SET a gene, **Set** translocation, myeloid leukaemia-associated, gene map locus 9q34.3, encodes a **SET domain** protein; *SET* contributes to the *SET-CAN* fusion gene formed by fusion of two genes at 9q34 in rare cases of acute myeloid leukaemia

SET domain a highly conserved protein motif implicated in the modulation of

Figure 67   Serum protein electrophoresis.
Serum protein electrophoresis in a control normal sample (lane 1) and in nine patients with a paraprotein (lanes 2–10). The normal sample shows, from above down, albumin and α1, α2, β1, β2 (faint) and γ globulins. The nine patients' samples show a paraprotein with mobility ranging from early to late γ; generally there is also a reduction of normal polyclonal immunoglobulins.

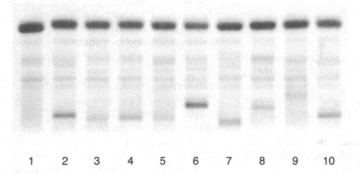

chromatin structure; originally identified *Drosophila* Su(var)3-9, 'Enhancer of zeste' and Trithorax proteins; a signature of proteins that regulate the remodelling of either transcriptionally active or repressed chromatin

severe combined immunodeficiency (SCID) a heterogeneous group of disorders leading to a severe defect in humoral and cell-mediated immunity, usually with an autosomal recessive inheritance but sometimes showing an X-linked recessive inheritance; some of the underlying defects are tabulated (Table 16)

severe congenital neutropenia a genetically heterogeneous group of conditions in which there is a severe congenital reduction in the neutrophil count, **Kostmann's syndrome**

sex chromatin the chromatin mass that represents the inactive X chromosome, present as a drumstick-shaped appendage in some granulocytes

sex chromosomes the X and Y chromosomes; normal females have two X chromosomes and normal males an X and a Y chromosome

sex-linked recessive a mode of inheritance in which a gene on an X chromosome leads to a disease or an inherited characteristic in hemizygous males or homozygous females (Fig. 68)

sexually transmitted disease (STD) a disease transmitted by sexual intercourse, a venereal disease

Sézary cell a neoplastic T lymphocyte with a characteristic convoluted or cerebriform nucleus, present in the blood in **Sézary syndrome** and sometimes in **mycosis fungoides**

Sézary syndrome a cutaneous T-cell lymphoma with circulating Sézary cells

SH-2 domain a protein motif found in cell surface and intracellular signal-transducing proteins which allows binding to phosphotyrosine-containing target proteins in a phosphorylation-dependent manner

SH2DIA a gene, also known as *SAP*, gene map locus Xq25, encoding SLAM-associated protein (SAP); mutation leads to the **X-linked lymphoproliferative syndrome** (*see also* **CDISO**)

SH3GL1 *see EEN*

SHIP a gene, SH2-containing Inositol Phosphatase, gene map locus 2q36-q37, encoding an enzyme involved in phosphoinositide turnover; it has a major role in negative signalling in lymphocytes and in the down-regulation of cytokine receptor-mediated signals in myeloid cells

Shwachman–Diamond syndrome or Shwachman syndrome an inherited disorder characterized by neutropenia,

Table 16 Some of the genetic causes of severe combined immunodeficiency.

Defect	Inheritance	Presence of T, B and NK cells
Deficiency of Janus-associated kinase 3	Autosomal recessive, *JAK3* gene at 19p13.1	T−B+NK−
Deficiency of common γ chain of receptors for IL-2, IL-4, IL-7, IL-9 and IL 15	X-linked recessive, gene at Xq13.1	T−B+NK−
Deficiency of α chain of IL-7 receptor	Autosomal recessive, gene at 5p13	T−B+NK+
Deficiency of β chain of IL-15 receptor	Autosomal recessive	T−B+NK−
Adenosine deaminase deficiency	Autosomal recessive, mutation in the adenosine deaminase gene at 20q13.2-q13.11	T−B−NK−
Deficiencies of recombinase activating gene products	Autosomal recessive, *RAG1* and *RAG2* genes at 6q21.3	T−B−NK+
Signalling defect	Autosomal recessive, mutation in p56^{lck} gene encoding a tyrosine kinase signalling molecule	T+B+NK+
CD45 deficiency	Autosomal recessive, mutation in gene for CD45 tyrosine phosphatase	T+B+NK+

Figure 68   Sex-linked recessive inheritance.
The transmission of haemophilia through the female line from Queen Victoria to her descendants. It will be seen that transmission occurs from carrier females to haemophiliac males and that known carrier females are the children of either haemophiliac males or carrier females.

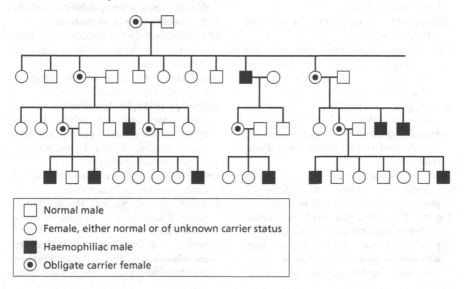

☐ Normal male
◯ Female, either normal or of unknown carrier status
■ Haemophiliac male
◉ Obligate carrier female

Figure 69   A sickle cell.
A scanning electron micrograph of a sickle cell.

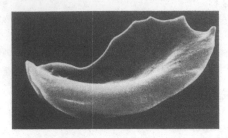

exocrine pancreatic insufficiency and dyschondroplasia

SI   units units of the **Système International d'Unités**

sickle cell an erythrocyte that becomes sickle or crescent-shaped as a result of polymerization of **haemoglobin S** (Fig. 69)

sickle cell anaemia the disease resulting from homozygosity for the β^S gene

sickle cell disease a heterogeneous group of diseases, including sickle cell anaemia and various compound heterozygous states, in which clinicopathological effects occur as a result of sickle cell formation

sickle cell trait heterozygosity for the β^S gene

sideline a cytogenetic term for a daughter clone identifiable because it shows karyotypic evolution

sideroblast an erythroblast containing **siderotic granules**

sideroblastic anaemia an inherited or acquired anaemia with the bone marrow having a significant proportion of **ring sideroblasts**

siderocyte an erythrocyte containing **siderotic granules**

siderotic granule an iron-containing granule that is identifiable by a **Perls' stain**

sign a disease feature that is visible, palpable or otherwise identifiable on physical examination (cf. **symptom**)

Signal Transduction and Activator of Transcription (STAT) proteins a family of at least 7 multi-domain **transcription factors** that are activated in response to ligand signalling in a variety of biological systems; dormant STATs exist in cytoplasmic multiprotein complexes; following ligand binding, receptor phosphorylation, either due to the action of **Janus kinases (JAKs)** or due to inherent receptor tyrosine kinase activity, allows docking of STATs to the receptor; this leads to STAT phosphorylation by JAKs; phosphorylated STATs are able to dimerize and are translocated to the nucleus where they can regulate gene expression by binding to STAT-responsive **enhancers**

single-strand conformation polymorphism analysis (SSCP) a method of detection of mutations in which a single strand of DNA, a **PCR** product, is radiolabelled and subjected to non-denaturing gel electrophoresis; mobility depends on conformation as well as size so that a single base substitution may alter the mobility, permitting the recognition of an abnormality

sinusoid a thin-walled relatively large bone marrow vessel through which blood cells enter the circulation

SLC4A1 an alternative name for the *AE1* gene encoding band 3 of the red cell membrane and the antigens of the Diego blood group system

SLC19A2 a gene at 1q23.2-23.3 encoding a high-affinity thiamine transporter; mutation in this gene is responsible for **thiamine-responsive megaloblastic anaemia**

SLE systemic lupus erythematosus

Sm expressed on the surface membrane of a cell, e.g. SmIg, surface membrane immunoglobulin

small cell carcinoma of the lung a neuroendocrine tumour of the lung

small lymphocytic lymphoma a low grade lymphoma with neoplastic cells that resemble those of chronic lymphocytic leukaemia both cytologically and immunophenotypically

smear cell a cell that has been crushed during spreading of a blood film

SMMHC a gene, **S**mooth **M**uscle **M**yosin **H**eavy **C**hain gene, an alternative name for *MYH11*

smooth endoplasmic reticulum **endoplasmic reticulum** that lacks granules and therefore appears smooth; the smooth endoplasmic reticulum serves to transport proteins from the rough endoplasmic reticulum to the **Golgi apparatus**; the smooth endoplasmic reticulum of some cells contains enzymes and can synthesize lipids

SNX sorting nexins

solute a substance that is dissolved in another substance

solvent a liquid in which something is dissolved

somatic cell any body cell except a **germ cell**

somatic hypermutation the process by which germinal centre B cells that have been exposed to antigens undergo somatic mutation so that they produce antibodies with a higher affinity for the relevant antigen; the cells producing the highest affinity antibodies are selected to survive, a process known a **affinity selection** (*see* **clonal selection**)

somatic mutation a mutation occurring in a somatic cell, i.e. in any cell except a germ cell; somatic mutation is a physiological process in lymphoid cells but in lymphoid and other cells certain somatic mutations can lead to the occurrence of malignant disease

somatic reversion correction of genetic defect in a clone of cells by a back mutation, mitotic recombination or by a second site mutation that alters the reading frame or leads to synthesis of a protein that is better tolerated than the original one

SOP standard operating procedure

sorting nexins (SNX) a family of PX domain-containing intracellular molecules involved in the intracellular trafficking of endocytosed proteins

South-east Asian ovalocytosis an inherited abnormality of the erythrocyte membrane leading, in heterozygotes, to the presence of macro-ovalocytes and stomatocytes, resulting from mutation in the *AE1* (band 3) gene

Southern blotting a method, named from its inventor (Professor Ed Southern), of identifying specific sequences of DNA by means of cleaving the molecule with a restriction enzyme, followed by size-fractionation by gel electrophoresis, then 'blotting' onto a nitrocellulose membrane; single-stranded DNA on the membrane is hybridized to a complementary sequence of single-stranded DNA that serves as a probe

specific granule neutrophilic, eosinophilic and basophilic granules

specificity the capacity of a test to detect an abnormality without giving positive results in the absence of an abnormality

spectrin an erythrocyte membrane protein composed of **dimers**, **tetramers** and higher **polymers** of α spectrin and β spectrin, encoded respectively by the *SPTA1* and *SPTB* genes

spermatozoon (plural spermatozoa) a **germ cell** produced in the testis of a male

spheroacanthocyte a spherical cell with a small number of irregularly disposed spicules

spherocyte a spherical or near-spherical erythrocyte

spherocytosis the presence of **spherocytes**

sphingomyelin lipidosis Niemann–Pick disease, an inherited disorder of metabolism in which there is a deficiency of sphingomyelinase

spiculated cell a cell with spicules, e.g. an **acanthocyte**, **echinocyte**, **keratocyte** or **schistocyte**

spicule (i) an elongated projection from an erythrocyte (ii) a narrow piece of bone

spleen a lymphoid organ which is also part of the **reticuloendothelial system**

splenectomy surgical removal of the spleen

splenic pertaining to the **spleen**

splenic atrophy regression of the **spleen**

splenic lymphoma with villous lymphocytes a low grade B-cell neoplasm which, in the **WHO classification**, is included in the category **splenic marginal zone lymphoma**

splenic marginal zone lymphoma a low grade B-cell lymphoma

splenic sequestration acute pooling of erythrocytes in the spleen in **sickle cell disease**

splenomegaly splenic enlargement

splicing the process by which RNA sequences, corresponding to **introns** in the

Figure 70   Staging of Hodgkin's disease.
A diagram showing the lymph node regions, as defined for the staging of Hodgkin's disease. Staging is carried out as shown in Table 17.

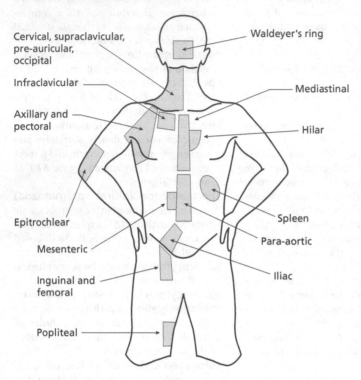

Cervical, supraclavicular, pre-auricular, occipital

Waldeyer's ring

Infraclavicular

Mediastinal

Axillary and pectoral

Hilar

Epitrochlear

Spleen

Mesenteric

Para-aortic

Inguinal and femoral

Iliac

Popliteal

gene, are removed during processing of RNA (*see* Fig. 65, p. 202)

sprue   a malabsorption syndrome

SPTA1   the gene at 1q21 encoding α spectrin, a component of the red cell membrane; mutation can result in **hereditary spherocytosis** or **hereditary elliptocytosis**

SPTB   the gene at 14q22-q23.2 encoding β spectrin, a component of the red cell membrane; mutation can result in **hereditary spherocytosis** or **hereditary elliptocytosis**

spur cell anaemia   haemolytic anaemia with **acanthocytes** occurring in severe liver disease

squamous cell carcinoma   a malignant tumour of epithelial cells

SRP20   a gene, **SR P**rotein **20**, gene map locus 6p21, encodes an adaptor protein kinase of the SR (Serine-Arginine) family that is involved in the nuclear export of

cellular mRNAs; contributed to a *SRP20-BCL6* fusion gene in a patient with transformed follicular lymphoma

SSCP   single-strand conformation polymorphism analysis

ssp   abbreviation for species, as in *Candida* ssp

stab cell   a **band form** or **non-segmented neutrophil**

stage   an expression of the extent of a malignant disease

staging   the process by which the stage of a disease is determined (Fig. 70 and Table 17)

standard deviation (SD)   a mathematical indication of the degree of dispersion of values around a **mean**

standard error of the mean   the mean divided by the square root of the number of observations

Table 17 Staging of Hodgkin's disease (Hodgkin lymphoma).
Each patient is given a composite stage e.g. IA. IIIB.

Stage	Criteria
I	Disease in one lymph node region (*see* Fig. 70) or lymphoid structure (e.g. thymus, spleen or Waldeyer's ring); stage I_E has limited contiguous extension beyond a lymph node but with this being encompassable in a radiotherapy field
II	Disease in two or more lymph node regions or structures but confined to one side of the diaphragm
III	Disease on both sides of the diaphragm but confined to lymph nodes and lymphoid structures
IV	Spread (other than limited contiguous extension) beyond lymph nodes and spleen, e.g. to liver, lung or bone marrow
A	Having no B symptoms
B	Having (i) loss of more than 10% of body weight in the preceding 6 months (ii) drenching night sweats (iii) fever

standard operating procedure (SOP)
a codified description of the procedure
for performing a laboratory test

'starry sky' a histological appearance in
Burkitt's lymphoma and other high grade
neoplasms in which macrophages are seen
as pale areas in a background of small
dark neoplastic cells

STAT proteins *see* **Signal Transduction
and Activator of Transcription (STAT)
proteins**

STAT5b a gene, **S**ignal **T**ransduction
and **A**ctivator of **T**ranscription **5b**, gene
map locus 17q11.2, encoding a STAT
protein which acts downstream of growth
hormone, IL3 and IL5 signalling; contributed to a *STAT5b-RARA* fusion gene
in a case of M1 acute myeloid leukaemia

statistical significance a statement of
the probability that an apparent difference or apparent relationship has arisen
by chance, expressed as a *P* value; a *P* value
of < 0.01 indicates that the likelihood of a
chance result is less than 1 in 100

STD **sexually transmitted disease**

stem cell a cell capable of both replacing
itself and giving rise to progeny

stem cell factor (SCF) the ligand for
c-KIT, a growth factor for haemopoietic
stem cells and a regulator of mast cell differentiation and function, encoded by the
SCF gene at 12q22-24

stem cell transplantation transplantation of **stem cells** harvested either from
the bone marrow or from the peripheral
blood

stem line a cytogenetic term for the
parent clone from which other karyotyp-
ically distinguishable daughter clones or
sidelines are derived

sternal pertaining to the **sternum**

sternum the breast bone, used for bone
marrow aspiration

STL a gene, **S**ix **T**welve **L**eukaemia gene,
gene map locus 6q23, encodes a very
small protein with no known homologies;
STL contributed to an *ETV6-STL* fusion
gene in a B-lineage acute lymphoblastic
leukaemia cell line with t(6;12)(q23;p13)

stochastic randomly determined

stoichiometric a reaction in which reactants combine with each other in a fixed
ratio, relating to their molecular weights

stomatitis inflammation of the mouth

stomatocyte an erythrocyte with a slit-
shaped opening (*see* Fig. 43, p. 125)

stomatocytosis the presence of
stomatocytes

storage cell a cell that has an increased
content of a metabolite and appears to
be storing it, e.g. a **Gaucher's cell** or a
foamy macrophage

storage diseases inherited metabolic
disorders in which normal cell metabo-

lites, which cannot be processed further because of a metabolic block, accumulate in cells and appear to be 'stored'

stress polycythaemia   *see* **pseudopolycythaemia**

stroma   the connective tissue supporting an organ such as the bone marrow

stromal   pertaining to the **stroma**

structural proteomics   the determination of structures of proteins that can only be defined in the context of their interactions with other proteins, polynucleotides, lipids or carbohydrates

subacute combined degeneration of the spinal cord (SACD)   degeneration of the posterior and lateral columns of the spinal cord as a consequence of **vitamin B$_{12}$ deficiency**

Sudan black B   a cytochemical stain which is taken up by the granules of myeloid cells

sulphaemoglobin   haemoglobin which has been irreversibly oxidized by drugs or chemicals with incorporation of a sulphur atom into the porphyrin ring

suppressor cell   a T cell that can suppress the activities of B cells, cytotoxic T cells and helper T cells

supravital stain   a stain performed on living, unfixed cells

surface area   an estimation of the total area of the body covered by skin, can be derived from a height and weight nomogram (Fig. 71), used for calculation of doses of anti-cancer drugs and for determining if an estimate of **red cell mass** and **plasma volume** is normal

survival curve   a graphical representation of the number of patients still alive plotted against time

Sweet's syndrome   acute neutrophilic dermatitis, can be a feature of **acute myeloid leukaemia** and the **myelodysplastic syndromes**

SYK   a gene, **S**pleen tyrosine **K**inase, gene map locus 9q22, encoding a non-receptor tyrosine kinase; *SYK* contributed to a *ETV6-SYK* fusion gene in a patient with a myeloproliferative–myelodysplastic syndrome; loss of *SYK* expression in breast cancer correlates with increased tumour load and invasiveness

Figure 71   Surface area nomogram.
A nomogram showing how surface area can be estimated from the height and weight of a patient. This permits drug doses to be calculated according to surface area. The surface area is more relevant than the weight alone to the effect of a certain dose of a drug.

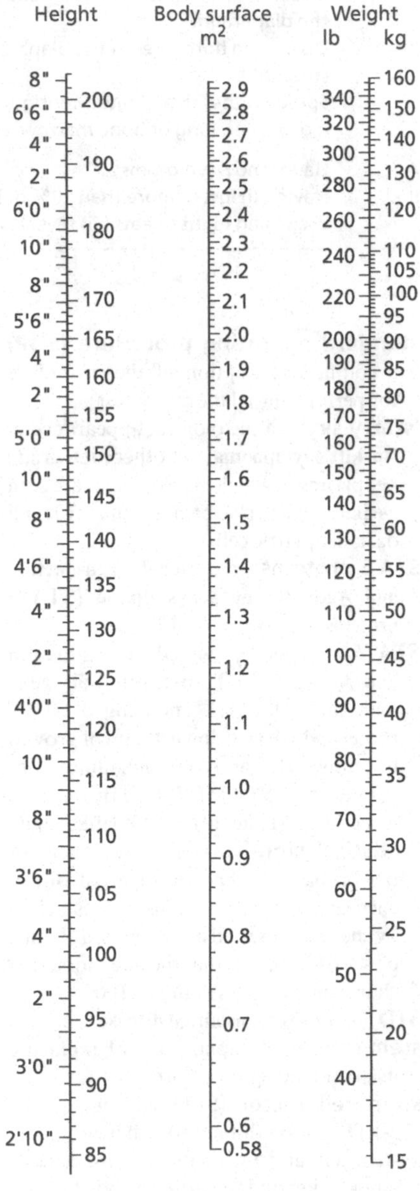

| Height | Body surface m^2 | Weight lb | kg |

symptom a feature of a disease that is experienced by the patient (cf. **sign**)

syngeneic genetically identical, e.g. an identical twin

syntenic of genes, thought to be on a single chromosome because they are lost concurrently with a specific marker gene that is known to be located on that chromosome

systemic lupus erythematosus a multi-system autoimmune disease which may cause **autoimmune haemolytic anaemia**, **autoimmune thrombocytopenic purpura** and the development of **antiphospholipid antibodies**, including the '**lupus anticoagulant**', associated with **acquired thrombophilia**

systemic mastocytosis a disseminated mast cell neoplasm

T

T an abbreviation for the pyrimidine, thymine

TAL1 a gene, T-cell Acute lymphocytic Leukaemia 1, also known as Stem Cell Leukaemia haemopoietic transcription factor, *SCL*, gene map locus 1p32, encodes a basic helix–loop–helix transcription factor that is essential for haemopoiesis and vasculogenesis; forms transcriptionally active heterodimers with any of the isoforms encoded by the *E2A* locus; its normal activity is regulated by interaction with **CBP** and **LIM domain** proteins; *TAL1* is dysregulated:
- by a small deletion, detectable only by molecular techniques, which fuses most of the gene with the promoter of the upstream *SIL* (SCL Interrupting Locus) gene, associated with T-lineage acute lymphoblastic leukaemia
- by proximity to the *TCRAD* (αδ) locus at 14q11 in T-lineage acute lymphoblastic leukaemia associated with t(1;14)(p32;q11)
- by proximity to the *TCRB* gene at 7q35 in T-lineage acute lymphoblastic leukaemia associated with t(1;7)(p32;q35)

TAL2 a gene, T-cell Acute lymphocytic Leukaemia 2, gene map locus 7q35, encodes a homologue of *TAL1* that is essential for embryonic brain development; dysregulated by proximity to the *TCRB* gene at 7q35 in T-lineage acute lymphoblastic leukaemia associated with t(7;9)(q35;p13)

TAN1 a gene, Translocation-Associated Notch homologue 1 (*Notch1*), gene map locus 9q34, encodes a transmembrane receptor homologue of the *Drosophila* notch protein; when notch proteins bind their ligands, (known as jagged and delta), the notch protein is cleaved to generate an intracellular protein (notch-IC) which activate the **RAS** signalling pathway; *Notch1* is truncated and loses its extracellular domain in T-lineage acute lymphoblastic leukaemia associated with t(7;9)(q34;q34); removal of the Notch extracellular domain results in a dominant gain-of-function Notch allele

TCF3 *see E2A*

TAM transient abnormal myelopoiesis

t-AML therapy-related acute myeloid leukaemia

TAP1* and *TAP2 Transporter-associated with Antigen Processing genes that encode proteins delivering peptides to developing HLA type I molecules; mutation of either gene can result in an immune deficiency syndrome (*see* **bare lymphocyte syndrome** and **HLA type I deficiency**)

Taq-Man™ a semi-quantitative **PCR** technique incorporating a target-sequence-specific fluorescent probe as well as the necessary primers; the probe is labelled with two fluorescent dyes, a reporter and a quencher; during the PCR, the exonuclease activity of Taq polymerase destroys the probe and releases the reporter dye, which fluoresces; the level of fluorescence reflects the amount of product generated, which is in turn dependent upon the amount of starting material (*see* Fig. 63, p. 197)

Taq polymerase a heat-stable **DNA polymerase** that is used for **PCR**

target cell an erythrocyte with haemoglobin concentrated in the centre of the cell, giving the appearance of a target

tartrate-resistant acid phosphatase (TRAP) an enzyme present in hairy cells and occasionally in cells of other types of non-Hodgkin's lymphoma; also expressed by osteoclasts

TAX the transforming protein encoded by human T-cell leukaemia virus type I (HTLV-I); constitutively activates NFκB (see also **REL**) by binding to and chronically activating IκB kinase (IκK), an enzyme complex that phosphorylates and inactivates IκB, thereby allowing NFκB to enter the nucleus

TBI total body irradiation

T cell a T lymphocyte

T-cell receptor surface membrane receptors in **T cells**; they are of two types, αβ and γδ; T cells with an αβ T-cell receptor are capable of recognizing and binding an antigen-derived peptide in the context of an autologous MHC (*HLA*-encoded) complex on the surface of an antigen-presenting cell; different T-cell receptor molecules recognize preferentially peptides in an HLA class I (with up-regulation of CD8 then occurring) or class II context (with up-regulation of CD4 then occurring)

T chronic lymphocytic leukaemia a term which has been variously used to designate large granular lymphocyte leukaemia, T prolymphocytic leukaemia and other entities; to avoid ambiguity, the use of this term is not recommended

TCL1a T-Cell Leukaemia/lymphoma 1a, gene map locus 14q32.1, encodes a coactivator of the **AKT** kinase which is normally expressed in primitive B and T lymphocytes; *TCL1* is dysregulated in inv(14)(q11q32) and t(14;14)(q11;q32) associated with T-cell prolymphocytic leukaemia; the dysregulation is consequent on the gene being brought into proximity to the *TCRAD* (αδ) locus at 14q11; in addition to *TCL1a*, three other genes normally expressed in primitive lymphoid cells and overexpressed in 14q32.1 rearrangements are present at this locus: *TCL1b* (T Cell Leukaemia/lymphoma 1b) encoding a homologue of *TCL1a*; *TNG1* (TCL1-Neighbouring Gene-1) and *TNG2* (TCL1-Neighbouring Gene-2) which encode proteins of unknown function; *TNG1* and *TNG2* are sometimes collectively referred to as *TCL6*

TCL1b *see TCL1a*

TCL3 *see HOX11*

TCL6 *see TCL1a*

TCR T-cell receptor

TCRAD (αδ) the T-Cell Receptor Alpha Delta (αδ) locus, gene map locus 14q11, where there are a cluster of genes encoding the alpha and delta chains of the T-cell receptor; the *TCRA* genes have V (variable), J (joining) and C (constant) gene segments; the *TCRD* genes have V (variable), D (diversity), J (joining) and C (constant) gene segments; the *TCRAD* locus contributes to oncogenesis by leading to the dysregulation of proto-oncogenes which are brought into proximity to it, a relatively common mechanism of leukaemogenesis in T-lineage acute lymphoblastic leukaemia

TCRB the T-Cell Receptor Beta gene, gene map locus 7q35, where there are a cluster of genes encoding the beta chain of the T-cell receptor; there are V (variable), D (diversity), J (joining) and C (constant) gene segments; the *TCRB* locus contributes to oncogenesis by leading to the dysregulation of proto-oncogenes which are brought into proximity to it; a relatively common mechanism of leukaemogenesis in T-lineage acute lymphoblastic leukaemia

TCRG the T-Cell Receptor Gamma locus on chromosome 7 where there are a cluster of genes encoding the gamma chain of the T-cell receptor; there are V (variable), J (joining) and C (constant) gene segments

TdT terminal deoxynucleotidyl transferase

teardrop poikilocyte a teardrop shaped erythrocyte, particularly a feature of **myelofibrosis** and of **megaloblastic anaemia**

TEL *see ETV6*

telangiectasia permanent dilation of superficial capillaries and venules of the skin or the mucous membrane which can lead to haemorrhage

telomerase an RNA-protein complex that is essential for maintaining nucleoprotein caps at the **telomeres**; it is composed of telomerase RNA (hTR) and a specialized reverse transcriptase (hTERT)

telomere one of the two ends of a chromosome

telophase the final stage of **mitosis** in which the chromosomes assemble at the two poles of the cell where they are surrounded by a nuclear membrane, following which the cytoplasm begins to divide (*see* Fig. 6, p. 14)

TEM **transmission electron microscopy**

temporal arteritis inflammation of the superficial temporal artery, usually associated with a high **erythrocyte sedimentation rate**, can cause blindness

teniposide an anti-cancer drug which interacts with **topoisomerase-II**

teratogen a substance that can cause fetal malformation when administered to a pregnant woman, e.g. coumarin anticoagulants

terminal deoxynucleotidyl transferase (TdT) a DNA **polymerase** that catalyses terminal incorporation of nucleotides into DNA, a marker of immature cells of lymphoid and, to a lesser extent, myeloid lineages

termination codon also known as a stop codon, a codon that causes termination of protein synthesis

tetramer a **polymer** composed of four **monomers**

tetraploid having 92 chromosomes

tetraploidy the presence of two sets of chromosomes in a cell so that there are 92 chromosomes

TF the gene encoding **transferrin**; mutations leading to **atransferrinaemia** cause **microcytic anaemia** with iron overload; a common polymorphism among European populations leads to a slight reduction in serum transferrin concentration and predisposes menstruating woman to iron deficiency anaemia

TFG a gene, *T̲RK-F̲used G̲ene*, also known as *TRKT3*, gene map locus 3q11-q12, encodes a ubiquitously expressed coiled-coil protein of uncertain function which normally exists as multimers; *TFG* contributes to one of two *TFG-ALK* fusion genes in occasional cases of anaplastic large cell lymphoma associated with t(2;3)(p23;q21); the chimaeric proteins carry the coiled-coil domain of TFG fused to the tyrosine kinase domain of ALK and are oligomerized leading to constitutive tyrosine kinase activity

TFR2 a gene at 7q22 encoding a **transferrin receptor**, mutation of which leads to a small minority of cases of **hereditary haemochromatosis**

TFRC the gene encoding the major **transferrin receptor**

TGFβ **transforming growth factor β**

TGFB a gene, gene map locus 19q13.1, encoding T̲ransforming G̲rowth F̲actor B̲eta; germ line mutations in *TGFB* are the cause of Camurati–Engelmann disease, an autosomal dominant disorder characterized by skeletal defects

Th1 a subset of **helper T cells** (type 1 helper T cells) that secrete **interleukin-2**, **interferon-γ** and **lymphotoxin** (tumour necrosis factor β) and promote cellular immune responses

Th2 a subset of **helper T cells** (type 2 helper T cells) that secrete **interleukin-4**, **interleukin-5** and **interleukin-6** and promote B-cell proliferation and antibody secretion

thalassaemia an inherited disorder in which one of the component chains of haemoglobin is synthesized at a reduced rate

thalassaemia intermedia a thalassaemic condition that is moderately severe but nevertheless does not require regular transfusions to sustain life

thalassaemia major thalassaemia that is incompatible with more than a short survival in the absence of blood transfusion

thalassaemia minor an asymptomatic thalassaemic condition

therapeutic of benefit in treatment of a disease

therapy treatment

therapy-related acute myeloid leukaemia (t-AML) acute myeloid leukaemia following the use of mutagenic drugs or radiotherapy and likely to be aetiologically related to such therapy

therapy-related myelodysplastic syndrome (t-MDS) a myelodysplastic syndrome following the use of mutagenic drugs or radiotherapy and likely to be aetiologically related to such therapy

thiamine-responsive megaloblastic anaemia a constitutional disorder with autosomal recessive inheritance, characterized by sensorineural deafness, diabetes mellitus and thiamine-responsive megaloblastic anaemia with ring sideroblasts, resulting from mutation in the *SLC19A2* gene

thrombasthenia a severe inherited defect in platelet function

thrombin the activated form of prothrombin that converts fibrinogen into fibrin (*see* Figs 17 and 18, pp. 77 and 78)

thrombin time (TT) the time needed for plasma to clot after the addition of thrombin, a test for fibrinogen concentration and function and for the presence of thrombin inhibitors such as heparin

thrombocythaemia an increased platelet count

thrombocytopenia a reduced platelet count

thrombocytopenic purpura subcutaneous bleeding caused by a low platelet count

thrombocytosis an increased platelet count

thromboembolism deep vein thrombosis and pulmonary embolism

thrombolysis lysis of a clot

thrombolytic therapy administration of a drug, e.g. streptokinase, in order to cause lysis of a clot

thrombomodulin an endothelial cell surface glycoprotein that interacts with thrombin to activate protein C; deficiency, which is very rare, is associated with an increased risk of thrombosis

thrombophilia an increased propensity to form thrombi, either arterial or venous

thrombophlebitis inflammation of veins

thrombophlebitis migrans venous thrombosis recurring over a short period of time at multiple sites, often indicative of underlying carcinoma

thromboplastin a substance that promotes blood clotting; thromboplastins used in the laboratory are divided into complete thromboplastins, which have

tissue factor activity, and incomplete thromboplastins, which can act as a platelet substitute in the intrinsic pathway of coagulation

thrombopoietin (TPO) a hormone that promotes thrombopoiesis

thrombosis the process of formation of a blood clot

thrombotic thrombocytopenic purpura (TTP) a consumptive coagulopathy leading to thrombocytopenic purpura, characterized by a clinical pentad of fever, neurological abnormalities, thrombocytopenia, microangiopathic haemolytic anaemia and renal impairment

thrombus (plural thrombi) a blood clot within a blood vessel

thrush candidiasis, usually of the mouth or vagina, a common condition in immunosuppressed patients

thymic pertaining to the thymus

thymine a nitrogenous base that pairs with adenine (a pyrimidine)

thymocyte a lymphoid cell in the thymus

thymoma a tumour of the thymus, can be associated with pure red cell aplasia

thymus a lymphoid organ in the mediastinum, important in the development of T-lineage lymphocytes

TIF2 a gene, Transcriptional Intermediary Factor 2, gene map locus 8q13, encodes a transcriptional activator which normally binds to CBP; *TIF2* contributes to the *MOZ-TIF2* fusion gene in acute myeloid leukaemia associated with inv(8)(p11q13)

tinzaparin a low molecular weight heparin

tissue an organized arrangement of cells

tissue factor altered or damaged tissue that is able to activate the extrinsic pathway of coagulation; may also be secreted by activated monocytes

tissue factor pathway inhibitor a lipoprotein-associated inhibitor of the factors VIIa and Xa; also know as extrinsic pathway inhibitor; the majority is bound to endothelial cells with the minority being in the plasma (*see* Fig. 56, p. 170)

tissue plasminogen activator (tPA) a substance secreted by various tissues that is able to convert plasminogen to plasmin

Figure 72   T cell development (opposite).
A diagrammatic representation of the development of T lymphocytes. The common lymphoid progenitor in the bone marrow gives rise to precursor T lymphoblasts, which traverse the blood stream as naïve CD4-negative CD8-negative T-cell precursors. After entering the cortex of the thymus, T-cell receptor genes (TCR) are rearranged and CD4 and CD8 are expressed. The thymocytes then undergoes positive selection, as a result of presentation of antigen-derived peptides by cortical epithelial cells; peptides presented are either endogenous peptides in an MHC class I context or exogenous peptides in an MHC class II context leading the thymocytes to express, respectively, CD8 alone or CD4 alone. The thymocytes then undergo negative selection with apoptosis of self-reactive cells occurring. Following presentation of the relevant antigen by an antigen-presenting cell, such as a dendritic cell or a macrophage, thymocytes mature into a T cells with cytotoxic or helper potential. These lymphocytes traverse the blood stream and enter lymphoid tissues where they may be presented with either processed endogenous antigen (e.g. derived from a tumour cell or a virus-infected cell) in an MHC class I context or processed exogenous antigen in an MHC class II context. Antigen-presenting cells are macrophages, dendritic cells or B cells, the latter having trapped antigen by means of surface membrane receptors. The CD8-positive T cells, if presented with endogenous antigen in the correct context, develop into cytotoxic effector T cells which can migrate to other tissues and cause apoptosis of cells bearing the antigen. The CD4-positive helper precursor (Th0) cells, if presented with antigen in an appropriate context, develop into one of two types of helper cell, either Th1 helper cells, which help cytotoxic T cells, activate NK cells and macrophages and mediate inflammatory responses, or Th2 helper cells which help B cells, promote eosinophil production and can mediate allergy. Both types of helper cell secrete cytokines which create a positive feedback loop, thus enhancing the specific type of helper response. In addition, interferon-γ secreted by Th1 cells suppresses Th2 cells and IL4 secreted by Th2 cells suppresses Th1 cells.

TLI   total lymphoid irradiation

T lineage   pertaining to **T lymphocytes** and their precursors

TLS   *see FUS*

T lymphocyte   (i) a lymphocyte that is capable of participating in cell-mediated immunity following antigen binding or (ii) an abnormal cell related to normal T lymphocytes (Fig. 72)

TNF   tumour necrosis factor

TNFα   tumour necrosis factor α

TNF-receptor-associated periodic syndrome   a dominantly inherited syndrome resulting from a mutation in the type 1 tumour necrosis factor receptor gene, leading to periodic fever, myalgia and erythema associated with **neutrophilia** and an **acute phase response**

TNFRSF6   the gene, previously known as *APT1*, that encodes fas (**CD95**), a protein important in lymphocyte **apoptosis**; mutation of *TNFRSF6* leads to the **autoimmune lymphoproliferative syndrome**

TNFSFS6   the gene encoding **fas ligand**, mutations of which underlie some cases of the **autoimmune lymphoproliferative syndrome gene** (type Ib)

tolerance   reduced ability to mount an immune response to specific antigens

toluidine blue   a metachromatic stain for identifying basophils and mast cells

TOP1   the DNA **Top**oisomerase **I** gene, gene map locus 20q11, which contributes to a *NUP98-TOP1* fusion gene in therapy-induced acute myeloid leukaemia or myelodysplastic syndrome associated with t(11;20)(p15;q11) (*see also* **topoisomerase I**)

TOP2A   the DNA **Top**oisomerase **IIα** gene, gene map locus 17q21-q22, that may be amplified in acute myeloid leukaemia; point mutations in this gene have been observed in leukaemic cell lines resistant to amsacrine (*see also* **topoisomerase II**)

topoisomerase   an enzyme that makes a transient break in a strand of DNA

topoisomerase I   an enzyme that makes a transient break in a single strand of DNA

topoisomerase II   an enzyme that makes a transient double-stranded break in a strand of DNA

topoisomerase II-interactive drugs   also known as topoisomerase II inhibitors, anti-cancer drugs that act by interfering with the action of topoisomerase II; they can also result in myelodysplastic syndromes or acute myeloid leukaemia

total body irradiation (TBI)   irradiation of the whole body, may be used as preparation for bone marrow transplantation

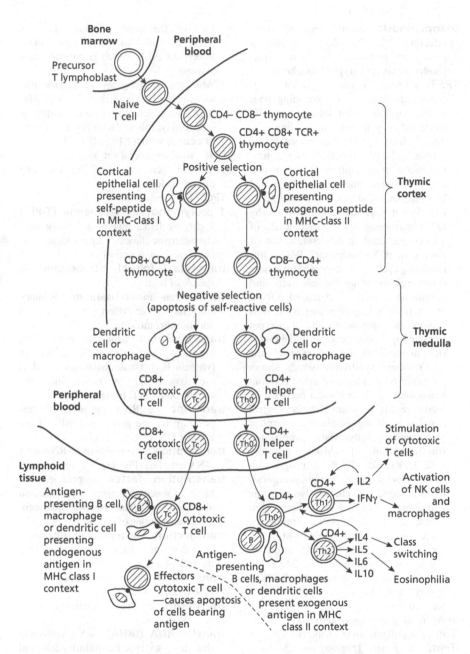

Bone marrow

Precursor T lymphoblast

Peripheral blood

Naive T cell

CD4– CD8– thymocyte

CD4+ CD8+ TCR+ thymocyte

Positive selection

Cortical epithelial cell presenting self-peptide in MHC-class I context

Cortical epithelial cell presenting exogenous peptide in MHC-class II context

Thymic cortex

CD8+ CD4– thymocyte

CD8– CD4+ thymocyte

Negative selection (apoptosis of self-reactive cells)

Dendritic cell or macrophage

Dendritic cell or macrophage

Thymic medulla

Peripheral blood

CD8+ cytotoxic T cell (Tc)

CD4+ helper T cell (Th0)

CD8+ cytotoxic T cell (Tc)

CD4+ helper T cell (Th0)

Stimulation of cytotoxic T cells

Lymphoid tissue

Antigen-presenting B cell, macrophage or dendritic cell presenting endogenous antigen in MHC class I context

CD8+ cytotoxic T cell

Effectors cytotoxic T cell —causes apoptosis of cells bearing antigen

Antigen-presenting B cells, macrophages or dendritic cells present exogenous antigen in MHC class II context

CD4+ (Th0)

CD4+ (Th1) IL2

IFNγ

Activation of NK cells and macrophages

CD4+ (Th2) IL4 IL5 IL6 IL10

Class switching

Eosinophilia

total iron-binding capacity the total capacity of serum or plasma to bind and transport iron

total lymphoid irradiation (TLI) irradiation of all major lymphoid organs, may be used as preparation for **bone marrow transplantation**

total parenteral nutrition (TPN) administration of all known necessary nutrients intravenously

toxic granulation increased staining of neutrophil granules occurring as a response to infection and inflammation but also as a physiological change during pregnancy

toxoplasmosis disease resulting from infection by *Toxoplasma gondii*, a protozoan parasite; may cause **lymphadenopathy** and **atypical lymphocytes**

TP53 a gene, Tumour Protein p53, gene map locus 17p13, encoding p53, a transcription factor that is normally expressed only in actively dividing cells but which is very abundant in most transformed cells; p53 functions as a homotetrameric transcription factor which activates many genes flanked by a p53 binding site, whilst repressing other genes that do not have such a site; induced by DNA damaging agents, high levels of normal p53 lead to cell cycle arrest or apoptosis; p53 up-regulates *WAF*, thus inhibiting cyclin–cyclin-dependent kinase complexes, arresting the cell cycle and permitting repair of damaged DNA; in addition, p53 up-regulates *BAX*, thus promoting **apoptosis**; an archetypal tumour suppressor gene, germline mutations in one allele of *TP53* are seen in the Li–Fraumeni syndrome (which shows an increased incidence of acute myeloid leukaemia); *TP53* mutation occurs as a second event in many haematological neoplasms, being implicated in poor prognosis myelodysplastic syndromes, transformation of chronic granulocytic leukaemia (20–30%), progression or transformation of lymphoproliferative disorders, e.g. chronic lymphocytic leukaemia (c. 15%) and Richter's syndrome (c. 40%), Burkitt's lymphoma, acute myeloid leukaemia (40–50%), Hodgkin's disease (60–80%), adult T-cell leukaemia/lymphoma (c. 24%) and some cases of multiple myeloma; hemizygously lost in acute lymphoblastic leukaemia with 17p–

tPA tissue plasminogen activator

T-PLL T prolymphocytic leukaemia

TPM3 a gene, Tropomyosin 3, gene map locus 1q25 encoding non-muscular tropomyosin, a ubiquitously expressed actin-binding protein; *TPM3* contributes to a *TPM3-ALK* fusion gene in t(1;2)(q25;p23), a variant translocation associated with anaplastic large cell lymphoma; the chimaeric protein consists of the oligomerization domains of TPM3 fused to the tyrosine kinase moiety of ALK which is constitutively activated

TPM4 a gene, Tropomyosin 4, gene map locus 19p13 that contributed to a *TPM4-ALK* fusion gene in a case of anaplastic large cell lymphoma with NK phenotype associated with t(2;19)(p23;p13)

TPN total parenteral nutrition

TPO the gene at 3q27-28, encoding **thrombopoietin**

TPO thrombopoietin

T prolymphocytic leukaemia (T-PLL) a chronic leukaemia of T lineage with characteristic clinical, haematological and cytogenetic characteristics

trabecula (plural trabeculae) a spicule of bone

TRALI transfusion-related acute lung injury

trans having an effect on a gene on another chromosome

transcobalamin a plasma protein that binds to, and transports, cobalamin (**vitamin B₁₂**); transcobalamins I and II are synthesized by neutrophils and transcobalamin II by hepatocytes

transcript an **RNA** molecule, corresponding to one gene, transcribed from nuclear DNA

transcription the synthesis of **RNA** on a **DNA** template (Fig. 73)

transcription factor a protein that binds to specific **enhancer** sequences and also to **RNA polymerase** and thus regulates **transcription** of specific genes

transduction the transfer of a bacterial gene from one bacterium to another by a bacteriophage

transfection the *in vitro* introduction of DNA into cells

transferrin a plasma protein that transports iron

transfer RNA (tRNA) RNA molecules that bind to specific amino acids and transport them to **ribosomes** for incorporation into peptide chains

transformation (i) the process by which a normal cell develops the phenotypic characteristics of a malignant or neoplastic cell (ii) evolution of a low grade to a high grade neoplasm

Figure 73   Transcription.
Transcription of RNA requires the presence of regulatory proteins (RPs), RNA polymerase II (RPOLII), general transcription factors (GTFs) and mediator proteins.
(a) RPOLII is a multi-subunit enzyme, which catalyses mRNA synthesis but is unable to recognize or bind promoter sequences itself. Instead it relies on GTFs, a group of accessory proteins, to recruit it to the transcriptional start site. Transcription is controlled by RPs which binding to enhancers. However RPOLII and GTFs alone cannot respond to RPs unless they bind to a multi-subunit complex of mediator proteins (M). The combination of M, GTFs and RPOLII constitutes the transcription initiation complex.
(b and c) The serine-rich carboxy-terminal domain (CTD) of the largest subunit of RPOLII is unmodified during transcriptional initiation, but is progressively and massively phosphorylated (P) as transcription progresses. Phosphorylation allows the CTD to act as a scaffold for the sequential attachment of RNA processing machinery to the nascent transcript, i.e. the capping enzymes (C), the spliceosome (S) and the cleavage/polyadenylation enzymes (X). Initial phosphorylation is by a GTF protein, TFIIH; subsequent phosphorylation is achieved by the recruitment of the kinase p-TEFb by the capping enzymes.

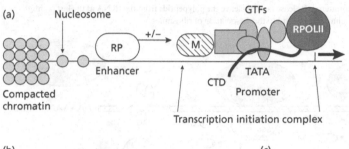

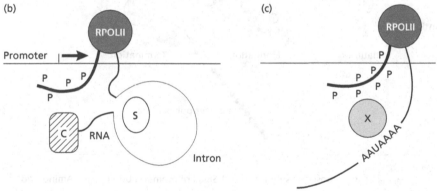

transforming growth factor β (TGFβ)
a multifunctional protein, encoded by ***TGFB***, gene map locus 19q31, that controls proliferation, differentiation, and other functions in many cell types; it has no sequence homology with transforming growth factor α; secreted by B cells, T cells, macrophages and mast cells; cells which synthesize TGFβ have specific receptors for it; TGFα and β are classes of transforming growth factors which act synergistically in inducing transformation.

transforming virus   a virus capable of inducing malignant transformation of animal cells in culture

transfusion   the introduction of blood or blood components into the bloodstream

transfusion-related acute lung injury (TRALI)   acute lung damage following shortly after blood transfusion, usually as a result on transfusion of blood containing high titre anti-leucocyte antibodies

transgene   a gene introduced into a **germ cell**, usually of another species

Figure 74 Translation.

Translation is the process by which the sequence of codons of a messenger RNA (mRNA) directs the synthesis of a polypeptide chain. The mRNA code is read in a 5′ to 3′ direction, directing protein synthesis in an amino-to carboxy- direction. It is a cytoplasmic event that takes place on large ribonucleoprotein complexes called ribosomes, which comprise large and small subunits. Amino acids enter the ribosome attached to transfer RNA (tRNA) molecules. Each tRNA is only able to recognize one amino acid (to which it is covalently linked) and contains a trinucleotide sequence (anticodon) complementary to the codon representing the amino acid that it carries. Translation starts at an initiation codon, which is usually AUG (encoding methionine). This codon is flanked by certain consensus sequences in the 5′ untranslated region (UTR) of the mRNA that are complementary to the 3′ end of the ribosomal RNA in the small subunit; this ensures that all methionine codons do not act as translational start sites. The small subunit binds mRNA and guides the anticodon sequences of incoming tRNAs to the mRNA codon currently being translated. The large subunit catalyses the transfer of the carboxy end of the nascent polypeptide chain, which is attached to the tRNA bound to the preceding codon, to the amino end of the amino acid attached to the incoming tRNA. Translational initiation and elongation are dependent upon GTPase accessory factors (initiation and release factors). Translational termination begins when a stop codon is encountered. Release factors cleave the polypeptide from the tRNA at the last coding codon and ribosome recycling factors lead to the dissociation of ribosomes.

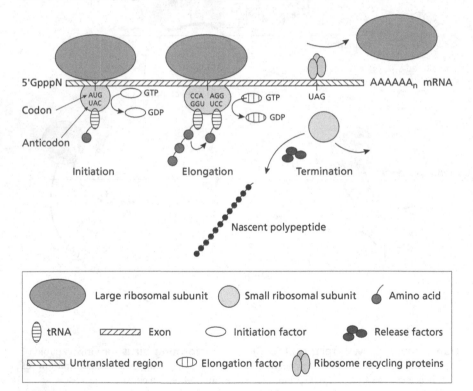

transgenic animal an animal, usually a mouse, expressing a gene of another species, which is introduced by injecting DNA containing the required gene into the pronucleus of a fertilized egg

transient abnormal myelopoiesis (TAM) a transient leukaemia occurring in neonates with **Down's syndrome**

translation the synthesis of protein from a mRNA template (Fig. 74)

translocation the transfer of part of a chromosome to another chromosome; may be reciprocal or non-reciprocal, balanced or unbalanced (Fig. 75)

transmission electron microscopy (TEM) an electron microscopy tech-

Figure 75 Translocation.
A translocation is a transfer of part of one chromosome to another; most often this is reciprocal. This figure contrasts an inversion of chromosome 3 with five translocations involving the same chromosome: (a) inv(3)(q21q26); (b) t(3;3)(q21;q26); (c) t(1;3)(p36;q21); (d) t(3;5)(q21;q31); t(3;12)(q26;p13); t(3;21)(q26;q22).

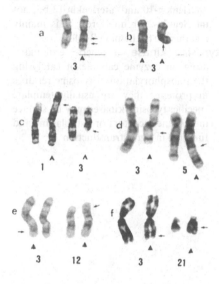

nique in which electrons pass through a thin section of a cell or tissue, revealing its internal structure (*see* Figs 12 and 14, pp. 29 and 31)

transplant tissue or cells deliberately transferred to another individual with the intention of achieving **engraftment**

transplantation the introduction into the body of viable cells from another individual with the intention of achieving **engraftment**

TRAP tartrate-resistant acid phosphatase

trephine a strong needle for performing a biopsy of bone and bone marrow

trephine biopsy (i) the procedure by which a biopsy specimen of bone and bone marrow is obtained, using a trephine (ii) jargon for a biopsy specimen obtained with a trephine

trilineage involving the granulocyte–monocyte, erythroid and megakaryocyte lineages

triploidy the presence of an extra copy of each chromosome in a cell so that there are a total of 69 chromosomes

trisomy the presence of three rather than two copies of a chromosome in a cell or clone

trisomy 21 (i) Down's syndrome (ii) the presence of an extra copy of chromosome 21 in a cell, a clone of cells or an individual

TRKC a gene, **T**yrosine **K**inase receptor 3, also known as **N**eurotrophic **T**yrosine **K**inase receptor **3**, *NTRK3*, gene map locus 15q25, encoding a receptor tyrosine kinase, that contributes to a *ETV6-TRKC* fusion gene in acute myeloid leukaemia associated with t(12;15)(p13;q25); the chimaeric protein is a constitutively activated tyrosine kinase

tRNA transfer RNA

tropical spastic paraparesis (TSP) a myelopathy caused by **HTLV-I**, the **retrovirus** which also causes **adult T-cell leukaemia/lymphoma**

tropical splenomegaly *see* **hyperreactive malarial splenomegaly**

TSP tropical spastic paraparesis

TTF a gene, RhoH/TTF- **T**ranslocation **T**hree **F**our, also known as **R**AS **H**omologue gene family member **H** (*ARHH*), gene map locus 4p13, encoding a haemopoietic-cell-specific small GTPase of the Rho subfamily of **RAS**-like molecules; is involved in cytoskeletal organization; the gene contributes to the *TTF-BCL6* fusion gene in B-lineage non-Hodgkin's lymphoma associated with t(3;4)(q27;p13) and was rearranged to the *IGH* locus in one case of multiple myeloma with t(4;14)(p13;q32)

TTP thrombotic thrombocytopenic purpura

tuberculosis a disease resulting from infection by *Mycobacterium tuberculosis*

tumour a solid mass of tissue, usually neoplastic in nature

tumour necrosis factor α **(TNFα)** an **acute phase reactant**, a cytokine secreted by macrophages, NK cells, T lymphocytes, B lymphocytes and mast cells, which promotes inflammation, encoded by a gene at 6p21.3; a monoclonal antibody to TNFα, infliximab, is available for therapeutic use

tumour necrosis factor β   *see* **lymphocytotoxin**

tumour suppressor gene a normal cellular gene, one of a subset of **proto-oncogenes**, which helps to control growth and proliferation of cells; the loss of function of tumour suppressor gene can contribute to either the development or the progression of a neoplastic tumour

type 1 blast a blast cell with no granules (**FAB** group definition)

type 2 blast a blast cell with scanty granules but without features of a **promyelocyte** such as a lower nucleocytoplasmic ratio, an eccentric nucleus and a Golgi zone (**FAB** group definition)

type 1 (Th1) helper T cell a CD4+ helper T cell that secretes **interleukin-2**, interferon-γ and **lymphocytotoxin** (tumour necrosis factor β) but not **interleukin-4**, **interleukin-5** or **interleukin-6**; it is mainly responsible for activation of macrophages and for T-cell mediated cytotoxicity

type 2 (Th2) helper T cell a CD4+ helper T cell that secretes **interleukin-4**, **interleukin-5**, **interleukin-6**, **interleukin-9**, **interleukin-10** and **interleukin-13** but not **interleukin-2** or interferon; it is mainly responsible for helping B cells

tyrosine kinase a generic term indicating an enzyme capable of catalysing the phosphorylation of tyrosine residues in proteins; they are usually template specific; tyrosine kinases may be surface membrane receptors or cytoplasmic and function in signal transduction

U

U an abbreviation for the pyrimidine, uracil

ubiquitin a small globular protein which exists throughout the cell (hence its name), either in a free form or conjugated to other proteins through a covalent bond between the glycine at its carboxy terminal end and the side chains of lysine on other proteins; encoded as either linear repeats (polyubiquitin) or fused to a ribosomal protein gene—after protein synthesis, the enzyme ubiquitin C-terminal hydrolase liberates individual protein units

ubiquitination the post-translational modification process whereby **ubiquitin** is conjugated to target protein; the process involves the sequential actions of activating (E1), conjugating (E2), and ligase (E3) enzymes; E3 proteins carry **RING fingers** and bind specific substrates through a structural motif known as a ubiquitination signal (degron); monoubiquitination targets proteins for endocytosis and nascent proteins for secretion; polyubiquitination marks proteins for destruction in **proteasomes**

UGT1 the gene encoding **U**DP **g**lucuronosyl **T**ransferase-**1**, a polymorphism in the promoter of which causes **Gilbert's syndrome**

UKCCG United Kingdom Cancer Cytogenetics Group

ultrasonography imaging parts of the body by means of sound waves of such a high frequency that they are inaudible to the human ear

ultrasound very high frequency sound

ultrastructure the features of a cell as ascertained by means of an electron microscope

unbalanced translocation a translocation in which there has been net gain or loss of part of one or both involved chromosomes (Fig. 76)

unconjugated bilirubin bilirubin that has not been conjugated to glucuronic acid by the liver; an increased concentration of unconjugated bilirubin occurs in haemolytic anaemia

unfractionated heparin heparin as extracted from animal tissues, with molecular weights ranging from 5000 to 30 000 daltons

universal donor a blood donor whose blood can be transfused into patients of any blood group, i.e. an O Rh D-negative donor (without a high titre of anti-A or anti-B antibodies)

universal precautions an approach to prevention of transmission of blood-borne pathogens by regarding every blood sample as potentially high risk

universal recipient a recipient of a blood transfusion who can receive blood of any group, i.e. an AB Rh D-positive individual

Upshaw–Schulman syndrome a recessively inherited syndrome of recurrent **thrombocytopenia** and **microangiopathic haemolytic anaemia** resulting from deficiency of **von Willebrand factor-cleaving protein**

uracil a **pyrimidine** that pairs with **adenine**

uraemia the presence in the blood of excessive amounts or urea and other nitrogenous compounds as a result of renal failure

urobilinogen a breakdown product of **bilirubin**, present in the faeces and urine

URO-D the gene encoding **UR**oporphyrinogen **D**ecarboxylase, mutation of which

Figure 76   Unbalanced translocation.
Most translocations are balanced, i.e. there is no loss
of chromosomal material detectable by standard
cytogenetic analysis. However there are some
translocations that are often unbalanced. One such
is t(1;19)(q23;p13), observed in B-lineage acute
lymphoblastic leukaemia. It can occur as a balanced
translocation (a) or as an unbalanced translocation
(b). In the unbalanced translocation, designated
der(19)t(1;19)(q23;p13) the derivative chromosome 1
(comprising a large part of chromosome 1 and a
small contribution from the short arm of
chromosome 19) is lost and is replaced by a second
copy of the normal chromosome 1. The derivative
chromosome 19 is not lost. Effectively there is
monosomy for a small part of 19p (which is lost with
the der(1)) and triploidy for a large part of 1p, which
is present in the two copies of a normal chromosome
1 and also in the der(19).

causes about a third of cases of familial
porphyria cutanea tarda
urokinase   a thrombolytic compound
present in the urine
urticaria pigmentosa   cutaneous mastocytosis
USP25   a gene, Ubiquitin-Specific Protease 25, gene map locus 21q11, encodes a
deubiquitinating enzyme which cleaves
free ubiquitin from ubiquitin precursors
and ubiquitinylated proteins; *USP25*
contributes to an *AML1-USP25* fusion
gene, encoding a truncated AML1 protein, in myelodysplastic syndromes

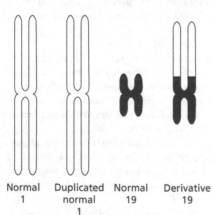

Normal   Derivative   Normal   Derivative
   1   1   19   19
(a) **Balanced translocation**
     t(1;19)(q23;p13)

Normal   Duplicated   Normal   Derivative
   1   normal   19   19
                1
(b) **Unbalanced translocation**
     der(19)t(1;19)(q23;p13)

V

vacuole a fluid-filled cavity within a cell which, in the case of phagocytes, is formed by invagination of the surface membrane

variable expressivity a variation in the expression of a **phenotype** between individuals with the same **genotype** (in contrast to **penetrance**, which is an all or none phenomenon)

variable number of tandem repeats (VNTR) a variable number of copies of a DNA sequence at a specific locus that can be used as a genetic marker

variance a number representing the dispersion of measured values around a mean expressed as SD^2

varicella-zoster a herpesvirus that causes chicken pox (varicella) and shingles (herpes zoster)

vasculitis inflammation of blood vessels

vegan an individual who eats no animal protein; veganism can cause **vitamin B$_{12}$ deficiency**

vegetarian an individual who abstains from the flesh of animals and may or may not eat fish, eggs and milk

vein a thin-walled vessel conducting blood back to the heart

venepuncture the puncturing of a vein in order to obtain a blood sample

venereal pertaining to or caused by sexual intercourse

venous pertaining to veins

venous thromboembolism deep vein thrombosis and pulmonary embolism

venule a small thin-walled vessel conducting blood towards the heart, connecting capillaries and veins

VHL the gene encoding <u>V</u>on <u>H</u>ippel <u>L</u>indau protein, which targets hypoxia-inducible protein 1α (HIP1α) for degradation; homozygosity for a mutation in this gene causes Chuvash **polycythaemia** and other rare familial polycythaemias, probably because impaired degradation of HIP1α leads to enhanced synthesis of **erythropoietin**; there is also enhanced synthesis of **transferrin** and **transferrin receptor**

vimentin an antigen expressed by rhabdomyosarcoma, Ewing's sarcoma and spindle cell carcinoma

vinblastine a plant alkaloid used in treating leukaemia, lymphoma and some solid tumours

vinca alkaloids alkaloids derived from plants of the Vinca genus, used as chemotherapeutic agents, e.g. **vincristine, vinblastine, vindesine**

vincristine a plant alkaloid used in treating leukaemia, lymphoma and some solid tumours

vindesine a plant alkaloid used in treating leukaemia, lymphoma and some solid tumours

viral pertaining to a **virus**

viral haemorrhagic fever one of a group of viral infections causing fever and haemorrhage (which is consequent on consumption of platelets), e.g. Lassa fever and Ebola fever

virus a very small micro-organism, not visible with a light microscope and capable of replicating only within a living plant or animal cell

viscera the internal organs

visceral pertaining to a **viscus**

viscosity the capacity of a fluid to flow more or less readily

viscus an internal organ

vital stain a stain applied to living cells

vitamin B$_6$ pyridoxine, a vitamin which may be useful in some cases of **sideroblastic anaemia**

Table 18   Characteristics of subtypes of type 2 von Willebrand's disease.

Subtype of 2	HMW multimers	Ristocetin-induced platelet aggregation	Factor-VIII binding capacity
2A	Absent	Decreased	Normal
2B*	Reduced/absent	Increased	Normal
2M	Normal	Decreased	Normal
2N†	Normal	Normal	Markedly reduced

* May have thrombocytopenia.
† Disease in homozygotes and compound heterozygotes for 2 A and 2 N types of mutation.

vitamin B$_{12}$ a vitamin essential for conversion of homocysteine to methionine and for conversion of methylmalonyl CoA to succinyl CoA

vitamin B$_{12}$ deficiency   an insufficiency of **vitamin B$_{12}$**, potentially leading to **megaloblastic anaemia, peripheral neuropathy, subacute degeneration of the spinal cord, optic atrophy** and **dementia**

vitamin D   a vitamin essential for the normal absorption of calcium

vitamin K   a vitamin which is essential for synthesis of the coagulation factors, **factor II, factor VII, factor IX** and **factor X**, and of the naturally occurring anticoagulants, **protein C** and **protein S**

vitamin K antagonist   an orally active **anticoagulant** that antagonizes the action of **vitamin K** by interfering with γ-carboxylation of precursors of **vitamin-K dependent proteins**

vitiligo   acquired patchy depigmentation of the skin; there is an association between **pernicious anaemia** and vitiligo

VNTR   variable number of tandem repeats

volunteer unrelated donor (VUD)   a bone marrow or haemopoietic stem cell donor who is unrelated to the recipient but has been matched for histocompatibility antigens

von Willebrand's disease   a haemorrhagic disorder consequent of **von Willebrand's factor** deficiency (*see also* **platelet-type von Willebrand's disease**), classified as:
• type I, quantitative, partial deficiency, autosomal dominant
• type 2, qualitative, functional deficiency, mainly autosomal dominant (Table 18)
• type 3, quantitative, complete deficiency, autosomal recessive (disease in compound heterozygotes or homozygotes)

von Willebrand's factor   a coagulation factor and adhesion molecule, encoded by the *VWF* gene, produced by endothelial cells and megakaryocytes: it is a carrier protein for factor VIII and is also necessary for normal platelet–endothelial cell interactions through its binding, predominantly, to platelet glycoprotein Ib/IX

von Willebrand's factor-cleaving protease   a metalloproteinase encoded by an *ADAMTS* family gene, *ADAMTS13*, at 9q34, which causes limited proteolysis of large multimers of von Willebrand's factor released from endothelial cells; inherited or acquired deficiency can cause **thrombotic thrombocytopenic purpura**

VWF   the gene at 12p13.3 that encodes **von Willebrand's factor**, mutation of which can lead to **autosomal dominant** or **autosomal recessive** von Willebrand's disease

VUD   volunteer unrelated donor

W

WAF1 an alternative name for **CDKN1A** the gene encoding p21^{WAF}, a protein that negatively regulates the cell cycle; *WAF* is up-regulated by the tumour suppressor gene, *TP53*

Waldenström's macroglobulinaemia a disease consequent on a lymphoplasmacytoid lymphoma with secretion of an IgM paraprotein, the latter leading to hyperviscosity

Waldeyer's ring the ring of lymphoid tissue, including the tonsils, encircling the pharynx

warfarin one of the coumarin anticoagulants

WASp a gene at Xp11.22-11.23, mutation of which is responsible for the **Wiskott–Aldrich syndrome** and **X-linked thrombocytopenia** in some families and, rarely, **severe congenital neutropenia**

WBC white blood cell count, **white cell count**

Western blot a modification of the **Southern blot**, used for identification of proteins; the name is a play on words

Whipple's disease a malabsorption syndrome resulting from infection by *Tropheryma whippelii*

white cell a leucocyte—a granulocyte, monocyte or lymphocyte

white cell count a quantification of the number of white cells in a defined volume of blood

WHO World Health Organization

WHO classification a comprehensive classification of haematological neoplasms published in its definitive form in 2001, see Tables 2, 4, 6, 7 and 10–14 and Fig. 55, pp. 7, 8, 127, 129, 137, 153, 157, 167 and 168, respectively

whole chromosome painting a technique for identifying individual chromosomes by the use of a combination of probes that bind with a high level of specificity to a single pair of chromosomes

whooping cough pertussis; the disease caused by infection by *Bordetella pertussis*

wild type gene the normal form of a gene, in contrast to a mutant gene

Wilson's disease an inherited metabolic disorder resulting from mutations in the copper transporting ATPase, *ATP7B*, leading to overloading of tissues with copper; **haemolytic anaemia** may occur as a presenting feature of late in the course of the disease

Wiskott–Aldrich syndrome a syndrome of thrombocytopenia, eczema and immune deficiency, resulting from mutation in the *WASp* gene

wnt a family of evolutionarily conserved genes which encode secreted glycoproteins homologous to *Drosophila* wingless; their cognate receptors are members of the fz (frizzled) family of transmembrane molecules; intracellular signalling is mediated via a variety of proteins including beta catenin

Wolfram syndrome a syndrome resulting from mutation of the *WFS1/wolframin* gene, gene map locus 4p16.1; *WFS1* encodes a widely expressed endoplasmic reticulum membrane protein; wolfram syndrome is characterized by diabetes insipidus, diabetes mellitus, optic atrophy and deafness (DIDMOAD); some patients also have **sideroblastic anaemia** and deletions of mitochondrial genes

Wolman's disease an inherited metabolic disorder, a juvenile form of cholesterol ester storage disease

Working Formulation a lymphoma classification which was superseded by the REAL and then the WHO classifications

World Health Organization (WHO) an international organization for the improvement of world health, source of the **WHO classification** of tumours of haemopoietic and lymphoid tissues

woven bone young bone which has not yet been organized into a lamellar structure

Wright's stain a **Romanowsky stain** which is the predominant stain used in the USA and Canada

WT1 a gene, **W**ilms **T**umour **1** gene, gene map locus 11p13, encodes a zinc finger transcription factor existing in four iso-forms; in addition is known to bind RNA and may form part of the spliceosome (*see* Fig. 65, p. 202); a candidate tumour suppressor gene, mutation of which is associated with an increased incidence of Wilms' tumour (and an increased incidence of acute myeloid leukaemia following Wilms' tumour and in relatives of patients with Wilms' tumour); encodes a transcription factor involved in growth and differentiation of various normal and neoplastic cells; expressed in normal CD34+ haemopoietic progenitor cells and overexpressed in CD34+ cells in acute myeloid leukaemia and chronic granulocytic leukaemia; expressed in blast cells of 88% of cases of acute lymphoblastic leukaemia and 97% of cases of acute myeloid leukaemia.

X

X the X chromosome, of which one copy is found in normal males and two copies in normal females

xanthoma a subcutaneous nodule or plaque containing cholesterol

xenograft a graft (transplant) from one species to another

xerocytosis an inherited defect of the erythrocyte membrane leading to increased cation flux, dehydration of cells and haemolytic anaemia

XG a gene at Xpter-22.32 encoding the Xg^a blood group antigen

XK a locus at Xp21.1-21.1 where there is a gene encoding Kx, a protein linked to the Kell blood group antigens; lack of Kx leads to the **McLeod phenotype**

X inactivation the inactivation of one of two copies of X chromosome genes in somatic cells of females (*see* **Lyon hypothesis** and **Lyonization**)

X-linked pertaining to characteristics or diseases transmitted by genes on the X chromosome, includes X-linked dominant and X-linked recessive; sex-linked is synonymous

X-linked agammaglobulinaemia a congenital X-linked deficiency in humoral immunity resulting from a mutation in the *BTK*, the gene encoding **B**ruton's **T**yrosine **K**inase, a cytoplasmic tyrosine kinase which is required for B lymphocyte development

X-linked lymphoproliferative disease an inherited susceptibility to severe disease following primary EBV infection, resulting from a mutation in the *SAP* gene (Signalling Lymphocyte Activation Molecule (SLAM)-associated protein) at Xq25, also known as *SH2D1A*, which encodes a NK and T-lymphocyte surface membrane protein that is part of the signalling pathway when these cells interact with virus-infected B cells; SAP on T cells interacts with SLAM (**CD150**) on both T cells and B cells and also with 2B4 (**CD244**) on NK cells

X-linked sideroblastic anaemia an inherited **sideroblastic anaemia** resulting from mutation in the erythroid-specific δ-amino laevulinic acid synthase gene, *ALAS2*; the condition mainly affects males but can occur in females as a result of skewed X chromosome inactivation

X-rays gamma irradiation, electromagnetic radiation of shorter wave length than visible light that is able to penetrate many tissues thus permitting the production of an image of a part of the body, applied therapeutically to destroy malignant tissues

Y

Y the Y chromosome, found in males but not in normal females

YAC yeast artificial chromosome

yeast artificial chromosome (YAC) yeast chromosomes that can incorporate large segments of foreign DNA, used in recombinant DNA technology; DNA sequences complementary to human DNA sequences serve a probe for those sequences

yellow marrow fatty bone marrow (cf. **red marrow**)

yolk sac part of an embryo, the initial site of formation of blood cells

Z

ζ the Greek letter, zeta; one of the two chains of haemoglobin Gower 1 and haemoglobin Portland

ZAP70 Zeta chain Associated Protein kinase 70, also known as *SRK* (Syk-Related tyrosine Kinase), gene map locus 2q12, encodes a nonreceptor tyrosine kinase expressed in T and NK cells which associates with the TCR zeta chain and is phosphorylated upon antigen stimulation; several germline mutations in this gene have been observed in kindreds with severe T-cell immunodeficiency (NK and B cells are normal)

zidovudine a drug used in the treatment of **AIDS** which can cause **megaloblastic anaemia** and **pancytopenia**

Ziehl–Neelsen a stain for Mycobacteria, which are acid-fast with this stain

Zieve's syndrome acute haemolytic anaemia with hyperlipidaemia occurring in patients with acute alcoholic liver disease

zinc finger a metal-binding protein motif that allows nucleic acid (DNA and RNA) binding and which is a key component of many transcription factors; there are estimated to be up to 800 zinc finger containing proteins in the human genome

ZNF198 a gene, Zinc Finger protein 198, also known as Rearranged in Atypical Myeloproliferative disorder (*RAMP*) and Fused In Myeloproliferative disorders (*FIM*); gene map locus 13q12, encodes a zinc finger protein; *ZNF198* contributes to a *ZNF198-FGFR1* fusion gene in a syndrome of chronic myelomonocytic leukaemia with eosinophilia/T-lineage lymphoblastic lymphoma (the **8p11 syndrome**); the fusion protein comprises the amino-terminal domains of ZNF198 fused to tyrosine kinase FGFR1 and is constitutively activated

zygote a fertilized ovum